THE CHALLENGE:
Despair and Hope in the
Conquest of Inner Space

RUDOLF EKSTEIN, Ph.D.

Director, Project: Childhood Psychosis
Reiss-Davis Child Study Center
Los Angeles, California

WITH CONTRIBUTIONS BY

Elaine Caruth, Ph.D.

Beatrice B. Cooper, M.S.

Seymour W. Friedman, M.D.

Joel M. Liebowitz, Ph.D.

Mortimer M. Meyer, Ph.D.

Leda W. Rosow, M.A.

Kenneth Rubin, M.D.

A REISS-DAVIS CHILD CENTER PUBLICATION

THE CHALLENGE: DESPAIR AND HOPE IN THE CONQUEST OF INNER SPACE

Further Studies of the Psychoanalytic Treatment of Severely Disturbed Children

BRUNNER/MAZEL Publishers • New York
BUTTERWORTHS • London

Copyright © 1971 by Rudolf Ekstein

published by
BRUNNER/MAZEL, INC.
64 University Place
New York, N. Y. 10003

Library of Congress Catalogue Card No. 70-156467

SBN 87630-044-1

MANUFACTURED IN THE UNITED STATES OF AMERICA

To the memory of my father,

ERNST EKSTEIN, 1883-1970,

WHO ENCOURAGED ME TO MEET SITUATIONS
OF ADVERSITY WITH ACTIVITIES OF HOPE

TABLE OF CONTENTS

TABLE OF CONTENTS (continued)

TABLE OF CONTENTS (continued)

ACKNOWLEDGMENTS

Whenever one is able to finish a larger piece of work, one would like to express one's gratitude and give due credit to the teachers and colleagues who have influenced one's education and work throughout the years. The work with psychotic and borderline conditions in childhood has occupied me now for more than twenty years, and I, of course, feel most grateful to the colleagues at *Southard School* and at the *Reiss-Davis Child Study Center*, many of whom have become co-authors in this volume and in the previous one on *Children of Time and Space, of Action and Impulse*. We always have tried to go beyond our little research islands, and we have been influenced greatly by a number of important developments elsewhere. I feel indebted to Anna Freud and the colleagues at *Hampstead* under her leadership; to Paula Elkisch and Margaret Mahler and the colleagues who have worked with them; and to Bruno Bettelheim and his co-workers at the *Orthogenic School*, who taught us as much as we could absorb about the use of a therapeutic environment for these children. Through the authors of the guiding themes heading chapters of this volume, I have indicated, in part at least, many other sources and authors from whom I have learned and been inspired.

During recent years I have had—in spite of immense difficulties—the loyal and understanding support of the clinical leaders of the Reiss-Davis Child Study Center: Dr. Rocco L. Motto, director of the organization; Dr. Seymour W. Friedman, director of Clinical Services; Miss Miriam C. Campbell, chief of Social Services; Dr. Mortimer Meyer, chief of Psychological Services; and Dr. Christoph Heinicke, acting director of Research. I also want to express my thanks to Mrs. Phyllis Vincent and to Mrs. Mildred Smoodin who have helped with the endless tasks in preparing the book manuscript.

In slightly different forms, "Levels of Verbal Communication in the Schizophrenic Child's Struggle against, for, and with the World of

Objects" and "Object Constancy and Psychotic Reconstruction" appeared in *The Psychoanalytic Study of the Child;* "The Orpheus and Eurydice Theme in Psychotherapy" in *Bulletin of the Menninger Clinic;* "The Dying and Living of Teresa Esperanza" in *Psychology Today;* "On Some Current Models in the Psychoanalytic Treatment of Childhood Psychosis" in *Handbuch der Kinderpsychotherapie;* "The Onion and the Moebius Strip: Rational and Irrational Models for the Secondary and Primary Process" in *The Psychoanalytic Review;* "Psychotic Adolescents and Their Quest for Goals" in C. Buhler and F. Massarik's *The Course of Human Life,* Springer; "The Psychotic Pursuit of Reality" in *Journal of Contemporary Psychotherapy;* "Cause of the Illness or Cause of the Cure" in *International Journal of Psychiatry;* "Certain Phenomenological Aspects of the Countertransference in the Treatment of Schizophrenic Children," "Reflections on the Need for a Working Alliance with Environmental Support Systems," "To Sleep but Not to Dream: On the Use of Electrical Tape Recording in Clinical Research," "The Relation of Ego Autonomy to Activity and Passivity in the Psychotherapy of Childhood Schizophrenia," "Inner and Outer Reality Testing on the Rorschach," "The Parallel Process as It Emerges in Casework," "The Trap: The Child's Emotional Illness as the External Organizer of the Family's Life," "One Step Beyond: Discussion of 'The Working Alliance with Angels, Good Spirits, and Deities,'" "Prolegomenon to a Psychoanalytic Technique in the Treatment of Childhood Schizophrenia," "Notes on the Treatment of Teresa: Assessment via Psychological Testing," "Relationship between Diagnosis and Mode of Intervention in States of Severe Impairment," "Differential Diagnostic Cues in the Severely Impaired Child," "Identity Formation in the Treatment of an Autistic Child," "The Working Alliance with Angels, Good Spirits, and Deities: Further Reflections on Object- and Self-Constancy," and "Casework with Psychotic Children and their Parents: Fusion, Separation, Individuation" in *Reiss-Davis Clinic Bulletin.*

This book is a Reiss-Davis Child Study Center Publication. It could not have been done without total staff involvement, without the help of our Research Seminar on Childhood Psychosis, and without the powerful support of the Board, the Volunteers and the contributors to this organization. And, finally, most thanks should go to the patients, their parents and relatives; collaborating institutions, psychiatric and educational; and many individuals who participated in this work. We only wish that our gratefulness to them for what we have learned from them could be translated more and more into effective and durable ways of helping.

RUDOLF EKSTEIN, PH.D.

THE CHALLENGE:
Despair and Hope in the Conquest of Inner Space

THE PROLOGUE: AN ADDRESS TO THE BOARD OF DIRECTORS

"Gentlemen—as you know, we have never prided ourselves
On the completeness and finality of our knowledge and capacity.
We are just as ready now as we were earlier to meet the
Imperfections of our understanding, to learn new things and to
Alter our methods in any way that can improve them."

SIGMUND FREUD, 1918

The Prologue: An Address to the Board of Directors*

I hope, of course, that my address will be more than the monologue of the invited guest speaker and that it will turn into a dialogue, a give and take so that we may see whether we can give each other strength in supporting our common undertaking, or if, perhaps, we are attempting an impossible task. How can I best describe to you the task assumed by those who work with severely disturbed children, be they autistic, psychotic, or suffering from severe borderline conditions of childhood and adolescence? As a matter of fact, we can be quite sure that people who work with these children are usually driven to it because of unusual circumstances; no one today accepts commitments of this kind unless he has—in addition to thorough training—also some inner reason for it, for that pursuit of the impossible dream. It is for this reason that I want to venture out and make a few autobiographical remarks in order to make you aware of the complexity of a person's professional choice.

Many years ago, when I was about ten years old growing up in Vienna, the family celebrated my birthday and I was quite surprised because on that occasion I received two gifts instead of the usual one. I opened the first package and it contained a book entitled, *German*

---

* I wish I could say that any similarity to the Board of Directors in real life and in real situations is merely coincidental and that all that I say here is fictitious. Actually, once or twice I have given an address such as the one that I use here. During one of these opportunities the address was taped and transcribed and I have just changed it sufficiently—as we do with our case histories—in order to protect the anonymity of that "Board of Directors."

3

Hero Myths, the kind of gift that ten-year olds enjoyed then—Teutonic heroes and ideals to emulate. But when I opened the second package, which came from a relative, I discovered to my dismay that it contained exactly the same book; I now had two volumes on German hero worship. I don't know what gave me the wisdom, because at that time I had no idea that some day the German "heroes" would drive me out of Austria, but I decided that one book on hero worship was enough, certainly on German hero worship. My father exchanged the second copy in a bookstore for three paperbound books, and it is about these three books that I want to talk.

They were Jules Verne's classic adventures, written some hundred years before our day: *20,000 Leagues Under the Sea, The Trip to the Moon,* and *The Trip Around the Moon.* There were three incidents detailed in them that I recalled throughout my life. The first incident, in *20,000 Leagues Under the Sea,* described how Captain Nemo and his strange crew fought a sea monster, and how one of the crew was suddenly in danger of being swallowed up by the monster. The reporter of that story, the only one who survived, was impressed by the fact that Captain Nemo and his crew spoke a special language he could not understand, so that it was impossible for him to guess their native land. As he watched the terrible struggle with the sea monster, he heard the man, in the agony of his despair, scream "Mother!" in French, and thus discovered the man's origins. That is the only incident that I recall from that book. As an analyst later on, I wondered why this particular incident had stuck in the mind of a ten-year-old boy. I will not go too far in confessing my own life, but you can draw your own conclusions. What impressed me most was that a person, an adult or child, who is desperate and helpless, screams for mother in his mother tongue.

The second incident took place in Jules Verne's *Trip to the Moon.* As you know, when I read it the book was considered an improbable fantasy; probably no one thought of it as a realistic account of the future. This book had a strange ending which was not only deeply upsetting to me but to most people at the time Jules Verne wrote it. In the story they succeeded in developing a cannonball which they shot to the moon, carrying the three heroes from the Florida coast (because of Yankee engineering, which Jules Verne thought was extraordinary). And he described the magnificent sights the heroes saw, except that having left the earth's gravity, they were now in the moon's orbit and would forever gravitate around the moon until the end of their lives. I was very much shaken by that ending, because it seemed a cruel punishment for initiative and curiosity, for the desire to find out and explore. So must have thought the people in France for whom the book was written, because they literally forced Jules Verne to revise the edition and to write a second book, *The Trip Around the Moon*. In it, Jules Verne described how the voyagers traveled around the moon but found a way to return to the gravity of the earth and then safely come back to Mother Earth once more.

Those are the three episodes that I recalled, and I have wondered ever since why I recalled these over the many others. By now, you probably realize I am describing a fantasy that is directly related to the problem we are concerned with. We all recall, during the recent moon-flight—now no longer a fantasy for a ten-year-old boy but the ambition of a whole nation determined to demonstrate something to the world —how all of us stayed glued to our television sets and wondered whether the flight would come off, whether it would be possible to get near the moon, whether it would be possible to fly around the moon.* And I believe the most unforgettable moments were those when we waited to learn whether the men in the space ship would be able to overcome the gravity of the moon, would be able to re-enter the earth's gravity and return. And I believe during the most recent moonflight we were concerned with an even more difficult problem, namely whether the ship designed to land on the moon could return to the *Mother Ship* and connect with the *Mother Ship* (the space engineers' choice of names, not mine) so that it could return to earth. The moonship was not equipped to go through the earth's atmosphere and was completely dependent on the Mother Ship, that is, on a support system, a loyal support system. By now, you know what I talk about. I am talking about the inner anxieties of a little boy who has problems about his mother and wonders what to do when he is in panic and screams for her but cannot find his way back to her. You understand now that I am talking about the magnificent identification of the American people with its heroes who venture into outer space and cause all of us to pray for their safe return, even though our concerns today obviously are much greater than whether these few men will return. It becomes clearer to me why our nation is the most willing of all nations to spend hundreds of millions of dollars to make it possible to bring about heroic achievements and not to allow the hero to die, but to ensure his return to Mother Earth. How different from my childhood book on German heroes; in those stories, there was nothing greater than to die in battle and go to Valhalla as someone who had "died with his boots on." It became clear to me that it is the double nature of man which makes him believe in books on hero worship, in war, in violence; but which

---

* The original address was offered prior to the Apollo's successful landing of astronauts on the moon on July 20, 1969.

also makes him want to read books in which the goal is to return to mother—or I should say the Godparents—to be heroic without being militant, to explore without being destructive, to be curious yet have a home base to return to. And it became clear to me that these books were terribly important in my own life because I began at that time to make a choice: I chose heroes who were explorers and scientists who were committed to the service of mankind, who were committed to bringing sick children back to life and back to their mothers, instead of heroes whose commitment was to conquest, to killing, to being killed and going to Valhalla. That was the ten-year-old's choice. It was shortly after that I decided I was going to work with children; I was very, very young when I made that decision. I became a teacher, then, later on, an analyst, and finally I specialized in training people for this profession as well as offering therapeutic services and engaging in research with very difficult, very sick children.

What are these sick children suffering from? They are children who have disconnected from their mother, if you like; who have not found safety so that they can live a life of their own, who are near the moon's gravity and have no gravity to Mother Earth and are therefore forced to remain out in space, to remain in their delusional psychotic world. They are children who need someone who knows enough to restore the gravity of reality for them, the gravity of life with mother and life with family and life with people. And this is what I have dedicated myself to restore.

But, of course, this kind of dedication, at first, is merely faith, and I have not come simply to appeal to you and make you feel sympathetic to a cause, because I know you are sympathetic. I have come to tell you about the concerns I have as an adult, not simply the ones that I had as a child who wanted to do something heroic for mankind. I want to tell you how I tried later to develop this basic faith in humanity and helping sick children, and the people who support the treatment of sick children; how I tried to develop it in a scientific, predictable, and truly professional way. Let me characterize that development from childhood faith to adult commitment through this episode in my life: when I was a young man studying philosophy, I came across the works of Emil du Bois-Reymond, who, in 1882, stated that there were a number of questions which science could never answer. One of these was: what was the far side of the moon like, how did it look? He thought it was utterly impossible; it would never be possible to answer that question. As a young student at the time I was deeply impressed with his comment and I felt that one should be realistic and ask only realistic questions that science could answer. Anyway my first attempts in our field of child psychology and analysis were to ask questions that one could answer. But I was restless, as young people should be, restless in a special way, and I wondered whether if I wanted to ask questions that I could answer, what kind of questions would these be? I wanted to go after that which was answerable, and I said to myself, a young man should be dedicated to the idea that if it was impossible to know what the far side of the moon looks like, I had better go and find out what the far side of the moon was like. We know now how the far side of the moon looks; what, in 1882, was an impossible question, according to du Bois-Reymond, is now a possible question. We have all the technology, all the scientific know-how. We are willing to take the risks and we have been able to organize millions of dollars, thousands of skillful men and women, to work together in a concerted effort to find out what the far side of the moon looks like. I believe, ladies and gentlemen, you now truly follow me; I am not really talking about the far side of the moon as if it were really that important to know. The space program that the United States has developed is not important simply because somebody landed on the moon; rather, the landing on the moon signified the concerted effort of many people to advance space science and space travel; it was the culmination of millions of other questions that brought scientists together—biologists, physicists, chemists, psychiatrists, psychologists, sociologists—to see how one can organize people in a concerted effort to find something out about truth and to make it possible to answer a question that, just a few decades before, seemed impossible.

Again, when I was a little boy, there was a story that intrigued me very much. It was a fairy tale by Wilhelm Hauff in which he described how one could open a person's chest and take out his heart and put in another heart—just a fairy tale. That fairy tale about *The Cold Stone Heart* was perhaps the first science fiction on heart transplants. The concerted efforts of science have now made it possible to open a man's chest, take out his heart, and put in another heart, to make it possible for him to live and possibly to overcome the problem of rejection of the transplant. Du Bois-Reymond, I am sure, would have said it was an impossible question that could never be answered. I suppose it is clear by now that I am committed to the notion that science makes sense and human effort makes sense only if, from time to time, they get together and try to do the impossible, to answer questions which were very, very hard to answer. It began when, as a child of ten, I suffered because Jules Verne's heroes could not come back from the moon to Mother Earth, and I hoped passionately they would be able some day to return to earth, to mother—which obviously reflects a personal experience, but one that everyone in this room understands, does he not? The synthesis between that early faith and the sophistication of science led me into analytic work, to the treatment of neurotic and psychotic people, to help them back to real life, back to mother, to family, to the peer group, to reality, to normal functioning. I guess by now I have given you more than a hint of what made me go into this field.

You see, essentially, the basic problem of the children we are treating here, the autistic and psychotic children, is one of having lost contact with mother in the truest sense of the word: they have lost contact with their fellow man and have been unable to reconnect with him. These children have sometimes no self, no capacity for normal relationships with other people. To them we frequently resemble monsters, like the sea monster of Jules Verne's fiction, or we seem like machines, like the spaceship that Jules Verne described. For them, the attempt to be reached by us has become a problem as impossible as the problem that Jules Verne posed one hundred years ago when he said that the moon gravity (that is, the gravity of psychosis, for we are speaking of psychosis, for we are speaking of lunatics) can never be overcome and we cannot bring "lunatics" back from the moon and back to Mother Earth. I am not surprised that space scientists happened to get interested in something which expresses, in spatial terms, the very problem we face when we treat psychotic children; that is, to make it possible for them to have normal relationships with people, normal relationships with themselves, and to recathect them, to reconnect them, to get together with them. Ladies and gentlemen, what are the technical problems if one wants to bring this about? They are enormous, and I hope that the question period will make it possible for me to discuss some of the obstacles we face; but essentially the main problem is that we deal with an illness that not only presents many puzzling aspects but that forces on us means of treatment, research, and training which are entirely out of the ordinary and are thus very much like the problems of space scientists. I believe the Apollo project has taken some ten years, but it looks now as if we will really reach the moon, doesn't it? It took ten years of dedicated work and support. It took many risks and dangers, even the loss of life. Do you also know that every six months or so, the space scientists had to face the interrogation of public accounting systems, asking: Why not this year? How long will it take? Who can wait that long—ten years, twenty years, five years, six months? There was not a year when there wasn't a question as to whether the Apollo project would continue—understandably, because in order to do this kind of research, one needs mass support, one needs the support of the total government and the resources of a nation. One needs to make decisions about priorities.

Of course, I am driving at the fact that in order to do the work that is done here in this wonderful clinical setting, one needs mass support which has to be constantly renewed. It becomes necessary to tell people what it is all about; one has to account to them. One cannot survive on blind faith, on arousing sympathy or guilt, but one has to prove over and over again that what one does is right. And of course this makes it very difficult because, if, let us say, I had to come to your Board every day in order to account for what I do, how would I find then time and energy, or the hope and courage and the faith to do my work? Imagine, for a moment, if all the space scientists had to appear every day in Congress in order to get their budget approved. Much of our public life (this is not only true in this clinical field, but it is true in any field) is wasted by the fact that there is a system of accounting which robs Boards of their energy, fund-raisers of their energies, scientists of their energy, and of course, has deprived many, many people of the services that would otherwise be available. But the reason that I am here is that I want to account to you for what we are doing, and show how useful it is to invest our, your strength in it. Of course, you are aware that the treatment takes endless time, and that each time treatment is interrupted, there is less chance to restore the situation because the sick children and their parents depend on the relationships that have grown out of treatment. Each time we lose a staff member, each time somebody travels away, each time we have to interrupt the treatment, we have a little less chance with that particular child, any specific patient. I would like to tell you that I have seen very few settings as organized as yours, that undertakes treatment for a certain number of children, and for twice as many adults, their parents, who also have to be in an intensive relationship with the treating team in order to continue the work; in other words, you deal at any given moment with that group of sick children, perhaps ten of them, and twenty of their parents, each of them individually, in a project that, in a small way, is as difficult as the Apollo project. As a matter of fact, it is even more risky than the Apollo project in that we constantly risk the life of the psychotic child and of the parents, if not their physical life, then their mental life. Therefore, we need guarantees, we need a support system that lasts. We cannot afford a situation where, after a successful "flight to the moon," to our goals with these children, we suddenly learn that we have lost our means for getting the child back to earth. In order to reach the psychosis, we have to go a long way, and when we finally have made contact with the psychotic core of the child, our task is now cut out for us; but if we have to interrupt it, if we have no support, we are lost—we cannot do it. Our work with psychotics is, I believe, very much against the present trend of the times. Why? The present trend is one where the overall crisis society makes us feel frequently that we ought to get away from emphasis on the individual, that we don't have enough time, energy, and wisdom to deal with just one person, with the mind of one person; that we ought to take care of mass problems and thus reduce our anxiety. To make an appeal for help for one particular individual—and that's really what it is—one is up against the fact that we are overwhelmed by the social problems of America. As I talk to you, I find myself really on an island of good will, surrounded by a sea of unrest, by a sea of social, political, and military problems which make us feel sometimes that what we do here makes no sense; and you may ask me, as well: does it make sense, does Freud make sense? Or, is such psychoanalytic work anachronistic? Outdated?

Freud had dedicated himself many, many years ago to the treatment of individuals, when there were masses of sufferers. Nevertheless, he did it because every single case that was treated successfully gave unbelievable insights which were then translated into the training of psychiatrists, social workers, psychologists, and psychoanalysts, and finally reached a core of our psychiatric services, so that today we no longer have dungeons in state hospitals, but have, in many parts of the country, state hospitals which offer psychotherapy, guidance, and many preventive services. Every psychotic child who is treated successfully means not only that we have salvaged one particular person, but that his treatment can become the means by which we can create an entirely different climate in the field of psychotherapy. I am thinking of one child I treated successfully, or rather I supervised the work and did the research on it. We called him the Space Child. You may find accounts on the treatment of that child in an early volume: *Children of Time and Space, of Action and Impulse* that describes the early work I did together with my co-workers. This boy lived in space, just as the travelers of Jules Verne except that he was psychotic. He traveled in space, he engaged in battles with monsters, he did not want to talk with people, he was isolated and far removed from the world. This child had ten years of treatment, ladies and gentlemen, at the Menninger Foundation, its Southard School. Today, he is a teacher of space science, a physicist and a mathematician. He is married and he has children. You may consider him a little odd, as professors of space science might appear around analysts or as we might appear to them, but indeed he has become a valuable human being. But the fact that he was cured is perhaps not the decisive point; what is decisive is that this patient helped me indirectly to pull hundreds of trainees to seminar after seminar; his case got into books that were translated into Spanish and German, into the psychiatric literature, and helped change the climate of the time. So that when I appeal to you, I am not appealing simply to say: "Please save these ten or twenty or thirty children! I am saying to you that much more is involved here. What is involved is that you are training a new generation of people who are willing to make commitments, individual commitments, commitments which will change the professions, will change the charitable work of the city, will change the research in the university; in other words, we conduct a model program which has immense meaning and significance. It is not the piece of rock that someone will bring back from the moon that makes us spend $300,000,000, but, rather, it is the fact that we can prove to the world that cooperative, peaceful enterprises—not wars in the Far East, the Middle East, the Near East, or Europe—have a chance for success. It is for this reason that I believe that, seen socially, ethically, researchwise, and in terms of direct service for the child, the work that we do is not only justified, but is a necessity, because if our society loses in the individual, liberty is done for, freedom is done for, and we will become a despotic totalitarian society. The best way to test whether you are interested in the individual is to measure the strength you have to dedicate to those fringe cases that I have just described that are so far away from us—near the moon, as it were, lunatics—where you can prove that you mean it.

I asked the chief of your clinic what kind of name you have chosen for yourselves. He told me that you have maintained a name from older, more sentimental days of charitable work and that you called yourselves, "The Godparents?" I suppose this name was developed at a time when you wanted to offer tangible services to children in need, perhaps children who had lost their parents, or who had incompetent parents, hospitalized mothers, etc. You could offer food baskets, direct services, and you could be in direct touch with the problem and understand it from living experience. But presently we cannot show you the babies and let you hold them, and we cannot help you distribute the food baskets, or take the children to your home. You have no living and direct experience to hold on to. How can we bring near to you what it means to work with children as sick as the ones that we describe? We need something much bigger than charity now. The appeal to the bleeding heart is not enough. We need *caritas*; we need a long-lasting love and investment to make it possible for a few space children to come back to earth, to be a part of us again. I have friends who escaped together with me from the Nazis in Europe. Their son, a musician who loves to play Bach, is now in Viet Nam; we want the children back who are in danger of being lost in another battle. Their battlefield is not in Viet Nam;* it is a battlefield of the mind. It is a cruel war because anyone who has ever understood the suffering of a psychotic person knows that it is even more beastly than a war in

---

* My friend's son was lucky enough to return after his service.

which people are being killed. It really is a killing war, a desperate war, and we want to make war on that war. In becoming the psychological peacemakers of these children we want to become the peacemakers of their minds.

We have learned now that heart surgery—open heart surgery—has perhaps an improving survival rate; anyone who needs to have heart surgery can go into it knowing that there is a good chance of survival. We now can also exchange a heart, and we have even a chance of surviving that. I think in the kind of work that we do with psychotic children we are doing just a little better, not very much better. Would you want to abolish heart surgery because the statistics are not good? Ours are not good yet, but the heart statistics will be much better five years from now. The kidney transplant statistics will be much better ten years from now, or one year from now. And in the treatment of psychotic children, if we have the opportunity for prolonged experience, if our work is committed, and if we have committed support, it may soon be possible to say that schizophrenia, childhood psychosis, and childhood autism are now treatable diseases of the mind; they are not hopeless any more. I am sure there are people among you with relatives who are hopelessly ill mentally. If we could have gotten them as children, I think, with the knowledge that we have today, they might not be hopelessly ill; they might have recovered to a large extent. I think if we are permitted another twenty-five years, childhood schizophrenia will be a treatable disease like a learning disorder. It will not always work; it is even true for mild diseases like learning disorders that we sometimes have no answers—after all, there is more to it than psychiatric treatment—but today it is within our reach. In order, however, to be successful, we need a support system which compares a bit to the support system that the astronauts need, doesn't it? In order to put three men into space and bring them back, you need hundreds of scientists, you need crews and battleships, you need a whole organization which is terribly expensive, not only in terms of money but in terms of coordination, human enterprise, human patience, and I am afraid that I have to confess to you that our work needs that kind of support system. It is unbelievable that each hour which a therapist conducts with these children—hopefully, a skilled therapist—takes endless support. I am not just speaking about your dollars; I mean the teachers we must train, the psychologists, the receptionist who must be capable of responding to people who telephone there and want help; the cook who is in steady contact with the children, the man who operates the elevator, the public relations people, the fund-raisers, the people who explain the nature of the illness to other people, the researchers, the trainers. All of them need to be a part of that support system. In other words, you are really taking on a private project, a pilot project that is about as difficult as going to the moon. It is, indeed it is. But then, ladies and gentlemen, would you want to come for the evening to our Board meeting if all you did was raise money for a few Easter baskets? Or is it more meaningful to invest yourself in a thoughtful experiment under thoughtful leadership that could have the kind of result that I described in the story of the Space Child? Let me end with one true story and I hope then we can open the discussion and I will try to answer every question and every thought you have as honestly as I can; and if I don't know, and often I will not, I will honestly tell you about the shortcomings and the failures of our work.

Another of my patients was a fourteen-year-old girl when she came to us, older than children with whom we usually start. She had suffered a schizophrenic break, become delusional and then homicidal; she tried to choke a girl in the classroom of her school and if two or three teachers hadn't pulled her off, the other child might have died. She thought she was married to Robin Hood; she had religious fantasies where she thought she was Jesus Christ. We had her in treatment four years with excellent results. She became the best student in her high school, received a university scholarship, and earned a Ph.D. in English. She married and had a child. At one crucial point in her life, she did not know whether she should continue her studies or have that child, and by chance her husband, a psychologist, brought home certain articles that he had found in the literature that had my name, and she instantly recognized that these articles, also published in the book I mentioned, were about her, even though I had carefully disguised the material. In one of these chapters I said that if my patient should ever discover the material, I know she would agree with me that, regardless of whether she might someday get sick again or not (because psychiatrists, like dentists, internists, or surgeons, cannot guarantee that their patients will remain well forever), she would be strong enough not to fall back into a delusional catastrophe but would be able to turn to other people for help. In other words, the contact between her and the helping person would never be broken. And she said that she found this statement such a challenge that she thought she ought to answer, and she wrote me an account of herself, some ten years after treatment. She said that there had been many critical times, and one or two moments when she thought she might fall back into illness; but during the greatest crisis, when she had to decide whether she was going to continue with her research or give it up to stay with the baby, she was able to sort out her commitments and decide that she would get a baby sitter from time to time so that she could still be a mother and, at the same time, continue her studies. She realized that, at times, she would have to be a part-time mother. But, she added, because of the treatment she had received and the insights she had gained, she knew she never would be a *part-mother*, as she felt her own mother had been to her.

I said to myself, I gave four years to this young person—four years, many hours of research, many seminar hours, many times when I asked myself: Will this seed come up? Not only did she overcome her own illness but she learned to be a mother; and her baby will never have to scream in French or English or any other language, "Mother, save me!" because she will have had a real mother. This is the project, this is the program we are engaged in. I realize, ladies and gentlemen, to discuss the nature of psychosis is extremely difficult, and I want you to be free to ask whatever questions you wish, whether they are sophisticated or whether you might consider them naive. Even the questions that we cannot answer are to unite us in a common cause and might bring us a little nearer to the point when we can perhaps say to a latter day du Bois-Reymond; "You were wrong. You thought that question could never be answered, but we can show you now that we have met the challenge, that we have responded to a situation of despair with activities of hope. Join us in that conquest of inner space."

Part One
DIAGNOSTIC ISSUES

For the analyst's inquiring mind, it is a second, vital objection that fact finding about assessment is at an end when the analytic method is not used. We need to be absolutely certain of the classification of a given case before taking the choice of therapeutic element away from the patient and into our own hands, i.e., before limiting the chances of therapy to one single factor. As our skill in assessment stands today, however, such accuracy of diagnostic judgment seems to me an ideal to be realized not in our present state of knowledge but in the distant future.

ANNA FREUD

CHAPTER ONE

Cause of the Illness or Cause of the Cure*

It is one of the most interesting paradoxes that Freud, who started with the determination to find out the mechanics of psychic life, discovered that the psychic life was full of meaning.

PAUL SCHILDER, 1933

From the 1930's to the present, the period of time covered by her review (1), Dr. Lauretta Bender has been identified with the multitudinous efforts to clarify and master by scientific, psychiatric means the perplexing but extremely challenging dilemma of childhood schizophrenia; indeed, she has been recognized in many quarters as the chief clinical exponent and theoretician of the illness. In a sense, the history of the expansion of our knowledge of childhood schizophrenia can be said to be Dr. Bender's professional history.

From the onset of her involvement with this clinical problem, she and her co-workers were in the unenviable predicament of assuming the responsibility for the care and treatment of children sent to Bellevue Hospital, and later to Creedmoor State Hospital, of whose illness they could only ask: "What is it, and what do we do with it?" Confronted with an illness that presented a confusing array of symptoms of severe emotional and organic dysfunction, often with an overlay of

---

* Seymour W. Friedman, M.D. is co-author of this chapter.

symptoms of mental retardation, an illness equivalent in numbers to epidemic proportions, they had to respond to urgent socio-medical-psychiatric pressures to treat. Their earliest therapeutic instruments, derived from the then known armamentarium of modified psychoanalytic theory, play and group therapy, puppetry and art therapy, and eventually supplemented by Metrazol shock therapy and other physiological therapies, were generally applicable to the broad categories of psychological and organic emotional illness. One even gets the impression that despite the urgent clinical commitment to treat, scientific interest and investment in the process of the treatment, as manifested in the literature, may have been masked as peripheral interest and curiosity, such as a paper on art therapy serving as a vehicle for publishing a complete case history of a schizophrenic child.

Drawing upon Schilder's experience of the failure of psychoanalysis of adult schizophrenics to bring to light relevant factors or traumata sufficient to account for the severity and malignancy of the illness, and supporting her views by similar disappointing results in the therapeutic work of Melanie Klein and her group, Bender concluded that psychoanalytic investigation of schizophrenic children had failed to provide adequate data to account for the severity of the illness. (The model for such thinking—oversimplified, we believe, even for the symptom neuroses—suggested that the discovery of the trauma, the "cause" of the illness, constituted its cure.) Regarding as futile the results of direct therapeutic efforts to clarify the mysterious nature of the illness, and moved by the need to understand it more precisely, Dr. Bender and her co-workers accordingly centered their clinical and investigative interest on the delineation of clinical patterns and diagnosis, at that time considered by many to be of lesser importance.

Dr. Bender turned to the broad areas of biology and psychology, with emphasis on key concepts derived from psychoanalytic and evolutionary theory, embryology and genetics, to comprehend the illness. In the evolution of her concept of childhood schizophrenia, she credits psychoanalytic theories of the genesis of personality, Gestalt psychology, Schilder's concept of biological and psychological interaction, Gesell's contribution to the embryology of behavior, and Kallmann's studies of genetic factors with the greatest influence. She drew upon these for the key concepts comprising her theory of a total organismic disorder with inherited vulnerability, characterized by a lag of maturation at the embryonic level resulting from evolutionary fixation; further resulting in embryonic plasticity and lack of pattern differentiation in all areas of bodily function; leading to decompensation, regression, and psychosis under physiological, organic, or psychological crisis or trauma; and bringing forth a core anxiety which evokes extreme defenses that determine the final clinical picture.

Dr. Bender's current formulation of childhood schizophrenia is most intriguing, comprehensive, and founded on accepted principles of biology and psychology. She is certainly justified in her confidence that she has an "idea of what causes schizophrenia." We find it regrettable, however, that after starting her extensive and significant work out of concern for treatment, she should finally have become involved with an investigation of its etiology and diagnostic nature that, unfortunately, added little to a foundation on which to base a more rational, reliable and appropriate method of treatment than was available at the beginning of her long and dedicated studies. Her concept of childhood schizophrenia is a masterful integration and synthesis of broad biological principles that attests to the global and total nature of this disorder, equivalent to the complexity of human personality development itself, and consistent with our recognition of its deep and pervasive complexity and powerful resistance to all forms of therapeutic intervention and influence. Her final formulation makes amply clear that in childhood schizophrenia we deal with an illness of utmost magnitude for which treatment can be expected to be equally difficult and complex. Paradoxically, however, the biological implications of Dr. Bender's valid diagnostic conclusions inevitably lead in the direction of the physiological and somatic therapies, which have so far failed to convincingly demonstrate a reliable effect on the illness itself. Her conceptions concerning etiology thus embody hidden prescriptions for treatment programs and directives for specific actions.

As we stated in an earlier paper (2), much research and clinical work in the area of childhood schizophrenia continues on many clinical islands, each developing its own special skills, its own theoretical strengths as well as biases. One is reminded of medieval guilds which did not share their trade secrets, their special ways of building cathedrals or of painting. Each guild, each little island, led usually by an outstanding individual, gave impetus to important work but often maintained typical insularity. Historically these guilds were not ready to get together on a master plan to tackle their problems. Are our "guilds" ready for such a master plan?

Assuming that Bender would not want to maintain a research island separated from the rest of the scientific community, we believe she will welcome our suggestion for bridges linking these various efforts. For this reason, to her review of work in childhood schizophrenia, we add other recent work of psychoanalytic orientation, itself at times not free of the insular orientation—a "childhood disease" so often true of clinical research, perhaps a professional replica of the very disease it tries to understand and treat. There is the work of Bettelheim at the Orthogenic School, of Anna Freud and her Hampstead group, of Mahler at the Masters Children's Center, of the late Beata Rank at the Putnam-Rank Center, each working in clinical settings with co-workers, to mention but a few of the psychoanalytic investigators who have devoted many years to this problem area. We refer to our own work, carried out during the last two decades at Menninger's Southard School and at Reiss-Davis Child Study Center, some of which has been described in our recent book (3), and based on direct psycho-analytic therapy of schizophrenic children, who are the subject and source of data of this research project.

Through the use of taped and recorded analytic interviews, re-peated psychological tests, careful diagnostic assessments, and concomi-tant work with parents and with community resources, we are deriving meaningful insights into diagnostic and psychotherapeutic treatment methods and techniques, as well as into the nature of the illness itself. A significant principle that has been repeatedly verified is the insepar-ability of diagnosis and treatment within both clinical practice and research methodology. Paraphrasing Kant's epigrammatic statement on the relationship between theory and experience, we say that *treatment without diagnosis is blind*, haphazard, and unsuccessful; conversely, *diagnosis without treatment is empty* and meaningless. In no clinical area does this hold more true than in childhood schizophrenia, where to divorce diagnosis from treatment is to arrive literally at a clinical depiction of the illness but not to reach or experience the illness itself. To separate treatment from diagnosis is to be left in the position of applying known and tried techniques of therapy to specific but iso-lated symptoms, behavior patterns, or physiological conditions, but not to the illness itself.

We are further confronted with the paradox, peculiar to the treat-ment of childhood schizophrenia but intrinsic in all psychological ill-ness, that the illness cannot be successfully treated by application of any technique, but only by means of a therapeutic process that transpires within the therapeutic relationship; i.e., only by treating the person with the illness, not the various manifestations or symptoms of the illness. Similarly, diagnostic understanding of the nature of childhood schizophrenia can be achieved only by knowing and coming to grips with the illness itself, which can be effected only by understanding the psychic structure and functioning of the person with the illness. Yet this understanding is derived only by treatment of the person, a process for which we believe classical psychoanalytic theory provides the basic model. The unique nature of childhood schizophrenia, however, re-quires modifications of psychotherapeutic technique, and these become at once the aim and the means of a search into childhood psychosis via psychoanalytic psychotherapy.

In evolving a concept of childhood schizophrenia, Dr. Bender leaves one with the impression that in turning away from psychological treatment as a source of data, she has instead turned to accepted generalized principles applicable to human life to explain the vast behavioral data that she wishes to synthesize into a coherent whole. In so doing she has admirably formulated her concept but has not synthesized the unique essence of schizophrenia; in fact, she may not actually be dealing with schizophrenia itself, but rather with the principles that could intellectually and logically explain the data by a coherent, integrated theory. One gets a similar impression from current efforts to explain the cause of schizophrenia by physiological and organic studies of the central nervous system, the autonomic nervous system, the endocrine system, and metabolic states: what is learned from these studies concerns the endocrine, metabolic, and nervous system functioning of schizophrenic individuals, rather than schizophrenia itself. Schizophrenia is not an abstract entity; it is a unique phenomenon in each individual, and is always more and other than the sum of its biological, physiological, and psychological processes. Only direct psychological involvement with the schizophrenic child as a participant observer— the use of oneself as an instrument—permits the synthesis of other clinical methods of investigation. Even diagnosis must be a process of involvement; and the key which opens the door to the inner world of the schizophrenic child is the empathic instrument of the trained observer and therapist.

The search for etiological factors as a basis for diagnostic representation, consistent with established scientific medical tradition, logically and practically leads to a rational basis for the treatment of causes and symptoms, but not of the illness itself. Schizophrenia is widely recognized as a total illness of the entire personality, a concept for which Dr. Bender, more than any other investigator, is scientifically responsible. Through and within the process of treatment of the schizophrenic person, etiology and diagnosis emerge as living, meaningful data which simultaneously explain the illness and provide necessary clues and directives for the formulation of a rational, appropriate philosophy of treatment.

Only when etiology, diagnosis, and treatment are inseparable functions of an integrated therapeutic purpose can etiology and diagnosis serve as interrelated, meaningful determinants for a rational and effective program of treatment. Divorced from each other, they reflect the fragmented, disintegrated and ineffectual process inherent in the schizophrenic illness itself. We suggest that it is precisely this phenomenon of fragmentation that has dialectically determined the development of scientific investigation into childhood schizophrenia, which originally started with the aim to treat as its thesis, switched to an investigation of the nature of the illness, and culminated in the antithesis: a rational and comprehensive theory of its etiology and diagnostic characteristics with no accompanying effective, enduring, and optimistic treatment program. We share with Dr. Bender her confidence that we know much better what childhood schizophrenia is and what causes it, and most of what we know, we learned from her; but we are still uncomfortable about our efforts to do something with and about it.

It is to this lack of synthesis that our research into childhood psychosis has directed its attention, in an effort to determine *not the cause of the illness but the cause of the cure.* To those who would regard this research methodology as a reversal of the accepted medical procedure of advancing from cause of illness to cure, rather than from cure to cause, we would respond that science should be identified with relevance, flexibility, and adaptability, and its methods must remain open to adaptation to whatever phenomenon it is committed to investigate and master.

From our study of the psychoanalytic treatment of childhood schizophrenia, we have learned that the primary process with its irrational psychic content can serve as the instrumentality of a process of change to a higher integration of psychic and personality functioning. In a like way, the peculiar characteristics of schizophrenia—the underlying principles of order governing its disorder—can direct research methodology in the service of achieving scientific rather than pseudo-rational control over its intrinsically irrational, fragmented identity.

We simply say that one does not understand childhood schizophrenia merely by comprehending its cause; one understands the process completely only if one discovers or invents techniques of change, interventions towards cure. Analytic work with schizophrenic children will not be the only road to the discovery of scientific methods of change. But Dr. Bender can accept that analytic treatment of schizophrenic children in the thirties is not the same as that of the late sixties. We hope our discussion will prove a bridge from island to island, just as the analytic treatment of these children attempts to create a lasting bridge between our world and the world of these children, who for so many years have been the passionate scientific concern of Dr. Bender.

Our task then—if we are some day to overcome the fragmentation of research in the field of childhood schizophrenia and permit the emergence of a wider plan that would gradually replace fragmentation with a division of labor—is to grant equal importance to diagnostic and therapeutic studies; to coordinate them with studies that unite biology and physiology with psychology and sociology; and to encompass, as well, the study of the human instrument—the researcher—as a participating observer, who discovers the deepest meanings of the schizophrenic child's mind, often through difficult and painful self-discovery.

Paul Schilder (3) must have had in mind such a unity of science and of scientific action. His words concerning all psychic life are indeed applicable to the psychic life of the schizophrenic child as well. He says:

> It is one of the most interesting paradoxes that Freud, who started with the determination to find out the mechanics of psychic life, discovered that the psychic life was full of meaning. He found this meaning not only in the purposeful actions of everyday life, in will, and determination, but also in psychic experiences which science and educated popular belief had so far considered as meaningless —in dreams, in delusions, in hallucinations, and in the pathology of everyday life, as slips of the tongue. Furthermore, he showed that the life of an individual forms a unit, that the earliest experiences of childhood as well as the later acquisitions not only remain in the psychic sphere but have a lasting influence in every phase of life. The total life of an individual becomes a dynamic unit. The terms "personality," "unity of the ego," and "psyche" were empty shells before his time; they have now the full richness of experiences of an accepted scientific methodology.

REFERENCES

1. Bender, L. "Childhood Schizophrenia: A Review," International Journal of Psychiatry, 1968, 5:3.
2. Ekstein, R., K. Bryant, and S. Friedman, "Childhood Schizophrenia and Allied Conditions." In Schizophrenia by L. Bellak. New York: Logos Press, 1958, pp. 555-693.
3. Ekstein, R. Children of Time and Space, of Action and Impulse. New York: Appleton-Century-Crofts, 1966.
4. Schilder, P. "Psychoanalysis and Philosophy," Psychoanalytic Review, 1933, 22: 244-287.

CHAPTER TWO

The Psychotic Pursuit of Reality*

The concept of reality testing is a central principle both in clinical theory and practice. This concept initially was defined as the capacity to judge the source of perception with reference to whether it came from within or without. Further refinement of this definition led to the concept of reality testing as a process wherein the individual checked his perception and thoughts to determine the appropriateness of his thoughts or actions and of the inferences he made from his perceptions. For such testing, it is posited that the individual uses some criteria against which to evaluate the reality of a perception, thought, or action. Under ordinary circumstances, these criteria are in the external world and accessible to consensual validation. In psychosis, however, as pointed out by Freud (1), the individual denies not only "fresh perceptions, but the importance (cathexis) of the inner world—that inner world which formerly reflected the outer world as an image of it—is withdrawn too." With such denial of the external world, the psychotic then obviously does not have reality testing available as based on the customary externally based cues. Shevrin and Toussieng (2) have postulated, on the basis of evidence that in the earliest period of life many schizophrenic children manifest unusual sensitivity to stimuli, that one way in which the individual can deal with the resultant threat of being flooded is to create a barrier against incoming stimuli. They go on to suggest that it is this defensive maneuver which may lead in varying degrees to preference for inner reality over outer reality. Psychoanalytic

* Mortimer M. Meyer, Ph.D. is the co-author of this chapter.

24

theory, however, has pointed out the importance of recognizing that the individual experiences not only the external environment as a reality, but his internal world as a reality, and that both the inner, unexpressed thought or behavior, as well as the expressed behavior, normally should be subjected to the reality testing process (3), (Ch. 4 this vol.).

The first step in the development of reality testing in the child is the gradual separation of the self from other objects, animate and inanimate, of the I from the not I. However, in completion of the process it is necessary that there develop stable internalized representation of the primary objects from whom the child has separated. Such a course of development, when it proceeds normally, lays the foundation for the child's being able to maintain an effective relationship between the inner and outer worlds. The outer reality object perceived on the basis of the inner reality becomes one with whom the child feels able to establish a safe and gratifying relationship. Thus, contact with reality becomes an established and autonomous function which does not require special effort to maintain a stable relationship. In the instances of extreme difficulty with the separation process, the child who is unable to establish any separation remains fused with the parent in a symbiotic relationship in which the lability of the contact with external reality destroys the capacity to differentiate between inner and outer worlds and thereby inner and outer reality. Paradoxically, the child who seemingly resorts to complete separation establishes an autistic position which, in fact, is rather complete isolation, as he has never developed recognition of another, separate object from whom to separate.

Such children have been described as having failed to develop a reality testing function, or else as having lost the reality testing function which once was present. Such children are thus considered to be floundering directionless and without guidance from any reality testing function. A modified view of this is one which suggests that it is not that reality testing as such is lost or absent, but rather that the individual, upon perceiving and testing the reality, for defensive reasons must alter the perceived reality to fit a frame of reference which will maintain a personal sense of integrity.

The above framework for viewing reality testing is based on the use of perception of the external environment as the only basis for a reality testing process in that the individual either uses external criteria as a basis of validity or has no such criteria. Such a hypothesis implies a single pole theory, in that there is only one focus for reality testing, that is, the external environment. On this basis, therapeutic efforts are bent in the direction of trying to assist the patient to cathect or re-cathect this single pole of reality, and experience has indicated the degree of difficulty which is involved in this reconstructive effort.

Careful consideration of the clinical material of schizophrenic children as seen in the Project on Childhood Psychosis (4, 5, 6) suggests an elaboration of this hypothesis and an additional interpretation. Although severely disturbed children appear to show little awareness of or contact with external reality, they have shown indication of an active internal life which represents a reality to them. Freud (1), in discussing the psychotic, pointed out that under such circumstances "the ego creates for itself in a lordly manner a new outer and inner world." These children behave as if their inner life is their critical reality and thus reverse the usual reality testing procedure. Normally, it is expected that the external environment will be used as the criterion against which to test the reality of an inner or outer percept. These children, instead, use their inner experience as criteria against which to test the validity of the outer experience. When external reality does not fit the criterion of their inner reality, it is disregarded or distorted. When external reality experiences in terms of their inner reality seem irrelevant to their inner needs, these are cast aside, just as the normal individual, who uses external criteria as a basis, may set aside inner reality experiences which do not fit the external criteria. Still further for these children, since external reality is experienced as a projection of the inner reality, many events take on special and terrifying meanings and, therefore, must be avoided at all costs.

USE OF INTERNAL CRITERIA

It is the use of these highly idiosyncratic internal criteria for validation, rather than the external criteria commonly used on the basis of consensual validation, that makes the psychotic so different and so difficult to understand. A thirteen and one-half year-old boy, with an underlying psychotic structure, reacted verbally to a situation in a manner which provides an opportunity to observe the way in which a psychotic can reverse the usual reality testing process. At the end of a game of checkers in which the therapist had clearly won, he burst out angrily, "I won. I won."

Taken by itself, this statement is blatantly psychotic denial of reality and bizarre. For this boy, who had been in treatment over four years, winning a game has been of fundamental importance to him as a defense against the catastrophe of losing. Losing means to him losing the whole self. Winning means being saved from the total destruction which he associates with losing, because losing means that his father, who constantly derogates him, is correct; and that he is, therefore, useless and "dispensable." Consequently, he cheats flagrantly, if necessary to win. On this occasion, Christmas week, his disturbance was exacerbated and he was very upset at losing a game of checkers. Thus, when it was evident to him that he had lost, he burst with the angry, "I won"—the denial of the reality. The therapist simply commented, "Okay." He then repeated more firmly, "I won." The therapist repeated gently, "Okay." Under ordinary circumstances, the person who cheats forfeits the game, and the other person wins. He went on to say that, by his rules, the therapist had cheated; because cheating was not cheating, and not cheating was cheating. His inner need to win was so crucial that he had to have the fact fit the need. Thus, he readapted the usual external criteria for winning. He had to change them and re-interpret the event to fit his needed inner reality, and thus reacted with psychotic denial. Ordinarily, we are not able to be a participant in the process, and only witness the resultant psychotic denial. He would then have been more like the classic psychotic, whose bizarre conclusions are evident and appear to have no logical process.

The importance of this illustration lies in the recognition that psychotic reality testing failure is not simply a matter of being unable to use the normal criteria for evaluation. The psychotic is not simply a disorganized person seeking organization, but a person with a system for evaluating that serves his inner reality far better than the organized approach to reality testing of the non-psychotic. Consequently, the "helping hand" initially may not be seen as a "helping hand," not only because it attempts to force the patient to face the threat of the avoided material, but also because it is seen as an attempt to destroy a laboriously achieved order and to substitute an alien basis for organization.

THE PSYCHOTIC CATHEXIS

The hypothesis offered here is that, whereas in the normal individual the cathexis is to external criteria as the basis of reality testing, in the psychotic the cathexis is to the inner world as the criteria for such evaluation. In the following material, rich in its communication on many levels, this patient treated in the Project reveals how tenaciously she wishes to stay in her inner world and to confirm its reality, rather than to move toward a world of external reality orientation.

"I know I am real, and I know I have a very pretty face like a doll's face . . . I have seen myself in the mirror, and I have seen that I have a very pretty face, and it looks like a doll's face . . . that's why I feel that I am not real . . . let's say, I'm like a doll. I feel I am so beautiful I am an angel." The patient goes on and talks about beautiful names such as Snow White and Cinderella, and then goes on to the beauty of Sleeping Beauty. "Because I look like a cartoon—my face looks like a doll's face. I don't look real, because I am so beautiful that I look like a cartoon." (Therapist interprets the patient's difficulty distinguishing whether she is real or not by pointing out that when she starts to think about herself, she quickly wanders off into the world of cartoons and imagination. He goes on to say, "You almost prefer to stay there, and whenever anyone tries to talk with you about real life, you talk about that part of yourself that goes with the fairy tale and the fantasy." "Right, Doctor, because I would call myself, I would be Snow White . . . I think more of myself. I am better than them. I am more beautiful than Snow White, Sleeping Beauty or Cinderella." As the patient pushes the therapist to tell about her beauty, she goes on to say, "Those are just examples I give you as of how, an example, I wish you would tell me of how beautiful I am." (Therapist comments, "Don't you think a deer is beautiful?") "Yes." ("But don't you think that a part of his beauty is that he is frightened?") "Well, let's forget that the deer is frightened. Now tell me what I would resemble, as beautiful as what?" (Therapist: "As beautiful as a Mexican girl that was to an American school.") ". . . Will you forget that! Forget that! Don't answer me those questions. Don't answer me, I'm as beautiful as a frightened deer or a Mexican girl. (Patient continues with increasing emphasis and irritation.) Forget that . . . answer me exactly the question I ask you. You are going to answer me the same as I ask you how beautiful is Sleeping Beauty, and you told me, well, she is as beautiful as when the sun rises . . . Am I as beautiful as a rose?" (Therapist: "No.") "No?" (Said with surprise.) (Therapist: "No.") "No?' (Said almost with astonishment.) ("You resemble a beautiful girl on a beach when the sun is warm and the ocean plays with the sand.") "What are you talking about anyway?" The passage above indicates how the patient struggles to maintain the pursuit of reality, but at this point still in the service of establishing the reality in terms of the inner world. To paraphrase Kris (7), it is progression of the ego in the service of the id.

The cathexis of external or internal reality, as basis for reality testing, should not, however, be thought of as discrete and dichotomized, but rather as the ends of a continuum. Such a continuum provides deepening insight into other observed clinical data. Thus, the much discussed "borderline psychotic" is not someone who is vaguely on the fringe of dealing with external reality, but rather an individual whose cathexis is fluctuating so that, with one foot in each realm, he straddles the distance in ever-changing, uncomfortable, and ineffective fashion. In some cases, this fluctuation involves an almost complete shift of cathexis from the use of external criteria for both outer and inner experiences to the use of inner criteria for both. In other cases, the cathexis is to external criteria for evaluating the inner experiences. In this way, the psychotic's inner world remains unchallenged. Thus far, the bi-polar concept of reality testing has been discussed in terms of the disturbed individual, but actually has helpful implications for the non-psychotic as well. Thus, Kris' (7) concept of "regression in the service of the ego" can be viewed as characterizing an individual whose cathexis to reality has that degree of security and richness, that regression to primary process is possible along this continuum without the danger that cathexis to inner reality will overwhelm the former.

ENTERING THE PSYCHOTIC'S WORLD

Numerous writers, in discussing the treatment of the psychotic, have talked about entering the psychotic's world. However, such discussion has always remained limited to entering the fantasy, the content, and assumed that the psychotic world was chaotic and unorganized, and therefore, difficult to follow. With a basis for understanding the psychotic's way of *organizing* his world, in terms of his *mode* of reality testing, his logic takes on more order and internal consistency. *The psychotic's thought disorder actually has an order.* It is but our value judgment that calls it "disorder." Such judgment can be likened to early beliefs that earthquakes had no order or scientific explanation because of their disruptive effect. It may be that it is as difficult and threatening a task for the psychotic to give up his well established logic as for the average normal individual to permit himself to give up his logic, as represented by retreat to primary process. In this sense, we have underestimated the task that therapy sets for the psychotic, as well as for the therapist.

Observation of psychotics, especially in treatment, reveals tentative efforts to reach out to incorporate the external reality. However, even with therapeutic help, this "pursuit of reality" is a very tenuous one, although a major aspect of the treatment. It is as if, for such people, external reality has all of the remoteness, threat, and confusion that primary process has for the non-psychotic, and must be avoided just as the non-psychotic tries to avoid the primary process. Thus, as Ekstein and Wallerstein (8) and Sechehaye (9) have pointed out, it becomes necessary for the therapist initially to retreat completely with the patient to his primary process world and ally himself with this frame of reference in order to establish communication. In contrast to the usual analytic approach with the neurotic, where the pursuit of material is in the service of restoring unconscious content—with the psychotic, the pursuit is to re-establish the wish to re-cathect reality episodes and advanced ego functions.

THE HALLUCINATORY WISH

The tenacity of the psychotic process can thus be understood in terms of the psychotic's basic belief that gratification can be obtained only through the inner reality, which serves as the basis for gratification through the hallucinatory wish. Because the content of the fantasies frequently uses material from a higher level, the therapist is inclined to lose sight of this underlying primitive and archaic mode of gratification. The psychotic, based on his early experiences, anticipates that external reality will always be frustrating and threatening. Therefore, depending upon the hallucinatory wish seems the more reliable and less dangerous approach. For the most regressed psychotics, even the admission of the external world into the hallucinatory wish system is too threatening. Thus, further distance is put between the self and the external world, by means of using only the self as content or permitting no content and thus no conscious fantasy.

In therapeutic work with neurotics, the need for intensive defense against archaic fantasies has been accepted and understood as part of the psychoanalytic treatment process. However, the external world-oriented therapist has not yet sufficiently recognized the fact that the external world can be as feared as the neurotic fears his internal world. The acceptance of the external world (that is, its internal representation) into the hallucinatory image tends to be misunderstood as representing more acceptance of the external world than is actually true. The psychotic's view of the external world can, perhaps, be best illustrated by the shadow-graph, in which the closer one moves the object from the screen to the source of light, the larger and more threatening becomes the object. As long as the psychotic can keep the object close to him and away from the source of light, in this case the external world, the threat is diminished. On the other hand, the more you must examine the internal image in terms of the external light, the more threatening the image becomes. The more the therapist is seen as an active part in the pursuit of external reality, the more threatening an object he becomes in geometric proportion. Whereas the neurotic is in close continuity with the external reality but experiences discontinuity with the unconscious, the psychotic is in close continuity with the primary processes and experiences discontinuity with the external reality, which results in the psychotic having only fragmentary islands of secondary process functioning. Thus, the therapist in working with a neurotic tries to bridge the discontinuity with the unconscious process. In working with the psychotic, on the other hand, the therapist must seek to help the patient bridge the discontinuity with the external reality. However, the basic stumbling block in working with the psychotic is the essential problem of creating the wish and need for external reality in such a patient. The pursuit of it must originate in the patient, and the therapist can only be an ally in this pursuit. The problem that develops when this need and wish have been stimulated in the patient is that, with such primitive psychic organization, this pursuit becomes an impulsive act which is in itself a failure in the attempt to achieve a reality orientation, because impulsivity represents the inability to delay and to cathect reality on a higher level of ego functioning. In addition, the impulsivity in such primitive psychic organization creates the situation in which the movement forward toward the pursuit of external reality brings with it impulsive acts that lack time for judgment, with resulting social emergencies that in turn jeopardize the therapeutic process itself.

BARRIER BETWEEN INNER AND OUTER WORLDS

This hypothesis has clinical importance, not only for the treatment process but for the development process as well. The orientation to inner world reality, as contrasted with orientation to outer world reality, can be likened to situations in which there is actual sensory deprivation, in that a barrier between external world and internal world has been erected. The difference is that in the former case, by turning away from the outer reality, the sensory deprivation, on a level of psychic process, is self-determined with resulting diminished intake and deformation. In the other situation, the deprivation is initiated on a physical level by an outside source, but also with accompanying psychic deformation. Research work with canal boat and gypsy children (10) has demonstrated clearly the stunting of mental growth and its irreversibility after a certain age. Where the allegiance to the stimulation from the external reality is present, although other defenses may operate, external experiences still have access to the inner world, and that aspect of the developmental growth dependent upon such stimulation can continue. The emptiness noted in the adult simple schizophrenic may, in part, be due to such self-imposed deprivation, and explain why with such people it is often possible to restore cathexis to the external world of reality, but not to eradicate the inner emptiness.

TWO ILLUSTRATIONS

Two patients being seen for intensive treatment in the Project provide illustrations of these processes. The first patient is a nineteen-year-old girl, who has been in treatment for about four years. In the diagnostic testing which has been repeated, she gave a Rorschach of a marked richness, which suggested not only the presence of highly differentiated fantasies, but of capacity for complex thought processes. Nevertheless, her performance on intelligence tests was in the range of borderline defective. The psychological tests suggested that she had a marked allegiance to her inner reality, which was highly organized, and that outer reality was conveniently woven into the inner reality so that she had the highly organized world which was based on the acceptance of inner reality as the central matrix. The apparent discrepancy can be explained by the emphasis given to the inner world which so blocked incoming stimuli that a self-imposed sensory deprivation occurred, with a resulting deformation.

In the treatment process, the same patterns reveal themselves. In her fantasies she showed a marked richness, highly differentiated thought, and yet a reality functioning on a very infantile and inadequate level. When attempts were made to help her orient herself more effectively to the external reality, she would defend markedly against it by denial and by indicating that her fantasies were always far superior to anything that the external reality could offer. Thus, the treatment was not only a matter of taking into account basic conflicts, but of a mode of life orientation which for her was so entrenched that attempting to make external reality a central matrix involved a total reorganization. She has become so habituated to and accepting of the schizophrenic process that for her there is no marked motivation to give it up. Rather, the motivation is to maintain at all odds the orientation she has achieved. In the treatment, for example, at one point she wanted the therapist to bring her some flowers, and there was a long detailed discussion with much obsessive indecisiveness on her part as to whether she wanted a real flower or an artificial one. The discussion involved comparison of the real rose with its beauty and fragrance but the presence of thorns, and the artificial rose lacking in fragrance and life, but without thorns. The patient thought that she wanted the real rose, but she wanted it without thorns like the artificial one. When the therapist, using metaphoric communication, pointed out that he could not provide her with a real rose without thorns, she insisted angrily that she wanted it, and finally concluded the discussion by saying, "Well, you bring me the real rose, and I'll take the thorns off," as if, in reply to the therapist's demands that she face the reality, she would distort the realities according to her needs by herself if he would not help her.

In contrast to this patient, is a sixteen-year-old boy with severe psychotic process. His Rorschach revealed severe schizophrenic thinking, but with little of the richness, elaboration, and well-differentiated fantasy of the other patient. His psychological test material suggested every evidence of his trying to cling to outer reality against the temptations of the inner world. However, his intelligence test score was within normal range. It was as if, in contrast to the previous patient, he was trying to maintain external reality as a focus of his orientation, although as a defense against facing the schizophrenic process within him. He used this orientation defensively, in that he did not attempt to use external reality as a basis for insight into or resolution of the conflict, but rather to help him deny his conflict and maintain connection with the outside world. This was evident in the marked motivation he showed to cope with external reality, to try to achieve in school, and to maintain himself on the outside by permitting his enjoyment of the inner world to emerge only when he was alone, and to maintain a facade of adjustment that hid the schizophrenia from the non-clinical eye. His treatment showed a corresponding difference from that of the previous patient. He is able to persevere in his commitment to treatment. He has been able to make marked improvement in his school work and to use therapeutic help to understand and resolve his conflict, rather than to cling to the inner world orientation. In more dynamic terms, one patient may be considered accessible and the other inaccessible to usual treatment modes. Recognition of the fact that both patients organize their psychic structure around adherence to a crucially different matrix makes it possible to understand dynamically why they present such different problems, although both have severe thought disorders.

It becomes evident that not only is there an inner reality experience and outer reality experience, and that each of these must be subjected to reality testing, but that both the inner and outer criteria are each possible bases for the reality testing process. Thus in the psychotic, the disturbance in the cathexis to the use of external criteria as a basis for reality testing has occurred and is crucial. In some instances this may be with respect to the testing of outer experiences, while in other instances it may occur with respect to the testing of inner experiences. In still others the disturbance may occur in both areas. Such variation helps explain both the difficulty in treating the psychotic and some of the marked variations in the social adaptiveness of psychotics.

REFERENCES

1. FREUD, S. Neurosis and Psychosis. In Collected Papers, 1924. Vol. II (Standard Edition, XIX). London: Hogarth Press, 252.
2. SHEVRIN, H., and TOUSSIENG, P. W. Vicissitudes of the Need for Tactile Stimulation in Instinctual Development. Psychoanalytic Study of the Child, 1960. Vol. XX, pp. 310-339. New York: International Universities Press.
3. HARTMANN, H. The Metapsychology of Schizophrenia. Psychoanalytic Study of the Child, 1953. Vol. III. New York: International Universities Press.
4. MEYER, M. M., and CARUTH, E. Project on Childhood Psychosis (Special Editors). Reiss-Davis Clinic Bulletin, 1964. 1, 2:54-108.

5. EKSTEIN, R. Children of Time & Space, of Action and Impulse, 1966. New York: Appleton-Century-Crofts.
6. EKSTEIN, R., and WALLERSTEIN, J. Choice of Interpretation in the Treatment of Borderline and Psychotic Children. Bulletin of the Menninger Clinic, 1957, 21:199-206.
7. KRIS, E. Psychoanalytic Explorations in Art, 1952. New York: International Universities Press, 177.
8. EKSTEIN, R., and WALLERSTEIN, J. Observations on the Psychotherapy of Borderline and Psychotic Children. Psychoanalytic Study of the Child, 1956. XI. New York: International Universities Press, 303-311.
9. SECHEHAYE, M. A. The Transference in Symbolic Realization. International Journal of Psychoanalysis, 1956. 37:270-277.
10. GORDON, H. Mental and Scholastic Tests among Retarded Children, 1923. London: Board of Education Pamphlet #44.

CHAPTER THREE

Relationship between Diagnosis Mode of Intervention in States and of Severe Impairment*

In order to deal with the topic of diagnosis and mode of intervention, it is necessary to start with a definition or description of diagnosis because there is much confusion between the concepts of diagnosis and nosology. The latter represents, essentially, a schema for cataloguing in terms of a terse shorthand. Diagnosis, on the other hand, represents a process in which information is obtained for purposes of treatment. This process, however, is one in which the information is not simply a matter of content, but content in the context of interaction. Content-within-interaction provides a basis of understanding both the needs that a patient will have in treatment and his style of using treatment. The professional attitude toward the relationship of diagnosis to treatment varies from the one extreme of the use of diagnosis as the total task to the other extreme wherein diagnosis is considered not only unnecessary, but hampering to treatment. In the work in the Project on Childhood Psychosis, both extremes seem to miss the full meaning of diagnosis as a process integrated into treatment and often the first step of treatment.

Mode of intervention, as used in this presentation, refers to the varied interventions within psychotherapy based on psychoanalytic theory. It is clearly unnecessary to discuss here the inappropriateness

---

* Mortimer M. Meyer, Ph.D. is the co-author of this chapter.

of treating all persons by the same mode of intervention. Equally un-necessary is an elaboration on the fact that the terse shorthand repre-sented in the final diagnosis covers varying patterns of behavior with varying methods of coping and defending.

Illustrating how the diagnostic process can serve to clarify the manner in which treatment will unfold and how communication can be estab-lished with an adolescent who can relate only in a psychotic, symbiotic style is the case of Teresa. Her case is presented in a chapter in Ekstein's recent book (1). This chapter discusses the diagnostic evaluation of the 15½-year-old, schizophrenic, Spanish-Mexican girl. It provides an ex-cellent illustration of the usefulness of the assessment including social history, clinical psychiatric interviews, a complete battery of tests, med-ical reports and other available records. Ekstein reports predictions about the therapeutic process developed from this collection of infor-mation and a proposed rationale for the predictions.

> The suggestion was made that the first transference develop-ment would show her as a small child coming to the rescue worker. The rescuer would bring about a miracle and make her well ma-gically. At the same time, he would allow her to remain in the forbidden childhood forever, thus creating a conflict between her and the aunt. This maternal figure Teresa saw as demanding that she grow and act normally, a goal which she would like to achieve, but which threatened the stability of her quasi-adjustment as a small, happy child. She would allow the therapist to be the pro-vider, and would constantly ask him to meet her anaclitic needs, the restoration of objects of her infantile world. . . . As she would attempt to allow herself a relationship with him, she would begin to see in him the dangerous object. She would thus fluctuate be-tween the quasi-hysterical position of the small child and the psychotic position of the adolescent. . . .
>
> Predictive formulations then suggested that the therapist would have to remain with the facade and the surface content at the same time that he would have to indicate his interest in her prob-lems and his desires to establish a way to help her. He would need to refrain from intruding into her inner thoughts, in part because the aunt, the parental person, had depicted him as a kind of father-confessor to whom the girl would have to tell all. (P. 79.)

The discussion illustrates further how the use of metaphoric com-munication served the demands of the situation. It permitted the pa-tient and therapist to talk as if they had no interest in dealing with the conflict even as they were dealing with it under the cover of metaphor.

The child instantly greeted me in the waiting-room with deep expressions of gratitude . . . someone . . . perhaps . . . sent by God in order to help her deep illness, which she described primarily as finding herself isolated on an island in an engulfing world of fantasy. (P. 80.)

Ekstein reports a little more of the girl's comments and then turns to his own reaction.

I very quickly caught on, I believe, to the metaphor quality of her language and attempted to let Teresa know that this treatment would consist in our attempting to get to know each other and each other's way of thinking. I spoke about building bridges or connections from the island on which she found herself to the rest of the world, so that she could venture out into the rest of the world if she wanted to. I hinted at the reason for her feeling isolated on an island when talking about the history of Mexico City, originally an island built for protection against surrounding hostile tribes, then developing into a magnificent city which dominated the country. The back and forth between Teresa and me indicated that she was eager for the connection, but time and time again she used allegories of space movies and television programs in order to show the danger of therapeutic contact. (P. 80.)

The function of the diagnostic process is the assessment of these patterns, since these are to be the essential parameters along which the treatment will engage. The frame of reference used is one in which diagnosis involves parameters, such as:

1) To what extent can the patient tolerate the existence of internal anxiety without seeking a mode of discharge;
2) What capacity does the individual have to use the anxiety toward constructive resolution;
3) When neither discharge nor constructive resolution is present, to what extent are there mechanisms for defending against experiencing or being paralyzed by anxiety;
4) To what extent are the mechanisms used syntonic or distonic;
5) To what extent do these mechanisms assist or interfere with the individual's ability to find a homeostatic way of life.

Such a concept of diagnosis is so integrated with treatment that the question of the existence of a relationship need not be given further consideration. It is the basic question of the character of the relationship between diagnosis and mode of intervention, with particular reference to states of severe impairment, which must be clarified. A basic differentiation arises immediately when one differentiates the severe from the less severe disorders. Therapeutic intervention in states of severe impairment, in one respect, requires a frame of reference which is markedly different in approach from therapeutic interventions where severe impairment is not present. For purposes of this discussion, psychological impairment can be considered as a continuum from the mildest to the most severe disorders. This continuum can be arbitrarily divided into those disorders ranging from the mildest to those which come close to but do not actually represent severe impairment. In the mildly disturbed, the integrative and reality-testing functions of ego process remain relatively intact. In the severe impairments, the integrative and reality-testing functions are disturbed to a varying degree and with varying degrees of overt evidence. As a consequence, although the content areas of difficulty and modes of defense may vary in the less disturbed, the basic mode of intervention remains essentially the same in that the therapist can anticipate a relationship in which reality-contact with the patient will always be present. With the severely disturbed patient, it is quite to the contrary.

In such cases, the therapist must always be prepared to find that the patient has lost reality-contact with the therapist. In contrast to the treatment with mildly disturbed patients, there are more periods of interruption of the usual treatment mode. These occur because of the difficulty resulting from the loss of reality-contact which requires a special mode of intervention to remain in contact with the patient. Another difference is present, as pointed out by Freud (2), in that the neurotic is in close continuity with the external reality, but experiences discontinuity with the unconscious. The psychotic is in close continuity with the primary process and experiences discontinuity with the external reality, with the result that in the psychotic there are only fragmentary islands of secondary-process functioning. Thus the therapist, in working with a neurotic, tries to bridge the discontinuity with the unconscious process. In working with the severely disturbed, on the other hand, the therapist must seek to help the patient bridge the discontinuity with the external reality.

With variation *within* the severely disturbed, like the *autistic child*, another mode of intervention is called for. This variation is the degree to which the individual has found his distortion of reality a more effective way of organizing his psychological life than using external reality for such ordering. The intervention where there is no motivation for allegiance to the external reality is markedly different from that where there is some toehold in terms of the patient's maintaining some degree of allegiance to the treatment. The therapist can anticipate which areas of conflict are more likely to stimulate movement in the patient toward the psychotic locus and which areas toward allegiance to appropriate reality. This becomes particularly critical in working with the severely impaired on an outpatient basis. At best, maintaining the patient in such treatment is extremely tenuous, especially since the material, as brought by the patient for a considerable amount of time, is so idiosyncratic and fragmented as to offer little insightful information for the therapist.

The following illustration is again taken from Ekstein's book in a chapter co-authored by Friedman (1).

> During the early interviews of the initial phase of treatment, the patient gave the impression that he was unable to make contact with the therapist. . . . In this sense, the apparent lack of capacity or wish to communicate was the very communication the child wished to express about himself. The therapist was experienced by Ted as an intruder and tolerated only if the patient could use him as an extension of himself, as a tool rather than as a partner in a therapeutic venture, and as a quasi-mechanical guidepost for his exploration of a world which was spatial and geographical, rather than populated by human beings. At this point, Ted's mode of relationship was primarily an autistic one. (P. 66.)

> As soon as the therapist, used as the impersonal, lifeless extension of the patient, wants to come to life and offer real help, the patient intensifies his insistence upon a tenuous gadget relationship rather than following through with a genuine interpersonal exchange. One has the impression that the child really speaks to himself as he wanders through the maze of this new situation, and even as he begins to play. Remarks directed to the psychotherapist are directed to the extension of himself. . . . To this phenomenon we wish to refer as the autistic position of the child in which the psychotherapist is tolerated only as the child's tool rather than as his partner. (P. 67.)

This information is translated into application into the treatment situation in many ways; one major descriptive pathway is through the concept of the coping process. From the information gained through the diagnostic evaluation, it is possible to make estimates of the patient's style of reacting in general and in specific areas. With this information, it is possible to enhance the effectiveness of therapeutic contacts. It is not only the simple matter of which areas of conflict are most urgently pressing—often the crucial criterion in the less disturbed —but also the question of whether the style of coping with such material results in attempts at constructive coping or in flight into psychosis. In view of the crucial need to create or re-create the ego-integrative capacities, it may be far more appropriate to reach the islands of secondary process before approaching the conflict material. The conflict material itself might advantageously be reached through indirect means such as the metaphor.

Another consideration is the importance of the parent as part of the diagnostic process for treatment. At times, in the treatment of the highly disturbed adult patient, the family is considered an essential part of the treatment. However, with children, the parents are not only essential to the treatment, but critical, if for no other reason than that the child is dependent upon the parents to get to treatment. Adults have reached a point in their development where they have a capacity to recognize consciously and to verbalize their need for help. Children rarely do, even in those cases where they are ready for such help. Children are realistically, in addition to psychologically, dependent upon the wishes, moods, attitudes of their parents. Since parents play such a critical part in the treatment process of the child, it has become quite clear to us that parents must be considered part of the diagnostic process. This is so not simply for the eliciting of information, but for evaluating with them their part in the problem and their commitment to the treatment process.

The question of parental commitment to treatment is a highly complicated one and goes far beyond the question of a commitment to bringing the child regularly and on time. The complication arises, in part, from the fact that in making a commitment to treatment, the parents make it on the basis of the current situation with certain notions of what the future situation will be like. The expectations are often not only inaccurate, but unheeding of the changes through which the child proceeds in the course of treatment and their effects. In the situation with the highly disturbed child, the parental commitment is even more crucial because of the long-term treatment required, with its concomitant demands on the parent. The opportunity for gratification from the child's improvement is very slow in coming, the ability of the parents to tolerate the child's pathology tends to diminish, and the treatment of the child threatens whatever homeostasis has been achieved in a highly pathological relationship. Consequently, the diagnostic process needs to evaluate the meaning of the current total situation to the parents. It needs also to estimate the degree to which changes in the child may impair the parents' ability to maintain a commitment which was both appropriate and sincere when it was made.

Evaluation of the parents has to take into account such factors as their degree of health, as well as psychopathology, and to observe, for example, how gratification at the child's developing health can offset the anxiety raised by the child's changes. The evaluation must attempt to provide information about the way in which the parent is likely to use adjunct treatment. This is important as a means of understanding both the new types of stresses which might arise and also whether the parents can resolve those attitudes which might result in impairment, disruption, or discontinuance of the child's treatment. The person providing the adjunct service must have information to understand what needs must be met through his service, so that the parent can be helped to develop attitudes to support the treatment, or—at least—not to interfere with it. Clearly, the implication is that the adjunct service in treatment of the highly disturbed child cannot be only an individually oriented therapeutic process for the parent; it must be in terms of planning for the treatment of the child.

With this perspective, the historical background takes on a different perspective from that where such background is used only as a means of understanding why the current situation is what it is. Within this framework, the historical background provides information to understand the part that the parent is likely to play in the treatment process, as the child develops in directions differing from the pattern of family relationship established in the past. It is not only in terms of maintaining the treatment, however, that the parents must be an integral part of the evaluation. Sometimes their participation becomes critical in understanding how to initiate the treatment so that it is within their capacity.

Friedman, in the diagnostic evaluation of Rena, an adolescent schizophrenic girl, describes this well. This paper illustrates pointedly the degree to which the diagnostic process is content within context, mentioned earlier, and how the diagnosis is integrated into the treatment. In this case, the mother and daughter had a symbiotic relationship in which

> destructive elements seemed to dominate the mother's relationship with her daughter. . . . The mother, accordingly, had no choice but to act out her positive impulses in hostile destructive action. (P. 58.)

The mother had sought psychiatric help previously because the daughter's symptoms had reached such a severe stage. Hospitalization—overtly a correct recommendation—twice resulted in almost immediate termination of the request for assistance. Friedman points out,

> Without this relationship, mother and daughter would lose all vestiges of ego identity, illusory as it was, and would collapse into a state of apathy. The mother's quasi-psychotic intuition that both would die was psychologically correct. It could be predicted that

the mother would collapse into a severe, possibly suicidal depression, while the daughter would regress into an inaccessible catatonia. The mother's manipulative effort opposing this recommendation constituted her desperate efforts to make the treatment situation possible. (P. 58.)

The immediate function of the diagnostic evaluation thus became the task of recognizing the emergency situation as the mother's emergency; of immediately engaging her in a process of evaluating, while coping with her own urgent conflicts. She had to be helped to mobilize her available strengths, to create a psychological atmosphere that would most effectively support her own treatment and Rena's. Allowing mother and daughter to remain undisturbed in their current relationship was recognition that their symbiosis provided the basic foundation and structure for the treatment situation. The situation was analogous to that of leaving the buttressing and pylons of an old bridge as the foundations for a new one.

The treatment recommendation most appropriate in this situation was, therefore, to introduce no immediate change in the mother-daughter relationship. "Mrs. R. accepted this arrangement and permitted Rena to start in therapy on the basis of three hours a week. The treatment continued in my office for a number of weeks." (P. 59.)

Finally, the time came when it became extremely difficult to maintain Rena in the home. The mother pressed to have the girl hospitalized and was furious with the therapist for not initiating the hospitalization. The therapist said "that it was a matter of great importance as to who took Rena to the hospital, and that it was of even greater importance how she was taken to the hospital." (P. 60.)

The evaluation had clearly indicated to the therapist that if he hospitalized the patient, both mother and daughter would see this as his move to separate them. He indicated further,

> What was most important was that she be able to convey to Rena that she, Mother, wanted her to go into the hospital and to continue her treatment; that she, Mother, could survive without Rena's presence at home, and that she, Mother, had confidence that Rena could also survive in a setting physically apart from her. For only by taking Rena herself, could she confirm and reassure her daughter that she did not hate her and would not kill her for leaving, that she was not afraid that both would die, and that her primary interest lay in genuinely accepting whatever was needed for Rena's recovery. (Pp. 60-61.)

This time, when the hospitalization took place, the treatment continued without interruption. This was accomplished because in the diagnosis the therapist had carefully evaluated the part that the mother would play in the treatment process.

In conclusion, it should be noted that this presentation is rooted in the concept that treatment is an organized but flexible process. It is not a stereotyped approach dependent upon the association of the moment, nor the limited meaning of the overt expressions of the patient and his family. This presentation is also based on the concept that for the treatment process to be most effective, it is important that the therapist have a frame of reference specific to the patient since general knowledge of personality theory and of treatment is not sufficient. To paraphrase Kant, diagnosis without treatment process is empty, and treatment without diagnostic process is blind.

REFERENCES

1. EKSTEIN, RUDOLF. *Children of Time and Space, of Action and Impulse: Clinical Studies on the Psychoanalytic Treatment of Severely Disturbed Children.* N.Y.: Appleton-Century-Crofts, 1966.
2. FREUD, SIGMUND. *Collected Papers* 2:277-282. Lon.: Hogarth Press, 1949.

CHAPTER FOUR

Inner and Outer Reality on the Rorschach*

The Rorschach has long been used as a means of evaluating the reality testing function of the ego. However, a comparison of the above two responses poses an interesting but heretofore unexplored aspect of the individual's relationship to reality as is reflected in his test performance.

In the first response, the subject uses appropriately the shape and boundary of the blot and integrates it correctly into the percept—"A bat." However, the inappropriate attribute of "eating people" ascribed to the percept represents a severe distortion of ideation. In the second response, the subject uses the shape and boundary of the blot inappropriately, although the content of the response is without evident distortion of inner ideation. Both of these responses are inappropriate but they differ in the manner in which they misuse the material. In each instance the relationship to reality is impaired in a different way. In the first response, "A bat, eating people," an unrealistic interpretation is assigned to a correctly perceived bit of reality. In the second instance —"A cat"—a realistic concept is arbitrarily assigned to a misperceived reality.

Examination of the nature of the difference between these two responses has led to the consideration that the concept of reality testing must be refined and elaborated. These two responses suggest that the ability to evaluate experiences which come from the outside must be differentiated from the ability to evaluate those experiences which come

---

* Mortimer M. Meyer and Elaine Caruth are the authors of this chapter.

from the inside. Clinically, such a distinction is implied by the recognition that there is both an inner and outer reality. Historically, however, philosophical and scientific psychology were primarily concerned with the acquisition of knowledge about external reality. Consequently, research was primarily focused upon such epistemological problems as the relationship between stimulus and reaction, and the means by which the psychic apparatus evaluated the stimuli from the environment.

CARD V

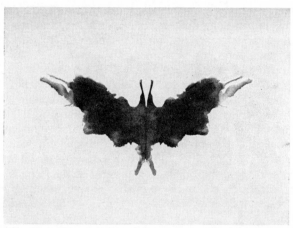

(Reprinted with permission of Hans Huber, Berne, Switzerland)

1—A bat, eating people. Vultures.   2—A cat.

Studies using techniques of introspection about the content of mental life were relatively rare before Freud. With the development of psychoanalysis, however, and particularly after Freud's discovery that the heretofore postulated sexual trauma were, in actuality, most often of fantasy origin, the emphasis upon the inner reality became paramount clinically. Currently, it would be truly a psychological anachronism to limit the definition of reality to those experiences which can be defined only in terms of their observable sources of stimulation. Nevertheless, residuals of this historically rooted reluctance to give full and equal weight to "the world within" as well as "the world without" are present to this day in the clinical use of the concept of reality testing. The theory and use of Rorschach technique for the purpose of evaluating reality testing have also continued to be tied to the original emphasis upon outer reality.

Reality testing was first described as the capacity to judge the source of perception with reference to whether it came from within or without. Freud's original formulation stated that perceptions which can be made to disappear by motor activity are recognized as "external, as reality, where such an action makes no difference, the perception originates within the subject's own body—it is not real" (1). Gross distortions of reality would, thus, be exemplified by hallucinations.

Reality testing, however, includes more than the ability merely to differentiate the subjective or objective nature of the source of the perception. It is generally only in the most gross disturbances that such a perceptual impairment does exist. Nevertheless, the relationship to reality can be defective even though the capacity to differentiate between inner and outer reality is relatively intact. A delusional system may not impair the perception but it will impair the interpretation of the perception and, thus, reflects a distorted relationship to reality. Hartmann has suggested such a distinction when he stated, "Actually, as mental phenomena are no less real in the outer world (although we often refer to the latter only in speaking of 'reality'), it might prove useful to include testing of the within as well as testing of the without . . . we could say that with the neurotic testing of inner, with the psychotic testing of outer reality is interfered with. However, a higher complexity is introduced by the fact that among others, that the two aspects of reality testing often interact" (3).

Subsequently, he elaborated this differentiation both between inner and outer reality as well as inner and reality testing: "Problems of acceptance, of distortion, of denial occur in relation to inner as well as outer reality—About the distorted picture of inner reality, . . . it seems reasonable to speak of a testing of the within, in addition to testing of the without—that is, to distinguish inner reality testing from outer reality testing" (4).

It has been less clearly recognized, though Hartmann seems to imply it, that these two aspects of the relationship to reality may vary independently of each other. The emergence of primary process in the content of the response has not generally been considered a discrete parameter of the reality testing function. Rather, the content of the responses has been considered merely as reflecting the individual's fantasy as it is projected onto the blot and therein giving evidence of the kind of ongoing internal life. Schafer, for example, describes the relatively low incidence of good form responses in schizophrenia as "indicative of the extent of the breakdown of reality testing and the suffusion of a perception with pathologically autistic thought content" (6), without considering the possibility that these two aspects should be dealt with separately.

Hartmann, however, was concerned primarily with the neurotic-psychotic dichotomy to which he had referred. In the understanding of patients whose pathology is characterized by fluctuating ego states, such as the borderline and schizophrenic patient, a knowledge of the vicissitudes and permutations of inner and outer reality testing might improve our understanding of how these patients experience their inner and outer worlds. Such understanding could give us greater insight into the nature of their particular ego disturbances.

We would like to suggest now a working definition of these two concepts. By outer reality testing, we refer to the process of perceiving external reality. By inner reality testing, we refer to the process of evaluating the accompanying fantasy in terms of its appropriateness to the circumstances involved and the realistic possibility of its fulfillment. Thus, an individual may indulge in many unrealistic fantasies, fed by either the primary or secondary process, but still retain the critical ego functions which make for recognition of their inappropriateness or unrealistic nature. On the other hand, an individual may indulge in the same fantasies but be unable to recognize their inappropriateness. In the latter circumstance, the inner reality testing is impaired, regardless of the effectiveness of the testing of outer reality. Where the fantasy has been guided by the primary process, we have evidence of the intrusion of a more chronic and pervasive thought disorder.

In differentiating between "the world within" and "the world without," it must be recognized that this is not a topological distinction. "The world within," is defined as the individual's world of thought and fantasies. The content of this world consists of the psychic representation of the individual's experience with outer reality, from which it is differentiated, although it follows certain parallel laws. The "world without" includes stimuli arising from the body of the individual so that distortions in bodily sensations, such as functional physical complaints, would be attributed to an impairment of outer reality testing. We are including the entire gamut of enteroceptive, properoceptive and exteroceptive input. This is opposed to the more usual distinction between enteroceptive and exteroceptive stimulation which is of significance in the development of the differentiation between "I" and "non-I," a differentiation which we usually refer to as *external* reality testing. Thus, disturbances of body *image* would be attributed to a distortion of inner reality. Obviously we deal here with a relative rather than an absolute distinction. Outer reality is perceived on the basis of the internal image, and the internal image is derived in part from outer reality. We might postulate that the experience of a fantasy limb is a product of a temporary impairment of both inner and outer reality testing. In this instance, sensations are misperceived as emanating from a non-existent piece of reality. At the same time, the psychic representation of the body image has not been readjusted to the new external reality of the change in the body. Loss of contact with reality can be similarly differentiated. Loss of contact with inner reality, such as feelings of depersonalization, may occur without concomitant external reality distortions. Loss of contact with outer reality, as exemplified by the "classic" bizarre-hallucinating schizophrenic, can occur in a patient firmly in contact with his inner reality, crazy though it may be.

Such a differentiated use of the concept of reality testing becomes of immense value when applied to the evaluation of the Rorschach. Here, too, reality testing has been traditionally regarded as a single entity which is reflected in the ability of the subject to perceive appropriately the boundary and shape of an object; that is, in Rorschach terminology, to use good form. The appropriateness with which the form of the blot is used is interpreted as the degree to which the individual pays appropriate attention to the boundaries of a reality situation in the environment. Thus, the handling of form reflects the readiness with which the individual perceives appropriately the external observable reality. Returning to the illustrative responses above, it becomes apparent that the subject making the first response was able to evaluate appropriately the external reality but permitted evidence of primary process functioning to emerge. By contrast, the subject making the second response misinterpreted the external reality but did not permit emergence of primary process functioning or distortion of inner ideation.

Within this frame of reference of two kinds of reality testing, it is suggested that a disturbance of outer reality testing would be evidenced by a misperception of the environment and would be reflected in the Rorschach by a disturbance in form. On the other hand, a disturbance of inner reality testing would be evidenced as an inability to judge the appropriateness of the fantasy and would be reflected in the Rorschach by the attribution of inappropriate or bizarre qualities to the percept.

Observing this differentiation in interpreting the Rorschach can contribute to a clearer understanding of the subject's potential for coping and adaptation. The subject who can maintain adequate form in spite of inappropriateness of content demonstrates an ability to relate to external tasks so that, objectively, his reality testing appears adequate. He can deal with that part of the task that can be separated from the inner image as if the reality testing were unimpaired even though the one aspect of reality testing is actually impaired, as evidenced by the inappropriate content. Such an intra-psychic constellation is observed in the ambulatory schizophrenic patient who is capable of maintaining a job in spite of peculiar and bizarre fantasies. This is the kind of patient who gets into difficulty primarily on the rare occasions when the external task makes demands upon internal imagery in order to complete the task.

The particular responses where the form, as well as the content, shows reality violation are then suggestive of those areas in which the patient is likely to experience the external environment as impinging upon the unrealistic imagery. This results in the impairment of outer as well as inner reality testing and concomitant failure in coping. This differentiation is thus particularly useful in understanding the seemingly erratic and shifting behavior of the borderline patient. It explains why at times he is able to behave as if there were no impairment in reality testing and at other times appears to be suffering from a complete breakdown of reality testing.

The records of children in the Project on Childhood Psychosis at Reiss-Davis Clinic furnish many examples of this kind of differentiation. Reproduced below are two different responses to Card IX from the protocols of two adolescent girls evaluated and treated in the Project.

CARD IX

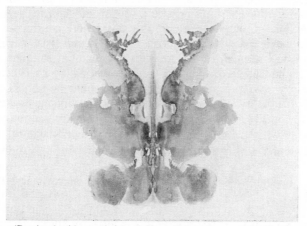

(Reprinted with permission of Hans Huber, Berne, Switzerland)

Subject A—"Two birdmen, formed of a carrot's body and a man's head bowing to each other."

Subject B—"Oh, I see another monster. This monster is scary . . . fat and big. Pink, two eyes, holes also. A long nose.

The first subject responded with two birdmen, formed of a carrot's body and a man's head, bowing to each other. This response reflects complete indifference to the ideational distortion inherent in this kind of contamination, yet there is careful documentation in the response with respect to form. This particular subject demonstrates clinically a similar discrepancy in her functioning. She was quite capable in her handling of reality, and the underlying thought disorder did not intrude into her handling of external reality. Eventually, however, the inroads of the pathology into her total personality organization led to a more acute overt break with reality.

The second patient, however, who was clinically unable to handle external as well as internal reality, responded to this card as, "Oh, I see another monster. This monster is scary . . . fat and big. Pink, two eyes, holes also. A long nose and hanging down. . . ." This response reflects complete indifference to the form of the stimulus. The content also is suggestive of some ideational distortion, although it is difficult to evaluate what would be a realistic description of a monster. For this particular patient, the monster within was occasionally projected and seen as a monster without. This patient also had difficulty differentiating inner from outer reality in a variety of other situations.

Certain aspects of the recent work in the area of sensory deprivation, or to use Kubie's more precise term, "afferent isolation" (5), may be interpreted within this proposed frame of reference of both an inner and an outer reality testing function. We would like to suggest some of the possible implications. In a study on sensory deprivation and interference with reality contact, it was stated: "Man is to a large extent dependent on continual commerce with his usual environment to maintain his highest level of thought functioning. Many of the effects of isolation may be understood as the emergence into awareness of a kind of thinking usually found in dreams, psychosis, and artistic creation" (2). We would like to suggest that this "continual commerce" might be thought of, to paraphrase Menninger, as a "vital balance" between inner and outer reality testing which is needed for the individual to maintain an optimal level of functioning. These studies suggest that when the opportunity for outer reality testing is minimal (except for those stimuli arriving through enteroceptive sensations), the individual will experience a breakdown in the inner reality testing and will evidence the intrusion of primary process functioning. In some instance he will undergo a breakdown in the outer reality testing and develop hallucinatory experiences. This need of the normal person for continued interaction between the external world and his inner world is reflected, perhaps, in the often reported phenomenon of psychological disintegration following retirement in many effective working people. It is also one of the problems that has to be faced in space-age aviation.

In closing, we would like to suggest that not only does what is real exist both internally as well externally, but what is unreal may be attributed to both the internal as well as the external.

REFERENCES

1. FREUD, S. "Instincts and Their Vicissitudes (1915)." *Collected Papers*, Vol. IV: 60-83: London: Hogarth Press, 1946.
2. GOLDBERGER, LEO, and ROBERT R. HOLT. "Experimental Interference with Reality Contact: Individual Differences." *Sensory Deprivation*: Symposium held at Harvard Medical School. Cambridge, Mass.: Harvard University Press, 1961.
3. HARTMANN, HEINZ. "Contribution to the Metapsychology of Schizophrenia." *Psychoanalytic Study of the Child*, 1953, 8:195.
4. ———. "Notes on the Reality Principle." *Psychoanalytic Study of the Child*, 1956, 11:50-51.
5. KUBIE, LAURENCE S. "Theoretical Aspects of Sensory Deprivation." *Sensory Deprivation*: Symposium held at Harvard Medical School. Cambridge, Mass.: Harvard University Press, 1961.
6. SCHAFER, ROY. *The Clinical Application of Psychological Tests*. New York: International Press, 1948, p. 69.

CHAPTER FIVE

Differential Diagnostic Cues in the Severely Impaired Child*

The problems in the diagnostic evaluation of the severely disturbed child are well known, and much has been written about them. Despite the many problems, psychologists are asked to use their skills to assist in evaluation although there are only limited formal techniques designed for such children. The questions of maturational problems vs. character deformation, neurological disturbance vs. schizophrenia, mental deficiency vs. emotional impairment of intellect are a few of the leading concerns. One of the approaches most consistently helpful in the diagnostic work at Reiss-Davis has been to use standard material, even for children without speech, but with a further frame of reference, which we are attempting to develop, added to the usual one for interpretation. This frame of reference, similar to that used by Weiner (5), is to approach the amount of material strictly from the functional point of view which permits more detailed inferences concerning strengths and weaknesses in such children. With these children, it is seldom a matter of how severe the disturbance is, but rather the area of greater or lesser disturbance, and, occasionally, the idiosyncratic meaning. The application of psychoanalytic principles is not new—it has been given much attention by such people as Schafer (4) and Holt (3)—but essentially it has been done more with the formal testing rather than to the schizophrenic and the autistic child. Mary Engel (2) and Eisenberg (1) deal with the problem more closely.

It should be quite clear that the suggestions offered below are in

---

* Mortimer M. Meyer is the author of this chapter.

terms of young children. They are not offered as scientific objective measures of autism or schizophrenia, but as extremely helpful clues when trying to select and understand children who may be taken into day treatment programs.

An examination starts, as all should, from the moment the examiner reaches the child's sight. However, it is important the examiner have some organized frame of reference for his observations, rather than simply picking up the random, confused assortment of clues which the child offers. These observations can be placed under such rubrics as reality testing, readiness for object relationships, body-image, capacity for drive for goal achievement, capacity for perseverance, and the like. Such observations when carefully evaluated become as a profile, differentiating one autistic or schizophrenic child from another, and provide important clues for approach to the treatment. The initial interchange can often help to distinguish the degree to which the child is ready to see the human as an object of convenience or as an object for interaction. The case of Alice, five years, six months, is a good example.

The examiner approached the seated child, who stared straight ahead as if completely oblivious to his arrival and presence. She kept meshing one hand in the other, alternately with putting one hand in front of her mouth and biting the palm. She appeared to be equally oblivious of her mother seated on her right. The examiner spoke of her red shoes and his red sweater, touching both in the process. She then touched the sweater and pushed slightly; thereupon, the examiner fell back and "popped up" again. She repeated the push so that it was directed into a game—an opportunity to infer that this seemingly autistic child had more awareness of people and readiness for them than might otherwise have been noted. When the examiner commented on her pretty red dress, the child immediately took the hem of the dress, put it into her mouth, and started to chew on it. Here was a gesture resulting from direct contact that could easily have been unobtained, yet it, too, carried the implication that the child was alert to and responsive to the examiner as a person for interaction. She then returned to her autistic-like behavior, whereupon the examiner indicated that it must be frightening for a child to have a strange person near her. He followed this remark with comments about wanting to play with her. She immediately pushed him, which could have been interpreted as pushing the examiner away, but in view of the earlier "game," was interpreted as her readiness to play. The examiner extended his hand and took hers, and she immediately passively got up with him and proceeded toward the examining room.

This same episode provided another suggestive inference. Her manner of relating was an aggressive one, as if her only way to relate on an initial contact was with an ambivalent "yes-no" move. She could either push aggressively or return to an autistic position. Such an inference can provide a first hypothesis: critical in her difficulties is her hostility to people as a defensive, protective measure which she, unlike some other severely disturbed children, is ready to have penetrated. The "yes-no," "aggression-passivity" was further noted in the way she walked along the hall. She would walk forward, suddenly stop, and then swing the examiner around and start to walk in the opposite direction. She would walk back and forth this way, although gradually making a forward approach. For a seemingly autistic child, Alice manifested a higher level of readiness for object relationships in an additional way. In walking back and forth along the hall, she would stop to look in every room with an open door. She would gravitate to the rubber puppets, the chief item of her play in the psychiatric interview which preceded the psychological testing, and want to take them with her. The search from room to room could thus probably represent her search for the previous object, the psychiatrist, and indicate a capacity to retain an object once pleasure had been derived from it.

A further source of information for the level of object relatedness is the style of contact. For example, Alice permitted the examiner to hold her hand and responded by voluntarily holding his. When she sat down on the floor to play, she chose to sit near him. In contrast is little Ronnie, five years, one month, who permitted the examiner to hold his hand but in a mechanical fashion only, and would sit in various places in the room as if the examiner did not exist. Another illustration of Alice's awareness of object relationships occurred when she discovered that there were two baby bottles. She immediately filled them both and brought one for the examiner and wanted him to drink from his as she drank from hers. Each time she refilled her bottle, she did the same for the examiner. Ronnie, in contrast, never showed any wish or recognition for sharing or participation. The implications for oral needs and wishes are clearly present, but will not be amplified here. Alice's actions made it quite apparent that she had reached a level in which another person had meaning for her in terms of usefulness and some kind of gratification, though little beyond this. In addition, people have some differentiation for her as observed from her ability to recall that the current examiner was separate from the previous one.

Evidences of the reality-testing function can be noted in the above material. Reality testing, as used here, represents not only the capacity to differentiate the within from the without, but also the difference of function of the many things in daily life. In the psychological situation, the materials available are more limited, and the test material for this purpose is not considered in terms of its direct measuring capacity, as much as for its evidence of the style of reality usage. Thus, Alice in the handling of the play materials related to the doll house appeared to find no purpose to the items. She not only handled them aimlessly but carelessly, as if things had no inherent meaningful purpose. Dolls, furniture and other paraphernalia were simply tossed on the floor, sometimes neatly, but not always. Yet, there was a marked contrast in her handling of the test materials when she was taken to the table for the actual formal testing. She was not only responsive to the performance-test material, but showed skill and care in handling it and showed concern about returning the material to the container. She often tried, sometimes with success and sometimes without, to put the cover back on each container when the material had been put in. Thus, she clearly manifested a capacity to differentiate which reflected the presence of a degree of reality testing. She differentiated the material which had specific task and purpose and was able to respond with a different set. This was, again, different from Ronnie. He would toss the doll material as if one piece were equivalent to the other, and pour one piece after the other down the stairway of the house. It was as if all the material were to be treated exactly alike regardless of its nature. People were thrown down the stairs, beds were thrown down the stairs, chairs, etc. When it came his turn to deal with the formal test material, it was much more difficult to get him to take the task seriously. When he did, he might complete the task, but had no interest in following through further. It was just something to be done and had none of the fuller reality values that Alice had shown. Not only the measurement of the material, but observing whether the child recognizes the appropriate associativeness of materials can indicate the capacity for reality testing.

A further facet of the handling of play materials that gives clues to traces of reality testing is the appropriateness of the use of play materials, whether organized play takes place or not. With organized play material, the level of reality testing is often very evident and of a relatively high level; however, when there is no organized play, the use of the materials can still give traces of the kind of reality testing which is present. Thus, Jill, six years, four months, liked to play with water, although with no evident purpose. She chose objects to fill with water. It was observed, however, that the choice of objects demonstrated a careful awareness of the use of objects. Instead of taking anything which would hold water, she chose a bathtub, a sink, baby bottles, and a toilet. She showed even further differentiation in that she drank from the baby bottles, but not from any of the other water-filled objects. This was in marked contrast with Ronnie who would line up play material, regardless of its significance, and sit rocking in the middle of it, making no use of the material at all, or mechanically throwing it down the doll house staircase as described earlier.

Another area of differentiation is that of goal-directedness which is often only observable through perserverance. This area has great significance because goal directedness, like perseverance, implies the presence of some degree of integration. The peg boards on the Merrill-Palmer, for example, can often be helpful in this discrimination. Thus, Alice, in spite of her many evidences of scattered behavior, was able to persevere through peg board A and peg board B, doing each three times as required. She had no hesitation in recognizing the task and seemed to gain some actual pleasure in it. Thus, there was evidence of ego development implied, not only in being able to follow directions, but in being able to follow an inward purpose. The actual test age may have some significance for other purposes, but for purposes of evaluating the presence of integration, it is the manner and style of the handling the task that become crucial. A contrasting example, given by Ronnie, is one on a lower level. This is a level where a child can remember from one session to the other things which gave special pleasure, but the integrated, motivated, purposeful pleasure is lacking. In this case, Ronnie had seen the penny on the Binet material and had wanted it. He persevered in wanting it but, of course, was not given it. In the next session he remembered it and still wanted it, even though it was not in sight. There was nothing he could do with it during the hour, nor was it part of any play maneuver or any direct physical accomplishment, yet it demonstrated a capacity to establish and retain a purpose, even though on a primitive level.

Last of these illustrations has to do with observations of body-image. Alice had almost no speech, and the speech which was present consisted of isolated words which were words of command. Her general coordination seemed excellent in terms of her handling of materials and her general movement. Yet a striking illustration that she did not have full command of body-image occurred when she wanted to sit down next to the examiner on the floor. She stood next to him, took the examiner's hand and repeated the word "sit" but without any additional indication of what she wanted. It was, therefore, not clear at first whether she was referring to the examiner's sitting on the floor, or whether she wanted to sit down herself. If it was the latter, there was nothing evident to prevent her from sitting. Finally, it became apparent that she wanted to manipulate the examiner and pushed him from sitting position to lying position on the floor and then back again. Then finally it was observed that, despite her good coordination in a variety of activities, "sit" this time meant that she wanted assistance from the examiner to help her sit down. It was as if she did not feel in control of a conscious, directed body movement of such gross change of position. Another illustration of poor recognition of body-image was demonstrated by Ronnie. He sat down against the wall and began rocking. His rocking movements were such that he not only hit the wall with his back, but at times hit the wall with his head with such severity that most children would have cried out in anguish. With him, it appeared as if he experienced no direct connection between his own body-image and its activities.

The above are clearly not exclusive, nor do they represent the limits of ways in which the examiner can use actions and materials for clues. But they do indicate some of the possibilities of devising locally useful modes for pertinent observations in diagnostic evaluation.

REFERENCES

1. Eisenberg, L. "The Classification of the Psychotic Disorders in Childhood." In Classification of Behavior Disorders. Leonard D. Eron, ed. Chi.: Aldine Pub. Co., 1966.
2. Engel, Mary. "Psychological Testing of Borderline Psychotic Children." Archives of General Psychiatry, 1963, 5:426.
3. Holt, R. R., and Joan Havel. "A Method of Assessing Primary and Secondary Process in the Rorschach." Rorschach Psychology. Maria A. Rickers-Ovsiankina, ed. N. Y.: John Wiley & Sons, 1960.
4. Schafer, Roy. Psychoanalytic Interpretation in Rorschach Testing. N. Y.: Grune and Stratton, 1954.
5. Weiner, I. B. Psychodiagnosis in Schizophrenia. N. Y.: John Wiley & Sons, 1966.

Part Two
TREATMENT ISSUES

Thus it is that I do not seek to define or defend what may be the "best" mode of therapy or to present "solutions" for the wide range of social-psychiatric patterns of behavior that come to be labeled schizophrenic, and concerning which there is much disagreement about diagnosis, etiology, course, prognosis, and suitable intervention. Often it is difficult to specify what one holds to be professionally desirable for the particular patient, when the unmet needs of so many others are apparent and currently beyond much, if any, help. Nonetheless, certain approaches limited to a few should not be abandoned simply because they are not readily available to, or suitable for, the many; the wise study of the single case can yield data applicable more or less directly to a multitude.

OTTO ALLEN WILL

Prolegomenon to a Psychoanalytic Technique in the Treatment of Childhood Schizophrenia*

Psychoanalytic therapy was originally devised to fit the need of adult neurotics and, likewise, the first adaptation of the method to children was made with the infantile neurosis in mind. Since then, in the adult field, the scope of analytic therapy has widened, and, with minor alterations, now serves, besides the neuroses, other categories of disturbances such as psychoses, perversions, addictions, delinquencies, etc. Again, child analysis followed suit extending its field of application in the same directions.

ANNA FREUD

As we consider the task of developing a general technique for the psychoanalytic treatment of psychotic children, we face the apparent paradox of using similar techniques for both psychotic and neurotic children. This poses many questions, inasmuch as this issue is intimately involved with the basic model of psychoanalytic treatment itself, whose limitations and limits, shortcomings, effectiveness, and possible improvement are constantly being tested as a valid model and instrument for the treatment of psychotic children.

---

* Seymour W. Friedman is the co-author of this chapter.

Freud's introduction of the concepts of the unconscious and the primary process led to a unified view of psychopathology in which normality, neurosis and psychosis were no longer regarded as essentially different and separate. In this unified view, the variety of part-aspects of so complex a disease as schizophrenia could be integrated and synthesized into a total disease condition manifesting itself in a variety of ways. Under the impetus of Freud's synthesis (7, 9) of the differences between neurosis and psychosis within a single conceptual framework of psychopathology, there emerged the essential elements for the outgrowth of a common treatment philsophy and model for dealing with both the psychotic and the neurotic child.

Freud's original topographic (8) and his later structural tripartite models (6) of the personality aptly served the model for classical psychoanalytic treatment of the stable patient whose psychic organization provides the structure for the therapeutic process. Here the significant elements of psychoanalytic treatment, as manifested in the unconscious becoming conscious, the conflict between impulse and defense, between the wish and the reality testing, and between impulsivity and delay functions, could be meaningfully utilized only by a personality of more advanced and stable neurotic psychic organization. The model of treatment consistent with these models of personality organization is the traditional structure in which the free association of the adult or the play activity and verbal productions of the child are met by the interpretive interventions of the therapist. The transference development of the patient is matched by a countertransference and empathy potential of the therapist.

With the neurotic child, the therapist's task is understanding, having like experiences, meeting the patient's controlled and relatively regulated regressions with his own countertransference regressions in the service of professional functioning, matching the patient's inner states with his own inner states, and effectively providing empathy to match the patient's need for psychological "mothering." This is made relatively and reasonably possible by the essential, basic similarity of their psychic functioning. The therapeutic process can proceed with reasonable hope of a successful outcome.

The psychotic child, however, confronts the therapist with a psychic organization of another order. With such a child neither topographic nor structural models of personality organization alone serve for treatment models. Instead, a modification which does not essentially alter the basic elements of these two models is required, one which, we suggest, can be achieved in their synthesis. For our understanding of the nature of the psychic organization of the psychotic child, we are especially indebted to Mahler (11). Her work has clarified the essential difference between autistic and symbiotic psychosis which, together, comprise childhood schizophrenia. By means of her insights we can reconstruct a model of the essential disorder in the development of object relations which characterizes these illnesses and is at the root of the total resultant psychic disturbance.

We can characterize infantile autistic psychosis essentially by its relative failure of affective cathexis of the mother as a human object. This creates a relatively empty inner human-object world over which the autistic child exerts complete and omnipotent control. Symbiotic psychosis can be characterized as a state of object- and self-cathexis but with failure to achieve separation and differentiation of self and object. The ego functions mainly by the delusion of omnipotence derived from the undifferentiated mother-object. We may disregard the primary autistic psychotic child whom we can consider as not existing in pure culture, as Kanner (10) at first held, but rather who always has relative elements of a symbiotic psychotic organization. We can then view the symbiotic psychotic child in either of two ways. In one, he is in a constant, dynamic, inner-turbulent state of movement between the symbiotic state and the stage of separation and individuation, for which symbiosis is the forerunner. In the second, he is regressively pulled toward the autistic position as a retreat from the threatening, devouring and engulfing dangers of the pathogenic symbiosis. For the infant who has had a pathogenic experience within the symbiotic matrix, separation deprives him of his needed delusional omnipotence derived from fusion with the mother. This leads to threatening collapse of the ego and to panic attempts to restore the symbiosis with the mother. In this state of separation and impotence outside the symbiosis, the psychosis serves as the adaptive means to restore ego functioning by restoring the symbiosis with the environment, external objects or therapist. Danger from engulfment by the parasitic mother-object, the negative symbiosis, however, leads to regressive retreat to the autistic position.

We can thus visualize the psychotic state as one in which self object representations are enclosed within the symbiotic sac, separated by a porous osmotic membrane. It is undergoing, without yet having achieved, separation, nor stable cathexis and differentiation of self and object. In this stage only primitive ego functioning exists. It is dominated by primary process and unstable impulse control, in which the thought disorder is characterized by the equations: thought = action; inner reality = outer reality; self = object.

For the psychotic organization we would then postulate a *three-dimensional model combining the topographic and structural models*, and conceive of the structural model as operating in depth. These various levels of consciousness may perhaps best be construed as different layers of psychic organization forming a hierarchy developing out of an undifferentiated archaic phase. In this can be found latent dispositions that will develop into the organizers of a more complex structure within the personality. Such an integrated model allows for a more refined and subtle description of the specific ego deviation suffered by psychotic children. It also permits the concept of fluctuating ego states at various levels of regression and progression. This is characteristic of the functioning of the psychotic psychic organization, which is correlated with the particular form of integration of id, ego and superego functions operating at a given moment and level.

Complementing this three-dimensional model is that of the *symbiotic sac* as the energizing force that fuels the ceaseless fluctuations or the quick, abrupt, deep regressions and the sudden reconstitutive progressions so characteristic of the functioning of such a child's psychic organization. With such models we can offer an explanation of the child's clinical behavior, therapeutic transference manifestations, and of the essence of his life adaptation. Familiar clinical observation indicates such a child's body-clinging and molding attitudes; his intense preoccupation with and grasping of objects, persons and parts of persons; his lightning-like shifts from libidinal to aggressive reactions, when a touch can suddenly deepen into a brutal penetration or tearing, and a kiss can turn into enraged, cannibalistic biting. In his encircling, engulfing, possessing and devouring of parts of the object and of the external environment, we see the id nature of the hungry search for part-objects. This reaching out and grasping of available part-objects reconstitute an autistic-like omnipotent control over a symbiosis which has to be maintained in order to avoid ego collapse and abysmal panic.

Paradoxically, omnipotent control over the symbiosis and the symbiotic partner is desperately needed in order to safeguard the delicate, developing filaments of self and object-differentiation that, overpowered by the dominant, devouring object, are threatened with obliteration. To maintain his precarious balance, to ward off destructive fusion and loss of self, the symbiotic psychotic child's psychic organization has no choice but to impose itself on all available objects. For such a child's only reality is its internal psychic reality, which it cannot fully distinguish from outer reality. Such a child must force its total environment into the mold and image of its own psychic organization, which is all it can master, as if to wipe out all semblance of difference and differentiation that threatens the symbiosis. He literally creates the world, or misperceives the object world, in his own inner image, and is committed to psychotic pantheism.

What seems to be the destruction and nullification of the environment by the deeply disturbed psychotic child is the expression of the savage onslaught of untamed instinctual drives unmediated by effective ego control. This can be understood as the psychotic adaptation of a personality that could not otherwise survive.

This model further enables us to see the forces in dynamic interplay. It highlights the essential similarity of the psychotic psychic organization and the normal neurotic organization, with the significant quantitative differences of ego, id and superego influence, and perhaps with qualitative differences which we cannot identify yet because of unexplored or unclarified areas of etiology (such as the biological, organic areas of heredity, constitution, etc.). Perhaps there is one essential quantitative difference leading to vast qualitative differences between these two basic organizations. This difference lies in the relatively greater effectiveness of the vicissitudes of the impulse-defense conflict in the formation of the neurotic organization, but with greater importance of the influence of a life-and-death struggle in the life of the psychotic personality. This is best depicted in his indecisive, ceaseless struggle for ego control over impulse, for differentiation of self and object, for achievement of ego autonomy through simultaneous differentiation and integration of its various functions. How this occurs depends on the effectiveness of its integrative and synthesizing function and the still unsolved task of neutralization or integration of energies. The psychotic is striving for mediation and integration of the self and external reality to become an effective human being capable of living successfully in the world. He is reaching for the fulfillment of the actuality principle, where trial thought may move towards appropriate action based on genuine option, that is, towards alloplastic behavior.

When we place in apposition to this psychic model the basic model for psychoanalytic treatment, we see the essential and major difference in the treatment of the psychotic child is the role of activity and technique by the therapist. The psychotic child, who is dominated by primary-process thinking, by impulse over delay, and by unstable self- and object-representations of an infinite degree, offers his productions and transferences. The therapist must meet them with his own secondary-process functioning and with a countertransference potential that is significantly challenged (13) (Chapters 8, 24 this volume).

He must competently meet the patient's transference developments with his own countertransference potential while confronted with an extremely difficult problem. He must meet the patient's unpredictable and alien regressions with his own controlled potential for regression; and, in effect, must match the patient's intrapsychic functioning, essentially foreign to him, with his own which is not only foreign but impossibly demanding to the patient. We might even speculate that the therapist is called on to undergo regression to the emotional experience of a symbiotic state that mirrors and reflects the inner symbiotic state of the patient's object relations. Thus enabled to accept the patient's need and demand for symbiosis, he can enter the patient's world but within himself. From there he can cue his response and attitude so that he is available to the patient's need at the same time that he maintains his self-identity; i.e., does not become truly psychotic himself. This enormous demand on the therapist for flexibility and accommodation may be all but impossible to meet; in which case no effective treatment occurs. Assuming that a treatment relationship with such children can be established, however, we cannot rely solely on what we already know about their treatment but must discover more through continued investigation.

The treatment of such children is replete with inherent dilemmas of the kind where the resources and ingredients indispensable to treatment are the very dangers that threaten and terrify the child. We are thus in the constant situation of having to make alliances with monsters of all varieties, nature and degree (2). Some of these unstable alliances are made with deities and mythical heroes. Among the psychotic child's most terrifying monsters are his own thoughts and thinking. At the same time that he cherishes, guards, and even plays with them, he fears them as if they were also alien monsters that can bring destruction to him and his needed objects. The child's thoughts and his thinking are, however, indispensable for the development of the treatment process, even if expressed in action or any non-verbal form of language. When we wish to treat him we also invite him to share and give us his thoughts, or at least invite him to have thoughts which he may or may not share with us, or may communicate in any language he commands. But in so doing we confront him with an immediate task that terrifies him and sets into operation mechanisms that may even destroy the initial treatment situation.

Not only are the child's thoughts potentially monstrous to him, they are often completely alien productions to the therapist, who at first may find them totally incomprehensible and therefore useless. We measure the primary process of the psychotic child's thinking against our own yardstick of secondary-process thinking and thought values and judge his thinking to be a thought disorder. In fact, observation of his thinking and language reveals a very meaningful order (Ch. 2, this vol.), although one based on primary-process language and rules of grammar (1) which reflect and represent the functioning of his psychotic psychic organization. Not only do his thinking and language have order, but meaning and purpose which, at least in part, we have come to see as being in the service of the restoration of or struggle against the symbiosis in order to maintain his optimal ego functioning. In effect, the therapist projects his own confusion onto the patient in speaking of the patient's thought disorder when he has not as yet conceived the hidden rules of the patient's thinking.

The patient's thoughts and language, by their private and foreign expression and form, invite the therapist to understand him only in a certain way. That way can be understood as an invitation to a symbiotic relationship. The therapist is to know the patient and his mind so well as to know his strange and foreign thoughts; to understand him on his own level of thinking; to share with him otherwise completely private thoughts and wishes; to maintain his omnipotent control while the symbiotic partner can thus fulfill his needs without even asking—the psychotic version of the non-verbal infant's needs being met by the mother's total empathy and understanding (12). The patient's thoughts, translated into action, are clearly seen as his instrument for consummating a symbiotic union with the external environment, from which he has not yet achieved clear differentiation and over which he must maintain control. His communications to the therapist, in order to be understood and responded to, demand that the therapist, too, think in primary-process language, give up his own secondary-process thinking, and enter into a thought and language symbiosis with the patient, where frequently communication regresses to communion.

The use of the metaphor (3) as an interpretive technique can, among other meanings, be understood in this way: as an entry into the patient's inner world via his language and thinking. The metaphor safeguards the patient's authority and control over the therapist's intrusion by stating the patient's terms. In using the metaphor, the therapist minimizes difference. While introducing himself as a representative of the external world, he does not demand that the patient accept that difference. Use of the metaphor permits the outer world to enter the patient's private world but without demands to cope with a foreign object which he cannot master. Useful and necessary initially and for large stretches of time during treatment, the metaphor outlives its therapeutic purpose as the patient outgrows his need for symbiosis and achieves a more stable and permanent separation and individuation of self from object.

Similarly, in the problem of regression we have another ally that is indispensable for treatment. Under optimal conditions, it serves its positive therapeutic function; out of control, as so readily occurs in the psychotic child, it becomes a monster that can destroy the therapeutic process and dissolve self- and object-cathexis. Here again, the

crucial feature is the maintenance of self- and object-cathexis, the optimal state of separation and symbiotic union, but with maintenance
of self-cathexis possible for that ego organization. In this situation,
the therapist would need to function like the psychological mother, his
empathy and understanding directing his distance and closeness to
the patient's inner state. He would meet the patient's regressions with
his own empathic regressions, like the mother who, for optimal mothering, can gauge the infant's need for dependence, support and need-
satisfaction while allowing for distance and stimuli to growth as the
infant is ready for these. The therapist's task is to meet empathically
the patient's regressive needs, and also his simultaneous or time-appro-
priate need for growth stimuli. He functions like the grain of sand
in the oyster shell which is the irritant that becomes the organizing
growth factor.

The therapist's interpretive activity is to adapt within this empathic
role. This brings us to a distinction between *interpretation* as the activity pertinent for stabilized self- and object-cathexis, i.e., between
two separate people; and *intra-pretation*, the therapist's mode of representing his function within the symbiotic sac, in order to maintain the
necessary optimal conditions of self and object separation and union
for continued ego functioning. In the relatively weakly differentiated
state of internal ego function and structure, thoughts and affects trigger
off psychological and motor acts that lead to loss of self and unreach-
able regressions. In the interpretation of affect to the patient, or of
demands for closeness, separation, dependence, or growth that the
ego cannot yet master, self-cathexis is lost and uncontrollable panic
regressions may occur. And in the interpretation to the patient of his
thoughts of fear, self-cathexis is lost. The patient experiences that the
therapist, by knowing his thoughts and fears, also has the same fears
and cannot protect him. The therapist is no longer a separate observer
but a participant in the patient's own self: the patient's self is now
lost in the therapist's mind. This leads to loss of object- and self-
cathexis and to regressions that may or may not lead to useful therapeutic purpose.

In "Object Constancy and Psychotic Reconstruction" (Ch. 14, this
vol.), we present the dilemma of *psychotic object constancy*. We
characterize this dilemma in terms of the ego's gross and quixotic distortion of reality testing in which the new or changing object was permitted
to exist only in terms of past negative images; i.e., the object existed
not as it was in reality but had to be what it was not, therefore being
delusional and unreal. To carry the point to an absurd extreme, we
can conceive of a similar, almost impossible dilemma confronting the
therapist who offers himself as a new object. He, too, must accept the

role of a mirror reflection of what the object must be to the self to the psychotic child, i.e., what it is not, and therefore to have to remain unreal. Further, he has simultaneously to remain within and without the symbiotic sac, to move back and forth and yet be at the same place with the patient's regressions and progressions. He has to speak his language, yet not speak but echo. He has simultaneously to be the self of the patient and object, yet remain himself at all times. In short, he has to engage in a host of primary-process maneuvers ad infinitum; a fantastic feat of psychic juggling which, if it were not feasible, could well-nigh make it impossible to treat such a child by means of psycho-analytic psychotherapy.

This may be the reality of analytic work with these children, after all, but this is the question that constantly confronts us. We would like to resolve it not by countertransference impotence or megalomania, but by the scientific curiosity and therapeutic commitment which motivates us in our research, as we develop techniques for treatment and training based on psychoanalytic understanding.

REFERENCES

1. EKSTEIN, RUDOLF. "From Echolalia to Echo: the Psychotic Child's Struggle against, for, and with Language." Summary in *J. Am. Psychoanal. Assoc.*, 1968, 1:117.
2. —— and E. CARUTH. "The Working Alliance with the Monster." *Bull. of Menninger Clin.*, 1965, 29:189.
3. —— and J. WALLERSTEIN. "Choice of Interpretation in the Treatment of Borderline and Psychotic Children." *Bull. of Menninger Clin.*, 1957, 21:199.
4. ——, J. WALLERSTEIN and A. MANDELBAUM. "Countertransference in the Residential Treatment of Children." *Psychoanalyt. Study of the Child*, 1959, 14:186.
5. FREUD, ANNA. *Normality and Pathology in Childhood. Assessments of Development.* N. Y.: Int'l. Univ. Press, 1965.
6. FREUD, S. *The Ego and the Id* (1923). *Std. Ed.*, XIX. Lon.: Hogarth Press, 1961.
7. ——. "Formulations Regarding the Two Principles of Mental Functioning" (1911). *Std. Ed.* XII. Lon.: Hogarth Press, 1961.
8. ——. *The Interpretation of Dreams* (1900). *Std. Ed.* IV. Lon.: Hogarth Press, 1953.
9. ——. "The Loss of Reality in Neurosis and Psychosis." *St. Ed.* XIX. Lon.: Hogarth Press, 1961.
10. KANNER, LEO. "Infantile Autism and the Schizophrenias." *Behavioral Science*, 1965, 4:412.
11. MAHLER, MARGARET. "On Child Psychosis and Schizophrenia: Autistic and Symbiotic Infantile Psychoses." *Psychoanalyt. Study of the Child*, 1952, 7:286.
12. SPITZ, RENE. *The First Year of Life.* N. Y.: Int'l. Univ. Press, 1965.
13. WINNICOTT, D. W. "Hate in the Countertransference." *Int. J. of Psychoanalysis*, 1949, 30:69.

CHAPTER SEVEN

Psychotic Adolescents and Their Quest for Goals

I suggested elsewhere that the frequent turmoil during puberty and adolescence hides a crisis about which it is frequently difficult to decide whether it expresses a sign of growth or is a symptom of pathology, particularly the pathology of schizophrenic and similar psychotic states (7).

Anna Freud, in a well-known paragraph from her classic text, *The Ego and the Mechanisms of Defense*, published as early as 1936, has summed up the dilemma with a few master strokes. She describes adolescents as:

> . . . excessively egoistic, regarding themselves as the center of the universe and the sole object of interest, and yet at no time in later life are they capable of so much self-sacrifice and devotion. They form the most passionate love relations, only to break them off as abruptly as they began them. On the one hand they throw themselves enthusiastically into the life of the community and, on the other, they have an overpowering longing for *solitude*. They oscillate between blind submission to some self-chosen leader and defiant rebellion against any and every authority. They are selfish and materially-minded and at the same time full of lofty idealism. They are esthetic but will suddenly plunge into instinctual indulgence of the most primitive character. At times their behavior to other people is rough and inconsiderate, yet they themselves are extremely touchy. Their moods veer between light-hearted optimism and the blackest pessimism. Sometimes they will work with indefatigable enthusiasm and, at other times, they are sluggish and apathetic (10).

About fifteen years later, Erikson (8) characterized the problem which the adolescent has to solve during this phase of development as the search for a permanent adult role, for occupational, social, religious, and personal commitments which lead him through an identity crisis which is insoluble unless society grants him a psychological and social moratorium. This moratorium releases inner organizing forces, enabling the adolescent to move toward young adulthood.

Pumpian-Mindlin (11) has described this phase of the search for commitment, the temporary role diffusion, the playing with and the acting out of future choices, in terms of omnipotentiality, the megalomaniclike belief of the adolescent that he can reach any goal while, at the same time, committing himself to nonpermanency. Potentially then, he can reach any goal or none, and during this phase the adaptive or maladaptive struggles of the adolescent will determine the outcome, while he is being watched with anxiety and envy by the parent generation.

Frequently these young people give us distorted pictures of pseudo-identification with the adult world. These distortions have been puzzling to the clinician and have encouraged the equally distorted pseudo-judgment that adolescence itself is a kind of illness. But it is true that often in this period one can hardly differentiate between psychopathology and normal growth crisis. However, some clear clinical syndromes can be delineated.

In what follows I wish to make remarks about the schizophrenic adolescent whose development parallels in many features that of the average adolescent. His psychopathological state, however, expresses itself in symptoms which, while remindful of the average adolescent crisis, carry in themselves the germs of destructive illness leading to the inability to solve such age-specific problems as the establishment of goals and purposes and the acquisition of skills by which to achieve these goals.

Charlotte Buhler's (2) lifelong studies of the human life cycle and the patterns of establishment of goals, which then, in themselves, become a motivating, organizing, and character-building force, have given us many guidelines. So, too, have Erikson's (9) discussions of the different life stages of man and his studies of ego virtues. These will be helpful as we attempt to throw some light on the schizophrenic adolescent's abortive struggle to develop life goals or *Lebensziele*.

In Charlotte Buhler's terms, the adolescent's attempts at setting life goals are first more experimental and programmatic than realistic. He sees and sometimes tries himself in various roles, but his commitments are temporary. While programming these adult roles, he projects himself in his phantasies into the future. All his moves in relating himself to the future realities of life, however, are provisional and preparatory rather than final. This probing by adolescents is bound up in existential-type conflicts. The question "Who am I?" plagues the thinking youth. He feels thrown into conflicts which he cannot resolve and in which he feels utterly alone. Not infrequently, his despair leads him to doubt his ability, his wish to cope with life, and makes him feel hopeless about himself and sometimes even suicidal.

All these problems occur in an exaggerated form in the case of the pathological development. The neurotic youth may tend either to make premature decisions and enter finite relationships, such as a very early marriage, or else he may luxuriate in fantasies of future glory and happiness. Thus a borderline schizophrenic and later homosexual girl, Edda, spent her free time at age 12 lying on her bed and dreaming about going to Hollywood with a suitcase full of brilliant plays, visiting and charming various famous actors and actresses, and becoming famous herself overnight. She prepared maps, studied roads to Los Angeles, put money aside, and packed a suitcase with clothes and some of her poems. However, it never got beyond that. (Case reported by C. Buhler in preparation.)

The psychotic youths described in the following paragraphs demonstrate four different forms in which their goal setting deviates from the normal, First, they have long-range fantasies, which, as such, are phase-characteristic but in their cases are completely unrealistic. Second, in reality they remain "stuck" in short-term goals, which may occur from childhood on or at any age, but which, in the psychotic case, appear as projects of major proportions. Third, they are unable to integrate themselves and to project a unified self from present to future. And fourth, they experience existential-type conflicts, which again, although they may be found in normal adolescents, in their case become serious struggles involving the question of life or death.

I invite the reader to follow me as I describe some clinical material illustrating these struggles in the psychotherapeutic work with a female schizophrenic adolescent, the vicissitudes of whose treatment I have previously described (6).

At first Teresa was hardly reachable and often out of contact. As she slowly ventured out of her autistic world and tried to join the world of her peers as well as that of the adults who were part of her social situation, she tried desperately to cope with a cata-tonic-like paralysis which kept her from putting into action whatever plans she was capable of developing. These plans seemed to remain forever part of her infantile, her primitive fantasy world. They reminded one of promises that small children offer their parents in an attempt to secure love but really are not meant to be kept. The difference, however, between the small child who offers the promise as a love-restoring device, and Teresa, our patient, is that the small child, as time passes, learns to deal with the promise in the fullest sense of the word and attempts to live up to it, while Teresa's promises could never be kept. They were but static symptoms of her regressed position. They were forgotten as soon as the psychotherapist was out of sight, and they could be compared to a repressed dream which one wishes to remember in order to report it to the therapist. When she finally remembered the promise, the mere recollection of it was experienced as if it were the fulfillment of the promise itself. However, as she continued on the slow road to recovery, frequently hardly noticeable, she learned to live up to small promises, which she could now fulfill on the installment plan, as it were.

Her practical life goals that she discussed during this phase of her psychotherapy concerned such issues as being able to leave the shower room, not after hours and hours of preoccupation with delusional fantasy activity while under the shower but after a specified time which would permit her to be on time for the volunteer worker who brought her to the clinic for the appointment. Somewhat later she experienced as a major achievement the newly gained capacity to take a bus by herself and to remember the number of the bus. This task occupied her mind for weeks and months until she could triumphantly report that she had reached this goal, which she saw as a magnificent achievement, although her performance was completely out of proportion to what would ordinarily be expected of a young person her age.

If one were to see these goals as the life goals she had set for herself, one would have to see them as no more and no less than very small, very tiny short-term goals. For instance, she described during an interview how her social and psychological paralysis finally abated after many weeks and how she was now "moving around a bit, helping the Sisters a bit" in the Catholic home where she then resided. Obviously, this very small investment in the world of reality, the world of social action and of actuality, indicated that much of her psychic energy was invested in other areas of her life. Her life goals, therefore, were of a different nature than the ones that make up the ambitions, the purposes, the activities of adolescents who belong in the ordinary range of psychopathology or normal behavior.

We will come back to Teresa later. First I want to offer similar material from other patients in order to stress certain interesting aspects of these small, short-term goals.

Another research patient was Donald, also a schizophrenic adolescent (Chaps. 8, 24, this vol.) (6). He was occupied in establishing his goal behavior with plans for the next few months, such as to be able to eat lunch together with the other children in the private school he attends. It took him months of mastering his anxiety and fear until he was capable of accomplishing this. Other actions concerned his fear of using the public bathroom, of joining children in a baseball game, or of eating and talking together with his parents. He was impelled to discuss these problems for hours and weeks with obsessive rigidity, and one gained the impression that a powerful struggle developed around a seemingly tiny issue.

A third patient, Danny, again an adolescent suffering from an adolescent schizophrenic character disorder, wanted to live up to the promises he thought he owed society and himself and to his ambition to become a musician, a songwriter. These promises to be fulfilled found practical expression in the attempt to finish a poem. He had written the opening lines and was able to complete it only after weeks and months of endless obsessions about it, accompanied by escapes into psychoticlike acting-out phases. His own enthusiastic response to the finished poem was temporary proof to him that he had a great future, but in the face of a minor frustration the enthusiasm vanished without a trace.

What and where are the true investments of such patients? The first patient, Theresa, is sometimes capable of establishing a feeble bridge between her inner world, her delusional preoccupation, and her attempts to communicate with the psychotherapist. She does this by means of what I have called *borrowed fantasies*. She can talk about herself only by metaphoric allegories borrowed from television shows or movies to which she is addicted. As she watches these shows, she sometimes remembers enough of one so that she can communicate the plot, frequently in a changed and bizarre form, and uses the show like a coat hanger on which she hangs her inner life during the transference struggle. The show becomes the brittle and unreliable bridge between her chaotic inner world and the vague desire to talk about that inner world.

During the hour (Ch. 24, this vol.) in which she attempted to report to her therapist that she was now successful in "moving around a bit," she used the screen play *Black Orpheus* in order to describe the vicissitudes of the current transference struggle. She saw herself as Eurydice who was involved with Orpheus, but who was, at the same time, also persecuted by the hateful, jealous, and revengeful Aristaeus. She dies a bitter death and Orpheus is to resurrect her. But as he turns around, spurning Pluto's injunction, and listens to her desperate pleas, he loses her again. She described, through her powerful identification with the heroine, her underlying basic philosophy, which then established the psychotic goal behavior of this patient. She considered herself as dead and, at the same time, miraculously alive. She lived through and died a thousand deaths and tried to become alive over and over again. She shared with the therapist the powerful and almost convincing fantasy that she was going to kill herself by the end of the year and, at the same time, told him that she has improved so much that she will never touch herself again, blurring the difference between masturbation and suicide. She has gained self-control and she wants to live. But then she projects the very suicidal and/or sexual fantasy into a homicidal or raping expectation, claiming that someone, some man, perhaps some woman, will kill her, attack her, by the end of the year. Her search for love and for acceptance, her struggle against death, are matched at the same time by the search for death. Her fear of death is matched by the fear of life, and like Eurydice, she moves backward and forward between the positions of life and death; and the helper, the beloved one, the rescuer, the therapist, at times is seen as the saviour and at other times as the crucifier, the dangerous murderer, the raper.

One can see then that underneath the conscious, the reality-oriented attempt to master small tasks and to be committed to short-term goals, is a powerful psychic system which is characterized by the inner struggle, the alternating commitment to life and to death. One well might say her goal is to stay alive. She does not search for goals which are going to make her life meaningful, but rather she struggles for existence itself. The meaning of her life is a life and death struggle.

She finds herself exposed to these powerful anxieties, these inner terrors, to such an extent that one well can say of her, if it is permitted to coin a new word, that she does not struggle with omnipotentiality but, rather, that she is beset by omni-impotentiality. She defends herself against the awareness of this omni-impotentiality, this utter helplessness, this terror of dying, by means of a defensive fantasy which changes the omni-impotentiality into megalomania. It is for this reason that, in spite of the fact that she does not do more than "move around a bit," learn to take the bus, learn to count money, and so on, she also speaks of goals such as of becoming a famous movie star, an outstanding singer, a great dancer, etc., goals that are indeed megalomanic because she can and does do nothing in order to move toward them. They are not goals but fantasies which are to cover up the helplessness, the fear of destruction, the terror of destructive impulses. They are promises to herself by which she tries to restore her self-love and to cope with self-destructive tendencies. These megalomanic fantasy goals are self-promises which are not meant to be kept; they are comparable to the promises of the small child to the parent, and just as the latter promises are made to restore the parent's love, these are to restore self-love, megalomanic narcissism. They are the psychotic version of what Schlesinger (12) called primary promises.

The same is true of our second patient, Don. He, too, even though his accomplishments sometimes move at a snail's pace and are characterized by obsessive repetitiveness which paralyzes him as well as the therapist who attempts to listen (Ch. 8, this vol.), establishes himself in fantasy as a powerful genius, a potential world leader, a great pianist, one who will impress the world with enormous success. But behind these megalomanic expectations looms large his omni-impotentiality, his utter helplessness, and his weakness, his fear of loss of self and loss of object, such as when he tells us that he needs proof that he exists. He sometimes looks at his therapist and wonders whether this experience he has refers to a real person or to a movie-screen picture of the therapist. He must then touch the therapist in order to establish for himself that there is reality. Sometimes he does not believe that he himself exists, since he cannot see himself. He would believe that he exists only if he could see his own image, and then he needs this evidence to prevent himself from being devoured by anxiety and terror. Descartes' *cogito ergo sum* is replaced by a "you touch me or let me touch you therefore I know that I am and that you are."

The third adolescent, Danny, when threatened by loss of object or self-experience, or with a kind of psychic death, tries to restore object and self-world by destructive acting out through wild aggressive attacks, through suicidal gestures, of which it is never quite clear, if one follows the meaning of the delusional material, whether they are to be understood as homicidal or suicidal.

We find then in these patients a variety of common denominators which all relate to the issue at hand: the quasi-search for goals in the psychotic adolescent. As we watch their rudimentary mastery of reality, we find that they have endless problems with social adjustment, school learning, work situations, and that they cannot master actuality, that is, apply reality testing to appropriate need-gratifying action. Even in those rare moments when islands of reality testing are comparatively intact, we realize that little energy is available for social mastery, for putting the reality testing into a context of actuality and organized achievement. We notice that small, short-term goals dominate their lives as far as realistic problem solutions are concerned. We find also that these patients, within their fantasy activities, see their power, their talents and their gifts, and their possibilities for success way out of proportion to the ordinary daydreams of adolescents. Unlike the successful artists, the writers, of whom Freud once said that they achieve through their fantasies what they have dreamed about in their fantasy, namely, honor, power and the love of women, these schizophrenic adolescents have not found the way to translate fantasies or daydreams into truly goal-directed behavior. But still, they see themselves, in spite of evidence to the contrary, as great persons, as world rulers, as creative artists, singers, millionaires, who must wait for the fantastic fulfillment of their wishes or live with the delusionary conviction that they have reached their goals, without ever having to relate these wishes or delusions to any kind of realistic behavior. The primary process does not lead to the secondary process but ends up in a dead-end street. They cannot see any relationship between these fantastic elaborations of their inner dreams and the very small investment they are able to make in their everyday dealing with social issues.

Their megalomanic fantasies, however, are not stable, are not constant, and give way frequently not only to underachievement and non-achievement but yield also to terror, to deep-seated anxieties, to the fear of death and annihilation. They fear that they and the world will perish, so that most of their inner investment does not constitute a struggle to find meaning in life, to initiate purposeful goal behavior, but rather results in a stay-alive struggle, the warding off of *Weltuntergangsphantasien* (fantasies of the world's end).

It must, of course, be emphasized that as these patients struggle for survival and struggle against self-destruction, their use of such existential notions must be understood within the context of schizophrenic thought disorder and disturbed schizophrenic object relations. When we refer to object relations, we do not have in mind the context of interpersonal relations, rather, we refer to the capacity or incapacity of patients to maintain object and self representations within themselves. Theresa, in her use of the theme of Eurydice, gave us a powerful picture of what keeps her from coming to the "upper world," the world of Orpheus and reality, of light and insight, and what keeps her from maintaining this world so that she can establish more than token purposes, more than short-term goals, and can really give meaning to life rather than having to remain committed compulsively to the only meaning she sees in life, the desperate struggle to stay alive, to not die. She struggles backward and forward, between the attempt to gain the object and to reestablish the self representation, and the regression in which she loses both and is paralyzed once more in a catatonic-like disaster.

From studies such as Spitz's (13) we know that the separation and individuation process in the small infant establishes the capacity to maintain self and object representations, an achievement which is then the basis upon which to build realistic goals in life. Adolescents who do not suffer from such weak object and self representation, who are in no danger of really losing them and have resolved this struggle, can move toward purposes in life, can change or maintain these purposes, can develop toward individuation and identity very much along the lines which have been described in the studies of Buhler and Erikson. They sometimes do give the impression that they are about to lose these achievements and, since the adolescent must give up the early objects' ties in the family and replace them with new ties, he lives through phases where these objects and self representations are on shaky ground. But, as we observe such patients during treatment, we see that they go through the ordinary vicissitudes of neurotic transference manifestations and that they utilize the object representation of the analyst in order to bring about reality-oriented life purposes and goals. This the schizophrenic adolescent is unable to do. He therefore develops transferences which are at times only of a neurotic order, but more frequently are actually psychotic transferences in which separation of self and nonself gives way to fusion-states where there is no clear-cut separation between self and object, between therapist and patient. Sometimes these transferences give way to quasi-separations in which either the self or object representation is maintained at the expense of the other. These are then the more autisticlike states in which patients seemingly cannot be reached during short phases of the therapeutic process.

We suggest, then, that the inability to maintain goals and goal-directed behavior, the incapacity to establish life purposes which are realistic, stem from the fact that schizophrenic adolescents are unable to maintain object constancy. Unlike their neurotic counterparts who suffer from omnipotentiality, these schizophrenic youngsters suffer from omni-impotentiality, a feeling of impotence which permeates all spheres of life, including the inability to maintain self and object representation. Their defense against this omni-impotentiality, this dread and this hopeless struggle for survival, this constant terror of death, is megalomania, which very frequently looks like the omnipotentiality of the ordinary adolescent but actually is but a forged, a nongenuine replica of it. Since most of their energy, then, must be used in order to reestablish some form of psychic equilibrium, their actual moves seem to be poverty-stricken, slow, token gestures, empty promises, tiny, short-term achievements.

Our stress on the issue of object constancy is to indicate the direction in which research in psychotherapy with such patients must proceed. Many case studies (6) in our research help us to establish new techniques utilizable in this struggle toward object constancy. The neurotic adolescent must learn to resolve the unconscious conflict with objects of the past and the present. But still, his is a conflict between separate individuals, between different representations of self, of past and present, and of objects of past and present. The psychotic adolescent offers us a pre-object world and a pre-self world, fused with the partial achievement of object and self representations. As long as there are unstable introjects, the purpose and the goal of life will be a desperate and hopeless struggle for existence, a compulsion to endlessly repeat past misery. But when object constancy is achieved, when capacity for object relations is developed, such existence will be the basis for new meanings and for permanent and realistic life goals, for the release and development of adaptive capacity toward self actualization and the positive use of reality as a source of challenge and nurture (6, 14).

REFERENCES

1. BUGENTAL, JAMES F. T. Values and Existential Unity, Chapter 22 in C. Buhler and F. Massarik, *The Course of Human Life*, New York: Springer, 1969, pp. 383-392.
2. BUHLER, C. *Der menschliche Lebenslauf als psychologisches Problem*, 2nd rev. ed., Göttingen: Verlag für Psychologie, 1959.
3. BUHLER, C. *Intentionality and Self-realization*, San Francisco: Jossey-Bass, in preparation.
4. BUHLER, C. & GOLDENBERG, H. Structural Aspects of the Individual's History, Chapter 3 in C. Buhler and F. Massarik, *The Course of Human Life*, New York: Springer, 1968, pp. 54-63.
5. BUHLER, C. & HORNER, A. J. The Role of Education in the Goal-Setting Process, Chapter 14 in C. Buhler and F. Massarik, *The Course of Human Life*, New York: Springer, 1968, pp. 231-245.
6. EKSTEIN, R. *Children of Time and Space, of Action and Impulse: Clinical Studies on the Psychoanalytic Treatment of Severely Disturbed Children.* New York: Appleton-Century-Crofts, 1966.
7. ————. Turmoil During Puberty and Adolescence: Crisis or Pathology? Reiss-Davis Reporter, 1966, 5:2.
8. ERIKSON, E. H. *Childhood and Society.* New York: W. W. Norton & Co., Inc., 1950.
9. ————. Reality and Actuality, *J. American Psychoanalytic Association*, 1962, 10, 451.
10. FREUD, A. *The Ego and the Mechanisms of Defence.* London: Hogarth Press, 1948.
11. PUMPIAN-MINDLIN, E. Omnipotentiality, Youth, and Commitment, *J. American Academy of Child Psychiatry*, 1965, 4:1, 1-18.
12. SCHLESINGER, H. J. A Contribution to a Theory of Promising: I: Primary and Secondary Promising. Unpublished, 1964.
13. SPITZ, R. A. *The First Year of Life.* New York: International Universities Press, 1965.
14. TOMLINSON, TOMMY M. The Psychotherapist as a Codeterminant in Client Goal-Setting, Chapter 13 in C. Buhler and F. Massarik, *The Course of Human Life.* New York: Springer, 1968, 212-228.

Certain Phenomenological Aspects of the Counter Transference in the Treatment of Schizophrenic Children*

*". . . to look at the phenomena so long until.
they seem to tell the story by themselves."*

JEAN MARTIN CHARCOT

In order to highlight the technical problems of the therapist in the treatment of schizophrenic children, we will start with the *copybooks* of the therapist rather than the case history of the patient.

The following are some extracts from the notes dictated by the therapist immediately following the hour with Don, his sixteen-year-old schizophrenic patient:

Hour No. 8: "As he droned on repetitively, a stereotyped smile on his face, without genuine contact with me or I with him, I found myself trying to ward off sleep. Much of what I did today was somehow attempting to be with him and to make remarks which were less of an interpretive nature and more of a facilitating nature . . . Sometimes, when I could not follow him, he went

* Elaine Caruth is the co-author of this chapter.

droning on almost as if he were talking to a machine and really did not need me."

Hour No. 10: "Again I was overwhelmed by the unusual drowsiness that this boy produces in me . . . It is particularly hard to cope, on the one hand, with the repetitiveness and, on the other, with the constant questioning which actually is a complete denial of the illness . . . He droned on . . . I think that my drowsiness is the correlate of the state of mind that he described later when he told me how he would be taken over right here in the hour by dizziness and drowsiness."

Hour No. 32: "My drowsiness started as the hour changed into a series of questions—obsessive renumerations which do not permit one to break through and bring the thought to an act . . . It makes me drowsy."

Hour No. 35: "This hour again was one of ceaseless questioning, such as what went wrong with him; what he could do about what went wrong with him; whether I would help him get well; could I explain to him what his illness meant; whether he was a mathematical genius; whether he was really crazy, etc. All of these are compulsive questions which really do not require an answer but rather use me as a kind of auxiliary ego who is to see for him, touch for him and act for him—like the little child who wants to find out about the world via the parents, who are to restore the reality world for him. Don gives the impression that he cannot get out of his dream world; rather he pulls me into his dream world. As I became more and more insistent about not answering questions, he spoke about himself waking up. He acted like a person who is in a half-dream, half-wake world who constantly wanted to use the other for orientation . . . He said to me that he was asleep and I should fall asleep with him—live with him in the irrational world of psychotic philosophy—while I constantly told him to wake up, look and test for himself."

These comments describe the subjective reactions of the therapist during the hour. Subsequently, when the electrically recorded tapes of these sessions were audited, the objective description of the therapist's behavior was that he spoke slowly and unspontaneously and had unusual difficulty hearing and understanding the patient. He appeared to be struggling to maintain contact and he seemed to be attempting to do so through mimetic devices of repeating phrases of the patient, the "facilitating remarks" referred to above by him. These gave the observer the impression of an echolaliclike quality to the communications.

Such clinical phenomena highlight the importance of the relationship between the role and the subjective experience of the therapist, and the nature of the object relations in the patient. It becomes apparent that the range and choice of effective therapeutic maneuvers are to some extent defined and delimited by the vicissitudes of the illness.

Here we would like to explore further the treatment of the kind of schizophrenic child whose disturbed object relations repeat in the transference the position of the small child who is still searching for the reassuring answering echo of the parent. Such children are struggling with the issue of differentiating themselves from the outside world, and their struggle for self-representation is developed against the background of the nature and quality of their introjects. Their interpersonal communications reflect an internal discourse and are fixated at a point where they are more of a monologue than a dialogue. These children seek to contact the therapist in a fashion which appears the reversal of the position of the autistic child who can only echo; these children can only hear the echo, as it were. They try to force the therapist into becoming a projected reverberation of their own unintegrated echo of the parent's earliest communications to them. They ply the therapist with questions which, in many ways, seem to be a variation of the theme "Little Sir Echo, who is the fairest one of all?" These questions implicitly demand of the therapist a symbiotic relationship which not only denies the presence of other objects but, even more important, denies the existence of the patient and the therapist as separate objects. Consequently, the therapist feels caught between the double bind of either saying to the patient, "You are the fairest one of all," or else replying, "There is one a thousand times more fair"; respectively, there is a reality and other objects. If the therapist replies in the latter fashion, the patient may experience it as such a narcissistic blow that he may retreat into a deeper psychotic regression, his tenuous hold on reality may be further weakened, he may lose control over his primitive aggressive drives and possibly act out through suicidal or homicidal gestures. If, metaphorically speaking, the therapist says, "You are the fairest one of all," he then reduces himself from the patient's standpoint to the echo who "is a nice little fellow but always so far away." The therapeutic problem in these instances is to develop technical interventions which have sufficient leverage to maintain contact and yet can still drive the therapeutic process forward.

We come now to Don, an eccentric bizarre-appearing youngster who is quite obviously emotionally ill. From birth onward Don has been described as either brain injured, retarded or epileptic; has required special schooling; but has never been treated as emotionally ill until recently when his complete inability to adjust to school situations and a family crisis brought about re-evaluation. To this day, neither parent has fully accepted or acknowledged the extent and severity of his illness. They continue to deny it to the boy as well as to themselves, despite the seemingly unavoidable contrast between his behavior and that of an older brotner, who is a brilliant biological researcher. The mother appears to have devoted much of her life to Don, which has helped him to develop a marginal manner of functioning on a reality level so that much of the psychotic symptomatology has been bound into the character formation. There appears to have been a deeply rooted symbiotic relationship between Don and his mother which, although it contributed to the strength of the minimal ego development, has also made it more difficult for Don to form healthier object relations with the father who himself is an emotionally ill person.

Clinical examination of this boy reveals a deeply ill schizophrenic youngster with a manifest thought disorder reflected in the emergence of primary process functioning. Delusional and hallucinatory experiences reveal his conflicts between omnipotence and impotence with grandiose fantasies related to intellectual achievement. He is constantly preoccupied with masturbation fantasies of a sado-masochistic nature which genetically can be related to the disturbed relationship with a paranoid father whose unpredictable episodic outbursts of hostile sadistic aggression intermingle with periods of loving warmth. Because of his own problems, the father also vacillates between periods of exceptional professional accomplishment and periods of incapacity to work. Don's image of his father is confused further by this extreme variability in the father's behavior.

Early in his treatment Don revealed to the therapist his preoccupation with sexual beating fantasies which were accompanied by incessant masturbatory activities. He spoke of a fantasy figure, Mr. P., short for Mr. Punishment, who would seduce him into sexual activities and would also become the annihilating sadistic figure. This boy's idiosyncratic version of "Pillow Talk" is literally to retreat to a darkened room and masturbate under a pillow mannequin fashioned to represent Mr. P. Shortly after the onset of treatment he developed a new fantasy figure, Dr. X., the introject of the therapist, Dr. Ekstein, whom he attempted to use in his efforts to counteract the seductions and the dangers of Mr. P. The vicissitudes of Don's object relations frequently could be inferred from his capacity to relate to the therapist as Dr. Ekstein or as Dr. X. When contact was minimal and when the boy was threatened by overwhelming psychotic panic, he would desperately call on Dr. X. for help. When contact was regained, he could begin to relate to the true object, Dr. Ekstein. A rather fascinating graphic illustration of this phenomenon was observed several times in his written communications to the therapist. Such communications, written during moments of panic, were frequently addressed to Dr. X. However, the letter inside the envelope was to Dr. Ekstein. The boy could describe the initial panic which motivated him to write the letter. At the same time he could report the subsidence of the panic as the vicarious contact with the therapist was restored through the written communication.

Don brings to the hour repetitive stereotyped questions, a kind of psychotic obsessionalism which avoids the thought but is tainted with the thought disorder. Communication is on a primitive and concrete level and the more abstract symbolic functions are not fully developed. Language is still a kind of act or acting out in the service of signal or expression functions (3) rather than communication. As he describes his sexual fantasies and attempts to engage the therapist into a discussion of the forbidden words, "punishment" and "spanking," which he himself dares not speak although he can listen to them, there develops a lascivious orgastic quality to his verbalizations. These reflect the need to turn the thought into the act, the discussion is thus experienced as a seduction. Because of the concretistic thinking, Don's signals require an "echo point" rather than a "counterpoint," as it were, as if he cannot abstract to a common language but can only hear and understand the concrete repetition of his own words.

Don's questions are of two kinds. First, there are the more primitive stereotyped ones which are basically variations of the underlying question, "Am I or am I not?" couched in the more advanced derivative form of "Am I a genius or am I crazy?"; respectively, "Am I so powerful I can overwhelm and destroy the world?" or "Am I so weak I can be overwhelmed and annihilated?" For Don, unlike Descartes' rational man, has not the psychic apparatus which would enable him to say, "I think—therefore I am." Rather he requires of the therapist that he echo endlessly the desired reassurance. He wants the therapist to become a projection of his own inner helpless reassuring agent, an echo of the parents' hollow reassurances to him. These reassurances were also, of course, to themselves in order to belie their underlying doubts.

And it is this role—of an echoing primitive introject—to which Don has assigned his therapist and against which the therapist has been struggling. To the extent that the therapist becomes the echoing introject and is drawn into Don's dream world, he becomes sleepy and groggy and can only sustain the kind of echolalic-like contact we see in the autistic child. And yet, unless he can allow himself some element of identification with such a role—allow himself to become Dr. X. so that he can then counteract Mr. P., the sadistic homosexually annihilating introject—he cannot treat this boy. He is somewhat in the position of a genie whom the boy keeps bottled up and yet derives strength from the very fact that he has a genie at his disposal, figuratively speaking. Therefore he must echo Don and yet change the nature of the echo sufficiently that Don can gradually permit him to become himself. To the extent that the therapist can become more spontaneous and alive, so can Don become freer of his paralyzing introjects. As the therapist becomes more of an introject and less an extroject he can begin to be perceived more realistically, and the strength derived from such contact helps the boy to fight against the older archaic and sadistic introjects such as Dr. P.

The questions also take another form. They constantly demand of the therapist that he tell the patient not "if he is" but rather "who and what he is." Such a patient is still struggling with the discovery of himself and the first step appears to be when the other person is a seeming echo of the pre-verbal feelings and perceptions; Johnny wants a bottle, Johnny is hungry, Johnny is wet, etc. The baby learns the spoken word through echoing and imitating the mother's seeming echo of his inner pre-verbal sensations and perceptions.

Actually, the good mother is not merely a true echo; rather she is what we might call an advanced creative echo—an interpreter—who, like the therapist, makes something new available to the child, for otherwise the infant could never become capable of a true dialogue, for which the recognition of a separate animate object is necessary. In similar fashion, the therapist might also be regarded as an advanced creative echo. He does not bring something new to the patient, but rather he attempts to make conscious and available to the patient that which has been conveyed to him, the therapist. Don, much in the fashion of the young infant, is still seeking only an inanimate undifferentiated echo—a wire mother, wired, as it were, for sound. He does not permit the therapist to become alive and separate, to become, metaphorically speaking, more of a mirror than an echo. In this context, we could say that the mirror has more autonomy than the echo; for it has the capacity of reflecting someone other than the self.

For Don, however, a mirror rather than an echo would be a terrorizing threat. It might then reflect his own infantile aggression and hostility, as was the case in *The Picture of Dorian Gray*, or else it might reflect the sadistically overpowering and devouring introjects like Mr. P. To continue the metaphor, we might conceptualize the *therapeutic problem as that to establish contact you must echo, but to develop leverage you must mirror.*

One must combine the echo with the mirror in such a way as to change gradually the nature of the echo without cracking the mirror —without destroying the primary narcissism and subjecting the patient helplessly to the terrors of his autistic world. The therapist must be like an observation-room mirror reflecting the reality of the outer world as well as revealing the feared inner world and how it distorts a patient's perception of the outer world. The therapist must, therefore, constantly confront the patient with the reality that he is ill and at the same time protect him from the terror inherent in facing his illness.

The relationship of mirror taboos to infantile narcissism has been described by Roheim (4). Mirror taboos are aimed at the level of children who are struggling with age-appropriate conflicts over giving up the primary narcissism. They convey to the child the idea that self-love is forbidden and dangerous. Similarly with the fairy tale; we hear the theme that self-love, one's image in the mirror, will eventually develop into object-love—the image of the future love that will appear in the mirror. The conditions for the future love to appear are thus depicted as the ability to give up the self-love and the need for the reassurance of the inanimate echo, and to allow the mirror to become alive and give its own answers. Relationships frequently develop thus from a narcissistic need for reassurance to mature object choice. When they fail to do so, we have the stepmother of Snow White—unable to tolerate in Snow White the representation of her own hated infantile self; and we have Don's mother—unable to become the animate mirror and let him know how sick he truly is because she, too, can only tolerate an inanimate echo of hollow and futile reassurances. This mother, long after the start of treatment, is unable to recognize the terror the boy experiences during the days when he is left alone and prefers this to the threat of exposure by placing him in a special school.

When we discuss the technical problems of the therapist in relationship to the position of the patient; how this defines the type of object the doctor is allowed to become; and the consequent available therapeutic maneuvers, we speak of an issue generic to all psychotherapy. Perhaps one of the distinguishing characteristics between child and adult therapy is that with children, the transference neurosis may frequently lead to an acting out not only of the child's intrapsychic conflicts but also, on the part of the therapist, of a counteraction, as it were, to the transference. With the adult patient, the transference neurosis may create feelings in the analyst which can be observed by him and understood but need not be acted upon. The child, however, who communicates via play and action rather than via the couch and reflection, can easily recreate the image of the internal parents and force the therapist into behavior that has some outward similarity to theirs. Thus, for example, the child who feels that he has never been given to can all too easily put the therapist in a similar position of denying and frustrating.

With the treatment of the schizophrenic child, however, there are certain unique complications which characterize the transference psychosis. First of all, the therapist may not have the leverage that the therapist of the neurotic child has since, faced with problems of contact and communication, he cannot utilize the strongest weapon in the therapeutic armamentarium; namely, interpretation. Furthermore, in order to establish and maintain contact with such a child, it may be necessary that he identify, at least initially, with the fantastically distorted role assigned to him by the patient's pathology. In Don's case, the therapist needed to identify with the role of the introject Dr. X. In treating the patient immersed in an autistic world peopled with primitive introjects, the therapist may be able to communicate and contact him only via the most primitive mechanism available to the autistic child himself. This may often be a kind of echolalia deriving from the very earliest primitive, undifferentiated methods of apprehending and preceiving that have been labeled "fascination" (1).

The role imposed upon the therapist in such instances is qualitatively quite different from that assumed by the therapist of the neurotic child, who may be forced, for example, into being the good or bad mother through the provocations of his subject. The latter is a role with which he can more easily identify and has considerable similarity to his basic personality structure. The therapist of the psychotic child, on the other hand, is forced to assume the identity created by a psychic apparatus which is functioning on an entirely different level.

There is truly a world of difference between the good and bad parent of the child operating on the level of the secondary process and the good fairy or the bad monster of the child operating on the level of the primary process. Both may be one in the unconscious and in the literature of the unconscious, such as the fairy tale, but they are not one to the therapist. To the therapist who must accept in part the role of omnipotence and omniscience, they present unique problems quite different from those of the therapist who struggles between the withholding and the giving parental roles. For example, the neurotic child in anger can ignore the therapist and try to act as if he were not there, via neurotic denial. The psychotic child, on the other hand, has within himself the capacity literally to have it be that the therapist is not there, psychologically speaking, via psychotic withdrawal. In a more fanciful vein, we might compare the differences to those in dealing with Dorothy, of The Wizard of Oz, in her normal state in Kansas, and Dorothy, momentarily psychotic because of, in this instance, organic trauma rather than emotional trauma. The healthy Dorothy can be told on a rational basis that she creates her own mean old women by permitting her dog to run loose; the dreaming Dorothy of Oz, however, is bedeviled by sorcery and can be rescued only by wizardry.

Techniques of treatment must be developed within the context that "that which already dwells within us seeks out and absorbs from the outer world whatever will give it sustenance and power" (2).

It is important to note, furthermore, that not only is the level of object relations constantly fluctuating, but it would appear that the nature of these shifts is far more sensitive than our present nomenclature indicates. The terms "extroject," "introject" and "object" are but gross classifications for the many gradations in finer shadings of all varying kinds of relationships. When we refer to an autistic or symbiotic position as a regression from more advanced levels of functioning, we must recognize that residuals from these higher levels of organization may make their appearance at the lower level of functioning. We do not deal with regression along a single parameter but rather with fragmentation and regression, with isolated islands of functioning and malfunctioning. Just as we know that intellectual functions may be selectively or momentarily impaired, we would like to suggest that object relations, in similar fashion, may be selectively distorted. Where the autistic or symbiotic position is the result of regression from more advanced levels of functioning, then the residuals from these levels of organization may make their appearance during periods of regression.

Thus a patient as sick as Don is still capable of moments of relating realistically to the therapist and of evaluating the desperate need that he has for treatment. He is able to function in certain intellectual areas at a fairly high level and, as we have seen, can shift his position momentarily as contact and communication with the therapist deepen.

We would like to turn now to this patient for a confirming echo of our speculations and use him as our reassuring agent alongside of the changing subjective experience of the therapist. With the development of insight into the meaning of the role to which he was assigned and how it led to the accompanying experience of sleepiness, the therapist could master the role of echo as a necessary tool in his technical armamentarium. The moments of sleepiness and grogginess became markedly briefer and rarer.

When the nature of this kind of contact was described to Don, he was able to acknowledge his need for the therapist completely to know his thoughts, to become an undifferentiated part of him and to echo only desired answers to his endless questions. He related his need for a constant reassuring yes to his questions to his intense fear of criticism. He recognized to some extent that Mr. P. was a part of himself. He saw the similarity between the kind of inner monologue between himself and Mr. P. and the kind of discourse he had sought to maintain with the therapist. There appears to be small but noticeable progress in which the echo quality changes from time to time into a real dialogue characterized by real contact with and relationship to the therapist. At the same time, the private autistic inner dialogue between the fragmented introjects continues and can be expected to continue for some time.

REFERENCES

1. BERNFELD, SIEGFRIED. "Uber Faszination (Concerning Fascination)." *Imago*, 1928, 14: 76-87.
2. BONAPARTE, MARIE. *The Life and Works of Edgar Allen Poe. A Psychoanalytic Interpretation*. Foreword by Sigmund Freud. John Rodker, translator. London: Imago Publishing Co., Ltd., 1949, p. 11.
3. EKSTEIN, RUDOLF. "On the Acquisition of Speech in the Autistic Child." Children of Time and Space, of Action and Impulse: Clinical Studies on the Psychoanalytic Treatment of Severely Disturbed Children. N. Y.: Appleton-Century-Crofts, 1966.
4. ROHEIM, GEZA. "Spiegelzauber (Mirror Magic)." *Imago*, 1917, 5: 63-120.

CHAPTER NINE

Concerning Psychotic Action

The 14th century monk, Buridan, defending the doctrine of free will, is said to have given us the story of the ass that died of hunger and thirst because it could not decide between a pail of food and a pail of water placed at equal distances from it. Caught between equally strong motives, Buridan's ass remained paralyzed and could not act. Actually, the story cannot be found in the medieval philosopher's writings but continues to serve as background for discussions concerning free choice; and the nature of the inability to act, to cope with reality and actuality, or to bring about action as a sequence to thought which Freud had characterized as trial thought.

If we were to see the ass as a victim of inner conflicts that did not allow for resolution and therefore prevented the solution of its task, we approach our clinical experiences with psychotic patients, whose actions often seem to have a kind of rationality about them although they do not actually serve the purposes of reality mastery—of adjustment and adaptation—but remain under the dominance of primary-process functioning. These psychotic acts then are not unlike the act of starvation of Buridan's creature when faced with a reality which actually offered opportunity for full satisfaction.

I should like to use a few sequences of activities—planned actions of a young patient of mine—to characterize different psychic levels of psychotic actions in his endless pursuit of reality mastery. These may serve as a magnified version of typical behavior during therapy, vacillating as it does between acting out—the reliving and trial recollection of past experience and past mental functioning—and the normal act that follows thoughtful preparation under the dominance of the secondary process and reality testing and serves the mastery of current realistic tasks.

The schizophrenic patient, now a young man who lives away from home in semi-independent fashion and tries to make a work adjustment in a sheltered workshop situation, came to me about the age of 15 having been obviously ill throughout most of his life and living at that time in an autistic world of his own. The parents had long since given up having him participate in any form of public education. He would remain at home, teaching himself at times with teaching machines, and waiting for the parent to come home after work. One of his most favored activities while alone, actually preceding the therapeutic work with me, was introduced by a carefully conceived, elaborately planned, and cautiously protected pattern of action. He would call up his mother to make sure she was at work and could not surprise him, carefully giving some contrived reasons for his telephone call. He would then proceed to close all the respective doors that might lead to his discovery, thus protecting himself against any kind of intruder. Finally, he would prepare the closet in his room for an encounter with his delusional object, Mr. P. (a fusion figure containing certain aspects of a gratifying and nurturing nature on the one hand, and an invading and destructive nature on the other, as perceived by him in both his parents). Out of pillows and pieces of cloth he would fashion this particular Mr. P. and dress him with clothing of his own. He and Mr. P. would then make love to each other, being involved in endless dialogues which really were delusional monologues, the lovemaking accompanied by reprimands, or sadistic fantasies of punishment (Mr. P. standing for Mr. Punishment), culminating in the orgastic masturbatory act. This love affair with the delusional object—merging with self-representations and substituting for the missed love objects—consisted of fantasies which he wove around the love doll and which permitted and set into motion sexual masturbatory gratification, well protected from intrusion. Sometimes the relationship with Mr. P. was merely punitive and sadistic—the patient, Don, always being the victim—as penalty for not doing a variety of errands which the mother had told Don to carry out in her absence.

As the time approached for her to come home, he would quickly try to remove all evidence of his private world and his intimate activities, and would become the stereotyped automaton who maintained a task-oriented facade in relation to the little things that he still could do in spite of his restricted and paralyzed life.

No doubt, there was reality testing in his actions, and many of the activities actually could be seen as bizarre replicas of actual relationships; but all of them actually led him away from outer reality towards his inner reality which he pursued with skill, with imagination, and with many hallmarks borrowed from our world: preparation, thinking out activities, testing dangers, protecting himself, and so forth. This activity, of course, can be understood better as psychotic play but might serve as the prototype illustration characterizing the nature of his psychic apparatus, against which we may then measure the change in the psychotic actions, the progress he is making as he pursues reality by coping with the reality of the pursuit of the psychotherapeutic task.

A few years later, he had succeeded in completing a high school program at approximately the same age as other youngsters; and after a futile attempt at college, he tried a variety of jobs, moved out of the parental home into a supervised boarding home, and started to supplement the help he received from home with part-time employment which required that he solicit newspaper subscriptions by telephone, a distant method of establishing some contact with people. He often spoke about his wish to use some of his earnings in order to visit his childhood home town, a western gambling center, where he hoped to contact old friends and families known to his own family. He spoke of that visit in nostalgic terms and thought of it not only as a place of fun but also as an opportunity to explore his own past, to find out more about himself and his parents so that he would understand himself better. He stressed that he would be careful to take just a limited amount of money along, to gamble just a little bit and for simple fun, and how he would make sure to stay within the limits of his well thought-out plan.

When I returned from the summer vacation, I learned that he had suddenly decided to use that first week, when our psychoanalytic therapy was to start again, to have the little vacation he had talked about. What follows now seems to have come from the theater of the absurd —a variety of weird episodes acted upon and arranged in several installments, characteristic of the kind of delayed transference reactions which patients of this kind act out and play out in order to illustrate through their action what the therapist's absence had meant to them, what the transference object is made into during long absences and interruption of treatment, and what the vicissitudes of the part-introjects would be as the treatment is resumed and again permits a struggle toward the recapture of reality and the kind of object constancy available to such patients.

As Don arrives in the western town, the old friends he contacts cannot put him up instantly, as he had hoped, and he must settle, like any stranger, in one of the small motels of the town. He meets a young man who poses as a war veteran and a cousin of "Nick the Greek," and he encourages Don to venture out with him on a gambling spree. At first they win, and Don seems to be assured of the fortune that was so often his dream when he did not want to rely on his own strength and work capacity but hoped that luck would be his lady tonight. He participates actively in all the necessary schemes, which then lead him back to Los Angeles to get money from his savings. He writes and signs the required papers, prepares the "proof" of some real estate undertaking for the bank, and literally disappears from sight. His friends in the gambling town cannot contact him, communication with the parental home and the clinic is broken off, and for a few days there is no trace of him. It is later discovered that he fell victim to a fraudulent scheme by an impostor and artful crook and that he had lost a few thousand dollars—an enormous amount in relation to the small earnings he had been collecting.

As he is finally found by his folks and returns to the therapeutic work, he at first believes that the trip to the old home town should be considered glorious proof that he had freed himself from his parents, that he could undertake what he wanted; and he underplays and underrates the destructive aspects of this episode—this resurrection, as it were, of the powerful Mr. Punishment of old to whom he surrendered in his helpless search for gratification that had started out as pursuit of independence—an action kept secret from the parents and prepared with much cunning. Only slowly does he become aware of how he had been the victim of an episode with much transference meaning in which he had acted out his thoughts and fears about, and his longing for, the therapist during his long absence, and his wishes to restore the object, to be involved with him in an act of faith and complete surrender. This episode also served to act out the feeling that the search for the father must inevitably end in disaster, must destroy all his means and self-esteem; and thus he was hinting that during the period of separation, he again had proof that trust in the therapist would end only in disappointment. Thus he was overwhelmed and destroyed by the untrustworthy stranger who never had any intention of helping him. And we find that the acting out of this bizarre transference fantasy ends up as a quasi-homosexual gambit in which he plays out the psychotic version of the oedipal conflict, and in which he paints the inevitable disaster that must befall him should he place trust in the male/father/therapist whom, at the same time, he desperately seeks and by whom he must inevitably be deceived, humiliated and destroyed.

All this insight comes only after the act, and we see once more that that psychotic action, like all acting out, is a kind of trial reflection— a substitute for thinking. Now that all of it is done, he reflects upon it, and ends up with the promise that the new insight will keep him from further mistakes of that kind. Again he pledges himself to the reality tasks of everyday life. Will that new pledge lead to fulfillment, or will it be but a primary promise to restore some temporary self-constancy?

From now on he will be very careful; indeed, he will check ahead of time before entering such a venture. And he finds himself on the Sunset Strip—the reward he feels he deserves after a day's work (at this moment he is employed eight hours a day in a sheltered workshop situation). There he meets a long-haired young hippie who introduces himself to Don as the real, live, and resurrected Brian Jones—mourned and idolized as the member of the Rolling Stones who allegedly had died by drowning a few months earlier. He claims that he was so much pressured by public adulation that he had to disappear and play dead, as it were. But Don has learned his lesson; he does not want naively to believe any longer but is now going to check on reality. He has learned, he feels, from psychotherapy that one must make sure before one acts, one must think and check ahead of time, and he wants to check out the story. On the one hand, he is convinced there must be truth to it, but whenever he comes back to his hour and is confronted with the therapist's remarks, his convictions are shaken. His testing of reality means no more or less to him than that he wants to prove the truth of the fantasy elaboration conveyed to him—a borrowed fantasy which he has now accepted as his private one. He had gone so far as to lend his car to the Sunset Strip hippie, and one gathers the impression that the car may have been used for transportation of illegal deliveries, perhaps of marijuana, etc.

In the seclusion of his room, isolated both from the therapeutic situation and the young man from the Sunset Strip, Don becomes absorbed in writing a letter addressed to the resurrected Rolling Stone, in which he confesses his doubts over the latter's identity as the true Brian Jones, and in which he beseeches forgiveness for doubting his identity, assuring him that he fully trusted his veracity and that he had no hostility towards him, but that he desperately needed reassurance lest he suffer a loss of faith similar to that which attended his disastrous experience in the gambling town. He also suggested that he needed support for his delusion in order to counter his doubts, evoked by "a top psychologist," who confronts him with the real possibility that he might be victimized once more by a hoax. He requests proof of his hero's identity: Could he play the guitar for him? Would he send him tickets for the next concert of the Rolling Stones, and would he take him backstage so that he could see by the response of the other Rolling Stones that his hero was real? He wants to compare his handwriting with the one shown on the recordings of Brian Jones, etc.

He manages to leave the letter on his mother's table on one of his visits—almost as if he wanted to be sure she would discover his fantasy and would confront him with the naivete of his psychotic judgment, having been made aware of his need for a trusted and loving object who, at times regarded as dead and missing, would inevitably come alive again and provide the nurturing he needs to re-establish his own identity.

As he moves from the Sunset Strip hippie, to the mother, and from her to the "top psychologist," he is driven to test out the reality of his delusions, and finally learns from the young man that all of it had been a hoax, that the missing Rolling Stone was really dead, and he is to grant forgiveness for the fraud. At that moment, the whole episode is denied, underplayed, forgotten, and thrown aside like the experience in the gambling town. He is restored temporarily to the reality concepts of his therapist, albeit no more than a quasi-identification with the therapist's reality accompanied by the peripheral recognition of his delusional objects as unreliable, as dismissable and less worthy of his faith than that "top psychologist" therapist, who once more prevails in his mind. It becomes clear, of course, that the young man from the Rolling Stones and the top psychologist are complementary object representations, equivalents of Don's psychotic object perception.

At times, Don is capable of reality testing and critical judgment, and he discusses valid criteria in order to establish the truth or falsity of his seducer's story, but the reality test, the critical judgment, the thinking as trial act—all are under the control of the illness rather than in control of the illness. Nevertheless, there is a difference between the first and second episodes. Both have the flavor of psychotic action. The first, however, is under the dominance of regression and object loss, while the second contains certain progressive features, such as the attempt to restore judgment and reality testing, and is under the dominance of reconstitution.

In the foster boarding home administered by a university teacher (also a "top man"), whenever Don is confronted with tasks which he considers unfair, he makes a bid for return to the protection and care of his mother. Nevertheless, he maintains his status in the foster home and also remains on his job, while suddenly making the fantastic discovery that he can walk around on college grounds and ask people for money to make a telephone call, and that he can get more money through panhandling in this way than he gets by working. He uses all manner of planning so that people will believe he is really telephoning: he dials the number of the telephone station he is using, and the money is returned to him because he has, of course, received a busy signal. In part at least, he has restored the mother who gives

without demands—although whenever he tries to telephone the pre-
tended object, he gets a busy signal; he has merely reached his own
number.

With the additional funds received from panhandling, he buys
beer and he and one of the young men in the boarding home get
mildly drunk. This foster sibling, a young Ph.D. candidate in philosophy, who allegedly speaks with an Austrian accent, becomes a friend
of Don. In their mildly drunken state they embrace each other, kiss,
and possibly masturbate each other. Don feels that he is strong and
can protect himself from sexual danger. Never would he really allow
fellatio experiences and intercourse, and he stresses how this newly
found friend is as fond of Don as Don is of him, and how the friend
tries to teach him good habits such as maintaining his job, getting
up early, not drinking too much beer, and keeping self-controlled.

This new episode, containing a search for a reliable object relationship and the struggle with homosexual temptation, is closer to reality
and to more neurotic transference meaning. It involves some reality
testing, the use of better judgment, and appears to be somewhat in
the nature of preparation and anticipation of the type of action that
would be considered neurotic or normal, rather than psychotic. Nevertheless, the tinge of his acts remains psychotic and in the service of
the restoration of his delusional world, which we pictured through
the initial episode involving the play with the puppet fashioned from
pillows, with Don receiving his psychic meaning from features of an
inner world in which introjects and self-representations are unstable,
shifting, unreliable, fusing and defusing, first granting pleasure and
reprieve, then threatening violence and annihilation.

Fairy tales and dreams have in common that their actions seemingly
start on a secondary-process level. The first lines of the fairy tale—
once upon a time there was . . . —can be seen against a background
of a world which is reality-oriented; the same is often true for dreams.
As the fairy tale proceeds, magic returns and people turn into monsters,
witches, and dangerous objects; the dream, too, may turn into the
nightmare dominated by primary-process thinking, both of them trav-
eling the path of regression.

The material I have offered from Don's psychotherapy strikes one
as a kind of fairy tale or dream in reverse. It is as if primary-process
dominance slowly moves toward secondary-process dominance. One
wonders whether Don will be able to move towards an awakening that
will not be a rude one but will constitute the happy acceptance of
reality and realistic action; or whether his adjustment must remain an
ambulatory schizophrenic one, in which the true Utopia for which
he lives rests with the primary rather than the secondary process, and

in which reality testing—the thought before the act—is only an unstable, unreliable achievement, forever in danger of destruction.

Much normal action is determined by ideals which merely represent the restoration of the Utopian past, but which nevertheless stimulate the capacity for adaptation and normal action. It remains an open question whether the psychotic's Utopias will ever encourage permanent adaptations, so that the story of Buridan's ass who refused hay and water will become inapplicable to the human species.

CHAPTER TEN

Identity Formation in the Treatment of an Autistic Child*

No one who has worked with autistic children will ever forget . . . how desperately they struggle to grasp the meaning of saying, "I" and "You." How impossible it is for them, for language presupposes the experience of a coherent I. Work with deeply disturbed young people confronts the worker with the awful awareness of the patient's incapacity to feel the "I" and "You" which are cognitively present and the fear that life may run out before such feelings may be experienced—in love.

ERIK H. ERIKSON

In the recent past, the phenomenon of infantile psychosis has increasingly become the subject of clinical and research studies. Whether the organic or psychogenic point of view is emphasized, the complexities are still too great to be certain about the etiology of this personality deficit. Nevertheless, there is a growing body of clinical evidence regarding the psychogenic nature of autism with special reference to certain typical psycho-dynamic conditions in the life experience of infants who develop such severe ego disturbances. One such condition is the absence of a positive emotional nurturant relationship with a mothering person in the early months of life.

---

* Leda W. Rosow is the author of this chapter.

The effects of such deprivation are especially important during the normal autistic and symbiotic phases of infancy. Mahler places emphasis on this period: "I believe it is from the symbiotic phase of the mother-infant dual unity that these expected precursors of individual beginnings are derived which together with inborn constitutional factors determine every human individual's unique somatic and psychological makeup" (9). The normal separation-individuation experience, she states further, is the first crucial prerequisite for the development and maintenance of a sense of identity.

This clinical presentation is concerned with the treatment of Kenny, whose development took place in an environment characterized by deprivation and trauma, resulting in the inhibition of speech and avoidance of human contact which comprise the autistic syndrome. The essential purpose of this paper is to focus on and delineate the achievement of a sense of identity and integration of the ego in this autistic child during the three and a half years of long-term psychoanalytic psychotherapy. "Identity" is used in the sense that Erikson found useful: to consider the sense of self or various selves as part of but different from the functions of the ego (5).

At four and a half, Kenny was a slight child who stood passively and silently, head to one side and one shoulder slightly raised. His head was bent so low that it was not possible at first to see his delicate, sad features. Kenny's symptoms included limited, primitive "scribble" speech alternating with mispronounced words; seeming inability to understand what was said to him; inability to make contact with other children or adults; and withdrawal from all activities except as a passive "victim" in sadomasochistic interaction with his brother, who was also extremely disturbed. On psychological testing in which he expressed no spontaneity at all nor interaction with the tester, who later became his therapist, his speech score was approximately below the age of two. However, on the form-board test he achieved scores approaching age level, characteristic of psychotic children whose behavior combines primitive arrested reactions with fleeting, more age-appropriate performances. His score fell in the retarded range of intelligence, but the scatter of his performance gave the impression that he had a potential for at least low normal functioning. The symptom pattern inevitably raised questions regarding the possibility of an anlage of brain damage or traumatic psychosis as important factors in Kenny's ego development. The diagnosis was that of infantile autism.

Kenny was born into a gravely troubled family that was incapacitated by severe emotional difficulties. The family consisted of the mother, father and the brother, Stuart, two years older, who had been in treatment for about two years when Kenny was brought to the

Clinic. Stuart's treatment had begun when he was three years, four months, because of symptoms including autistic-like withdrawal alternating with fits of maniacal rage, and long periods of uninterrupted screaming. His speech consisted of grunting, growling noises, and his parents were not certain whether he understood what was said to him. His diagnosis was "atypical childhood psychosis." His father had punished him by beatings and forcible ejection from the house. The parents, in their own childhood, had experienced beatings, seductiveness, forcible enemas and cleaning of the genitals in the service of "good hygiene." The mother suffered beatings from her husband and criticisms from her own mother as being unworthy to have attractive children. She thus lived in the center of a whirlwind of emotional and physical violence, and became literally paralyzed in her attempt to be an adequate mother. On the day of Kenny's birth, she was warned that another screaming baby would not be tolerated. Throughout the years of treatment it was not possible to recover precise details of Kenny's early days. All the parents remembered was that at birth he was a quiet baby and had a gentle cry. He did not sit up until ten months old, provoking the father's concern about his slow development which, however, was judged to be normal by the pediatrician.

Throughout his first year, Kenny was left very much to himself, the family being preoccupied with Stuart's problems. Kenny's crib became a sounding board for the screaming and primitive rages of his brother. When the parents realized that Stuart would poke his fingers into Kenny's eyes, ears and mouth as well as attack his body, they locked him out of the nursery, leaving him standing outside screaming endlessly. Kenny was left alone "to cry it out." The children's screams upset the father to such a degree that at seven months of age Kenny was beaten about the face.

In a psychic environment of constant screaming terror, physical assault and non-availability of a nurturant person, trauma was added to isolation. This phase in Kenny's life corresponds generally to the normal child's emergence from the symbiotic phase as described by Mahler. Although the mother could describe Kenny with empathy, in actual fact she was not able to show such feeling overtly. She was a rigid, deep-feeling, seemingly emotionless woman who worked incredibly hard, seemed to give endlessly of herself but in essence could not express warmth.

During his second and third years, Kenny was left with a succession of baby-sitters who were reported to have either neglected or mistreated him. Kenny developed autistic defenses to cope with these unbearable tensions. He remained on the periphery of the family milieu except when he permitted himself to be a passive victim for the hostility of others. When he came into treatment he was toilet trained, could partly dress and feed himself, and managed to remain in a small nursery school mainly by not participating in any of the activities.

STRUGGLE TO SURVIVE

Several months after the diagnostic evaluation, Kenny and the therapist started out on an odyssey into his inner life which, in effect, turned out to be a search for his identity. It was soon apparent that he was not a child whose extreme mechanical withdrawal is associated with failure to perceive emotionally, i.e., cathect the mother from birth. The initial treatment hours revealed autistic as well as symbiotic characteristics. These are highlighted in the following excerpts from the first therapy hours.

First hour: Kenny came quickly into the room, ran around touching everything quickly. He jumped from the desk, the chairs, the play table over and over paying no attention to me. He tried to pull things from the wall, broke crayons and threw everything out of the boxes, etc., until it was time to go. At times he perched himself in a very precarious position so that I had to follow him around to protect him. I stayed with him, told him I did not want to see him hurt. If I offered him anything to play with, he promptly threw it up at the electric fixture. At no time did he behave as if he had ever seen me before.

Fourth hour: Kenny appeared on a warm day wearing a very heavy jacket. He would not allow me to unzip it and he would not take it off himself, although he appeared hot. (This jacket, which he wore to every session, unfailingly, was not removed for another year and a half.) After frantically playing out a scene with dolls in which the boy doll was injured, Kenny quickly left the table, turned away completely and walked to a corner where he found a toy milk bottle which he filled full of marbles and began sucking on it. It was as if symbolically he had indicated that he got rocks instead of milk. He found a toy toilet and immediately left the room saying, "Bapoo," his word for bathroom.

Twelfth hour: Kenny was more relaxed today. He stayed very close to me almost as if he would melt into my body if he could. He grabbed my hand and then my fingers, pushing them in a hurtful way toward my arm. He jumped down from the table over and over. Once he got tired of that he found a piece of a plane which he had broken previously when he had thrown clay on it. He glanced at it and began to pound himself over the head. He found a toy train which he had broken and once more said, "Bapoo." It appeared that this word had a dual meaning: bathroom and broken.

These first hours revealed the range of ego states available to Kenny. They revealed the silent, hyperactive, non-speaking child who does not seem to perceive or relate to the therapist as if "inherently autistic." The fact that "bathroom" and "broken" were associated in his own language, revealed a very crucial fact about him: he felt broken or damaged and wanted to be fed like an infant. Although it seemed that he could function on higher levels of psychic organization, as suggested by the "instant play" with the dolls, it soon became clear that such levels were only fleetingly available to him. Although he wanted contact he could not bear to have it, and although he wished to be completely defended in his autistic state, he could not maintain it. He was thus in a chronic state of tension, and panic states erupted almost constantly. Ritualistic play with water, the toilet and mechanical toys and objects, as well as complete withdrawal, seemed to serve as defenses against his impulses, ineffectually controlled by fluctuating ego states.

An important factor in the early weeks of treatment concerned his reactions to his brother who was in treatment at the same time. One day as he permitted himself to come near the therapist, he heard his brother yell in the hall and immediately scratched the therapist's arm. It was as if he had momentarily fused with the aggressive screaming brother. He threw my phone on the floor. When I gave him a toy phone, he made a sound into it and threw it away. He made garbled sounds of all kinds, to which I responded by repeating some of them. I hoped to let him know in this way that he was not alone in his terror and that we could build an empathic bridge. His voice became louder and he tried out various sounds and even what seemed like snatches of song. He was using sound to contact the therapist rather than words. As I repeated everything he did, he became more excited. He lay down on the floor, seemed to withdraw into rapt isolation and began to make infantile sounds. I said "Now Kenny is a little baby," and handed him a toy milk bottle. He began to suck on it and I noticed his lips moved soundlessly as if he were saying "La, la, la" (his word for milk, I learned later). From then on each successive sound became more and more infantile until he was gurgling. It is possible that the soundless lalling may have indicated that precursors of speech had progressed this far in his first weeks of life. He seemed to be far away, not hearing anything I said, when suddenly, with a fierce expression on his face, he got up, grabbed hold of my arm in a vehement gesture and ran out. This significant treatment event revealed that he seemed to respond to whatever cue was given him and to take off from there as if he himself had no inner direction, and was not a separate being. The danger of becoming separate was constantly expressed in impulsive erratic behavior, as well as in reaction to the danger of relating to the therapist. He seemed to borrow the identity of anything or anybody within his vicinity which led to changes in the direction of what preoccupied him.

Kenny was constantly filling himself full of water and going into the bathroom. His apparently senseless activity in the bathroom gradually revealed the meaning of his struggle. I am reminded here of a wonderful title given to a paper by Alice Balint, "On Being Empty of One's Self." Indeed as Kenny drank and immediately seemed to empty himself, one wondered what remained with him. The struggle of the "self vs. the non-self" as Bettelheim (2) puts it, was constantly expressed in this kind of activity. It was on the lowest level of body function, that of taking in liquid and emptying oneself in the bathroom, where his awareness of himself was most dominant at that time. The minute the water would gush down, Kenny would be in terror as if he felt he would go down also. It was only at moments of such total fear of annihilation that he could tolerate the therapist's nearness.

The first year of treatment was characterized by Kenny's constant struggle to dare to exist. Every hour was filled with restitutive maneuvers to ward off a chronic anticipation of fragmentation. He moved around in the treatment hours constantly watching for the possible unleashing of destructive forces around him. He always seemed to be looking for external reassurances that if objects were in good working order, so would he be. One day, on his way back from the bathroom, he noticed that a cooler fan was not connected. He immediately muttered "Bapoo." I connected the fan and showed him it was not broken. He turned away from me and looked up at the picture on the wall. When we had first walked down the hall, I had shown him these pictures. He was now using this remembered experience to contact the therapist as if to indicate his relief. But having come so close to the therapist, he became anxious and so another form of defensive repetitive play was introduced. This was a game of "knock-knock" (so named by me). It entailed pushing the therapist out into the hall and then permitting her to come in. Later, he would go out and return. His object relationships seemed to be characteristic of the first level of separation of the infant from the mother, at an emerging minimal level of self-awareness.

Later, as he further identified himself with a cooler operated by a fan and water-filled system, he revealed that inanimate as well as animate objects were fused in his own inner experience. One day when he was unusually tense he ran through the Clinic searching for his mother. When he could not find her he drank enormous quantities of cold water and blew at the therapist like the fan. Having lost his mother, he substituted transitional objects, fountain and fan; with these he reconstituted himself to avoid the agony of feeling fragmented. This play, continuing for hours on end, emphasized the need of his primitive ego to be concerned only with defense. He was both frightened and fascinated by the fan, and became very excited when he learned that he could make it go and stop. I played a game with him saying, "Go," and then connected the fan. I would say "Stop," when we disconnected it. This became a ritual. However, one day when *his* saying, "Go," coincided with the actual rotation of the fan, he ran up and down the hall in terror as if he fantasied that his word, i.e., his impulse, had unleashed destructive forces. I had another clue regarding his inhibitions against talking. Kenny maintained his autistic defense by fusing with mechanical objects in his world, since this permitted him to remain silent and to keep his impulses unexpressed but, nevertheless, alive. By introjecting the power of mechanical objects, Kenny was able to cope with his sense of helplessness by using a kind of mechanical auxiliary ego.

In relationship with his brother, however, these defenses did not hold. Then he was forced to express affect through cue-taking from his brother. This was revealed one day when Stuart, in a bad mood, yelled at me, "Shut up," as soon as he saw me with Kenny. This strongly agitated Kenny. With great rapidity he hit me, broke crayons, wrote on the wall and rattled the water cooler. It was as if he had actually become his brother, fused with him and hated me through him. When he ran to the fan and tried to push his fingers between the rotating blades, I stopped him, and he hit me again. I could not understand the intensity of his rage, but I soon found out that previous to this hour, Stuart had told Kenny that I was going to leave him. It seemed that although other people could not get through to Kenny, Stuart always could.

Self-destructive behavior persisted throughout the treatment in the beginning years whenever he felt enraged or "bad." When I managed to convey to Kenny that I knew how he felt, that it was not true I was leaving him, once more he sent me away to play the game "knock-knock." He suddenly ran off to the bathroom and then came back. For the first time he had used the toilet and invited me in to show me his "anal gift" which he called "doo." It was as if he indicated that he wished to keep the therapist from going away by getting rid of his bad self (12). However, having dared to give up part of himself, he became frightened once more. He ran from one fan to another to make sure they weren't disconnected. Through this expression of his need for the therapist, it became apparent that Kenny had made an important step in the process of his own self-awareness.

In approximately the third month of treatment I realized Kenny warded off contact by becoming completely mute and ignoring me whenever I used the first or second personal pronouns regarding myself or him. I habitually began to refer to both of us in the third person. This defense made it possible for him to feel safe in an intensive pursuit of a symbiotic relationship with his mother, which was also brought into the treatment relationship. For his fifth birthday, I gave Kenny a toy car and a birthday card. He immediately left for the lobby to show this to his mother. When she did not look up, he stood there and showed her the card again. She glanced at it briefly and went back to her reading. His passive appeal was ignored and he came shuffling back slowly. He regressed and became silent, very restless and destructive, and he was not to be reached at all for the rest of the hour. He did not touch the gift I gave him, as if now both it and he were worthless. During this incident his behavior was reminiscent of Mahler's (10) description of the shadowing of the mother in the separation-individuation phase, i.e., a desperate appeal to and wooing of the mother which he carried on persistently at home in his wild and provocative behavior. He flushed the toilet endlessly in such fury that it seemed he would break it. He did break the radio in the car, the symbol of his hopeless attempt to reach his mother. He was severely punished and felt overwhelmed by the enormity of what he had done. His increased use of "broken" revealed that he felt not only that he was destructive, but also that his mother's anger annihilated him.

Shortly after, a favorite family cat was accidentally killed. This threw Kenny into unrestrained panic. He turned on all the electric lights and once more drank water so frantically he could barely swallow. During this time his mother reported that while in a store, Kenny noted that a band-aid display usually in motion was not working. He screamed uncontrollably until this display was turned on once more. Thus, following the death of the family cat who had become his central, libidinal object, Kenny created the role of a "band-aid" mother who would not let him get killed. He felt magically restored and a new phrase appeared in his vocabulary. He brought a little box from home and asked me to "fikit" (fix it). He would repeat the word followed by my name, saying "fikit-fafow," over and over. He felt clearly that the therapist now had become his auxiliary ego and he fantasied her as having a purpose in his life as a need-gratifying object and as the "fixer" who would repair the broken boy.

However, the fragile state of his tenuous identity was clearly high lighted in the following incident around the time of the cat's death.

At Halloween time, Kenny "to be like other kids," was dresse up to go "trick and treating." He came to this interview hou after a school party dressed in a clown costume, with makeup on his face. His normally pale countenance was now chalk white. H was completely disoriented, with a vague lost expression, as if h literally no longer knew who he was but was "moving in a tranc of agonized anonymity . . . As if he became almost impersona as if the escape from selfhood was complete" (14). Kenny's in voluntary "escape from selfhood" was his reaction to the fact tha the cat had died and he felt his fragmentation to be imminent An effort was made to include him in the production of a littl clay cat, hoping this would induce him to express how he felt, bu there was no response. He really was completely lost within him self. I then started to talk to him about Halloween. I told hin that the clown suit did not belong to him and that when h would go home he would take it off and would be Kenny again There was a burst of incomprehensible sounds. Although I mad some empathic response to him, Kenny withdrew completely. Thi time he revealed that understanding of his affects by the therapis was not enough. When the hour was over, he went as he ha come, shuffling his feet, walking slowly down the hall, one shoul der higher than the other, his tall hat askew on his head, a ver sad, grotesque little figure in a clown suit.

Fused identification with the dead cat as the victim and the de stroyer made him extremely vulnerable at this time to triggering-of stimuli. One day when Kenny heard Stuart screaming outside th treatment office, he immediately resonated with his brother's terror a well as his own. He ran up and down the hall destroying everythin in sight and then retreated to the usual water and bathroom pla His identification with his brother's wildness and rage soon reveale that the most acute sense of self concerned being bad and guilty. Th word "bapoo" was now replaced by "boy, do da," a repetitive declara tion of omnipotent and omnipresent destructiveness. One day Kenn saw an accident on the freeway where two trucks had collided. H came into the Clinic and with a burst of speech exclaimed, "Mot twuck go boom, boy do da?" The mother also was quite frightened b the accident and Kenny shared this emotion with her. As she stoo by listening to him, she wondered why he was always saying that. explained that Kenny felt that in some way he had caused the acc dent. She expressed her regrets that she had not understood, since sh had felt this way when she was little. She said sympathetically, " wanted so much to help him." Kenny heard his mother and now entered another progressive step in his development. It was no wonder that for Kenny merely to exist had been so dangerous. It had been impossible for him to identify clearly whose rage he feared, having been unable to distinguish between his own destructiveness and that of the external environment.

Now, people in his life could be presented in their different roles and he gradually began to show me the frightening as well as the supportive aspects of his home life. He used the clay dog and cat that I made for him and had them fight. He fed the cat giving it more and more water and tested the temperature of the water with his finger, identifying with the function of a mother who was taking care of her sick child. He thus signified that he had deepened the symbiotic relationship with the therapist. She evoked his panic when he felt punished as the aggressor, but also she restored his identity in the role he assigned to her as the fixer and maker of things who could restore the dog's tail, or make a cardboard gun on Kenny's demand. He yelled excitedly, "Ya fafoo," (therapist's name) as if she had at this instant become magic. As the magical protecting object via the things she made him, she clearly was being incorporated. Signs that he could accept delay and anticipate the future appeared when he was able to wait for a promised ride. In the past, it was reported by his mother that Kenny would have "screamed and been in a crazy panic all day."

APPEARANCE OF A TRANSITIONAL IDENTITY

Having restored the need-satisfying symbiotic object, the therapist, Kenny now seemed literally to integrate into a new identity "under the eyes of the therapist" (1). I had given Kenny a toy wagon for Christmas, his father helped him assemble it, and Kenny felt accepted. He brought the toy to the Clinic and wanted to play with it, tried very hard to do it himself, and finally succeeded. I exclaimed, "Why Kenny, you fixed it," to which he replied, "No Cluddy!" It gradually became apparent that Kenny had taken on a seemingly transitional identity (8), who could do and feel things that Kenny was afraid of or could not do. As Cluddy, he started a new kind of building play with blocks. High walls were built with nothing between them, the symbolic representation of his perception that his ego boundaries or the shell of his self was being restored and constructed. This step in psychic integration has been described by Mahler: "As the child begins to retrieve the symbiotic object and cathect its representation with libido, we observe more ego filled moods and emotions. These manifestations mark the first state of giving up and replacing autistic defenses. They also mark the ego emergence as a functional structure of the personality" (9).

The fluid shifting of ego states and ego functions continued for many more months of treatment. During the tenth month, the effect of heightened annihilation anxiety on perceptual distortions was graphically revealed after Kenny had been harshly punished for his increasingly provocative behavior at home. In this hour he was unusually pale, with deep circles under his eyes. Once more he seemingly found that all the things were broken. He sat listlessly, looking at pictures of railroads and engines. He pointed to a blue fence (which he had seen before) calling it water. It was as if he had regressed once more to an undifferentiated state. Gradually he began, as if reintegrating, to recognize the inanimate figures and objects in the book. However when he came to the picture of a movable, open guard rail on the railroad track, he became very tense and cried out, "Bapoo" (broken). He kept turning to the next page where the closed guard rail was shown. He did this over and over to reassure himself that it was not really broken. He kept putting my finger on the broken part as if this would restore it (himself). He insisted that my finger remain there. This seemed to reduce his anxiety. I tried to help him talk about the beating that he had received. There was no response. To the question, "Did you cry?" Kenny answered, "Cluddy cwy." Neither tears nor affect were permitted to Kenny, but for Cluddy, his blossoming identity and "stand-in," hopefully they could be risked without absolute threat of annihilation. Once more he returned to the open guard rail and since he realized that putting my finger there did not actually restore it, nor had it prevented him from being beaten, he tried another tack. He had me put a band-aid on his heel, which was not sore at all. In his magical, delusional thinking this restored both him and me—as a "fikit" object—and he went out, limping, with satisfaction.

Kenny had now begun to learn to swim. When I talked about it to him, he said "Cluddy afwaid." It was as if he now began to be aware of his own feelings, but was able to let me know only by projecting them onto his alter-self, instead of the machines that formerly had been his vehicle for such communications. Now we had another sign that his psychic organization had integrated to a somewhat higher level. One dramatic day it became obvious he was approaching an acceptance of Cluddy as himself. He noticed that there was some scribbling on a checker board that we had played with in the past and he called out, "Keeky do da, Cluddy do da?" Cluddy served as that part of himself that tentatively tried to reach out to the world and dare to face reality. Ego mastery was also attributed to Cluddy in "art" products made at school. Panic states no longer appeared as frequently, since, through Cluddy, he was able to express his feelings.

Therese Gouin-Decarie (7), writing on the relevancy of Piaget's theories for clinical child psychology, emphasized that the "maternally deprived child is also inevitably a sensory-motor deprived individual . . . although physically intact, the play of assimilation and accommodation will remain defective." Kenny's behavior certainly bore this out. His defenses served mainly to protect the ego from being overwhelmed, at the cost of depriving the ego of its cathexis for various functions. In the service of his autistic defense system, Kenny had successfully blocked or retarded the functions of affect and perception. With the unfolding of his self-awareness, energies were released for exploration of his world.

In one of the interview hours he became aware of and responded to different metallic sounds. This became an act of discovery that was infused with pleasure and was followed by actively sought sensory and perceptual experiences. "It was as if the frozen deanimated wall" (1) was removed. Explorations of inner and outer aspects of the Clinic building and of my car occupied him almost exclusively. One day when he was given a candy life saver, he looked at the hole and said very slowly, "Do-nut." In the past he had put a candy in his mouth without looking at it and would more often than not refuse to take it. He was now making associations and links between his perceptual experiences and motoric executive implementations. There was a noticeable decrease in his hyperactive, aimless behavior and his activities became more focused.

Although he was now almost six, his responses in some areas were reminiscent of an infant's. The concrete nature of his thinking appeared when he began to distinguish colors, as when he was busily turning the gears of a plastic toy. I helped him associate the names of the colors with the different gears, but he could only name the colors by calling, "White, paper; green, bathroom." He seemed unable to maintain an abstract concept of color without associating it to some firm facet of his experience. Kenny continued to present himself as helpless and needing care, as being unable to function except in the presence of an auxiliary ego, thus slowing down the process of separation from the symbiotic object. One day he asked me to sing. When he was invited to sing also, he said "No, Cluddy sing," and began to clean the dollhouse and arrange things neatly, involving me in this activity. In this behavior Kenny revealed that speech was still dangerous; it was associated with being a messy child who deserved punishment. What he seemed to say symbolically was, "If I am put in order, perhaps I can sing-talk." Kenny informed me through symbolic action rather than speech that he felt disarranged.

The central meaning of this little vignette, however, was that he seemed to be inviting the "good mother," as in a happy primary relationship, to be part of the experiencing duo. He suddenly got up from the play table and began to go through a learned set of gestures he had been taught in school. As I sang to him I watched his rigid movements, so like the dance of a marionette pulled by strings. Nevertheless, for the first time, his face was alive, his eyes shining with an intense expression of concentration while he performed his awkward little dance.

STRUGGLE TO SPEAK

Although Kenny began to use speech more freely, he still maintained his rigid defensiveness. He was now able to express rage through screaming, especially towards his brother. This release of aggression was usually followed by a further integration of ego functions. One day at the start of an hour, in the second year of therapy, he sat quietly, racing cars very vigorously.

I greeted him saying, "How are you, Kenny?" He replied, "Am fine!" I expressed my delight to which he quickly responded, "No, Cluddy talk." (I had been too intrusive and had not respected his defenses.) I asked, "Can't Kenny talk?" He said, "Fafoo afwaid." Suddenly a siren sounded outside and he sped to the window as if he were propelled, perhaps fearing punishment. On the way back he picked up a doll turned it around, looked at its face, put his hand on its mouth and screamed, "Shut ut." I interpreted his fear of getting hurt when he screamed, as if someone is going to come to hurt him, whereupon Kenny let out a sharp scream with a piercing panicky sound to it. He kept screaming for the longest time, yelling "Shut ut, shut ut." His face became infused with blood, the veins in his neck stood out, the sound of his voice became increasingly guttural. He stopped suddenly, completely worn out. I remarked, "Now I see why you are so afraid to talk. You're afraid that whenever you make a sound, someone will hurt you and now you're screaming and screaming to let me know." Kenny immediately ran to fill himself full of water. Before he left, he took the baby bottle with him but indicated that I was not to come.

The intrusive therapist had become dangerous by interpreting instead of offering herself as a symbiotic partner. However, through a conciliatory gesture, Kenny offered me the Fixit book to read. As I told him the story via the pictures, Kenny acted it out as if once more he could use his thought processes to tell me his inner meaning. He acted out the crying of the child in the story in such a realistic way that I could hear how Kenny must have sounded after crying for a long time. He made sounds of sobbing which became fainter and fainter with an increasing tone of abandonment appearing in his voice. He acted out his loneliness by projecting it onto the picture child. When he came to the picture of a boy who was watching a slashed tire being fixed he said, "Boy goof?" (Am I guilty?) At the end of the story he held the book for a moment. He sighed, stopped abruptly as if his breath were suddenly cut short, and then let out the remainder of a long deep sigh. His act had made his inner feelings visible. He seemed to be communicating a memory that had suddenly arisen to the surface (3).

This dramatic event revealed the disorganizing effect of trauma on his developing function of speech. The cry, the infant's first means of influencing the environment, had become negatively cathected so that to be vocal was to invite disaster and become helpless. During this hour the eruption of painful experiences associated with his crying in infancy was graphically play-acted. Concurrently he was also being punished at home for being so noisy, and probably it was Kenny's way of communicating something about his present experiences as well. Up to this time, Kenny could organize his experiences only with act, gesture and pantomime, but now vocalization was added.

With each discovery in the outside world, further separation of self indicated that he was beginning to feel unified. He would pull me out to the parking lot to show me the place of absent cars by saying, "One, one, one." When he was helped to grasp the concept that more than one, that many absent cars and people would come back, he eagerly began to count his fingers and toes and mine as well. It was quite moving to watch him make "his discoveries." For the first time since therapy began one and a half years before, Kenny took off his heavy jacket.

He now actively expressed the wish to be made whole. Whereas formerly the fountain and fan served as vehicles to express his need for survival, now he used the talking machine, the ediphone, to express his feelings about wishing to talk. At the beginning of a new kindergarten semester, he brought a photo of himself with this mouth open as if to speak. He denied this and said, "Boton"—a new version of "broken." He turned to me asked, "Me, you fix?" But with the heaviness of basic distrust still weighing him down, he turned from me to the machine and said "Do da,"—turn it on. He was encouraged to talk into it and tell about the picture which he called "teeto." The therapist verbalized his feelings and he listened as the conversation was played back. He responded to the machine as if it had become the therapist in reality and reacted with great excitement as he recognized our voices. He picked up his picture put it in front of the machine and said, "You see teeto, you see teeto."

The animate and the inanimate, the therapist and machine, were still fused by him and he endowed human as well as mechanical attributes to both. It was clear that Kenny was very much excited about deliberately wanting to talk. It also became clear to him that he could not voluntarily make the sounds that he wanted to. When he did try to talk, each word had to be forced out and the muscles on one side of his face would draw back in a tic-like facial movement. His voice tended to be a little flat, each word was separated by an effortful pause before the next one appeared.

One day he came in very angry and said, "You no fen me"—you are not my friend—"no fix words." It was characteristic of him that he would suddenly say or do something that seemed to reflect the existence of a more complex psychic structure than his behavior indicated. At school he had become aggressive and troublesome, and the teacher was beginning to ask questions about the level of his intelligence. He knew about this and started the hour by picking up a gun and shooting at me. He ran out of the room and started shooting into the hall. At that moment a woman walked down the hall and he said in fear, "Na shoo lady." I interpreted his anger toward me for not fixing his words. I told him that I knew he was angry and shooting his gun because he couldn't say his words. Kenny became angrier. Suddenly he stopped shooting, put the gun down and began slowly to prowl around the room, gradually becoming more and more active and excited. He picked up all the books and papers from my desk, looked underneath and went to the cupboard, picked up everything in his search for some unknown thing. When I asked him what he was looking for he said, "Look for word!" I told him that he had not shot his words out with a gun, they were still inside of him and that he would find a way to say them. His wish to speak led to added awareness of his own experiences and his responsiveness to them (13).

A very important aspect of his burgeoning ego was revealed in his growing body awareness. He had been subjected to abusive sexual play, but this had not been brought into treatment. However, he had had an accident at school one day and in his inimitable style, with a great deal of encouragement, was able to say: "Faw dow, hut head, fleet bed. Cold ladel." (Fall down, hurt head, sleep in bed. Cold water.) He pointed to his head where he had been hurt. The next hour revealed that another source of body concern had to do with sexual differences. In all the time he had been coming to the Clinic he had seemed to ignore totally or avoid the girls' bathroom. Now he pulled me into it and indicated that he was afraid to go in. He pulled back into the treatment-room and play-acted a "seduction" scene by inviting me to stroke his genitals. He had experienced this with someone else and it was with a strong sense of excitement that he tried to communicate it. Kenny was busily sorting out all the dangers in his life but this time the emphasis was on body functioning. One day just as he was about to say something he passed flatus which he called "poo sou." He did not seem to be frightened by this so I remarked that he could make noises with his behind and that his mouth could make sounds too. His response to this was "No nay noit." (My mouth doesn't make noise.) He told me that he made poo sounds but that was all. It was obviously still too dangerous for him to make any sounds vocally. In fact, he had behaved in the past as if all his body emissions were bad. However, the fact that he could make anal noises pleased him very much. I laughed. He immediately took the cue, looked delighted and, for the first time, Kenny and therapist laughed together.

He could now come to the Clinic with greater ease. One day he tore off his shirt in a great hurry. When he tried to put it back on he kept forcing his elbow into the sleeve. I offered to help him, but at first he wouldn't let me. Suddenly he looked directly at my face and asked, "Anri?" I said, "No I'm just trying to help you put on your shirt." At this Kenny looked at me directly and said, "Oh." He had become aware that non-verbal cues from the human face could now be visually engaged without fear.

At this time the school counselor called to report that although Kenny had completed his second year in kindergarten, he did not seem to know what was going on and that he had become more aggressive, less inhibited and less fearful of the children. The counselor raised the question of mental retardation. He suggested that Kenny would do much better in a school for mentally retarded children. However, the counselor accepted the explanation that Kenny's behavior was a kind of defensive pseudo-stupidity and he was permitted to enter a special class in the same school. Because of the co-operation of the school counselor, Kenny was able to continue in an encouraging educational environment (4). Learning inhibition at school reflected that he did not feel as yet that he could function as a separate self. Although autism as a defense was not so rigidly maintained, inactivity was another expression of it. To function alone was to destroy the possibility of return to symbiosis. This was vividly apparent when he was encouraged to fashion a clay animal. He insisted that he couldn't do it. To help him start the process I put my hand on top of his. As this happened, his hand seemed literally to fuse with mine as if he could function only in this way. Gradually his own muscles took over and he uttered a cry of satisfaction at his success. He felt as if he were now infused with power.

In spite of the primitive nature of his functioning he recognized that he was a failure at school and in desperation searched for another identity. One day he announced, "No call me Cluddy, no call me Kenny, call me Hal." This particular borrowed identity belonged to a real boy, his brother's friend. This was soon given up, since the magic was not sustained, but it was obvious that Kenny was separating his essential self from his part identifications. He would still savor his brother's triumph as if it were his own and still use him as an auxiliary ego to express his own anger. As the process of identification continued he internalized the brother's strength and power through the experience of the brother's absence. The brother was no longer coming to the Clinic when Kenny was. One day the confusion about who he was appeared when he played the "knock-knock" game and after opening the door said, "Tuie?" (Am I Stuart?) I reassured him that he was Kenny, not Stuart who was away at school. Concomitantly his building structures began to have better planning and coherence and very slowly the synthetic functions of the ego began to integrate.

Towards the end of the second year of treatment the interview hours became full of material about a new baby accompanied by self punitive activity. When Kenny voiced his apprehension, the mother denied that she was pregnant. She said that she was concerned about the fact that he sat about at home undressed all day. In the past he was the one "who always was independent." It was Kenny's way of telling his mother that he wished to be the baby, to be cared for. In spite of the mother's denials, Kenny's fantasies about the baby proved to be true. Anticipation of the new infant was very upsetting to everyone in the family. Outbursts of mutual hatred heightened the two boys' aggressive behavior. They reacted as if the baby were already there and chose each other as the objects of their jealousy. In imitation of his brother, Kenny acted out what seemed to be negative transference reactions in the treatment. When he became aware that he was being led to express hate directly to me, he became very frightened. However he also seemed to be aware that I was not the true object of his rage and he yelled, "Throw a baby dead, throw a mommy dead."

The mother reported that he was having "morning sickness" like herself and would go to the bathroom many times to try to throw up. Worries about her own condition were projected on to her disappointment in Kenny's improvement. For the first time she expressed dismay about the slow appearance of understandable speech. There now began a round of visits to doctors and dentists. At this point, contrary to the therapist's advice, Kenny was enrolled in a speech class. Once more, autistic defenses were fully evident so that at times it seemed that he literally could not hear, although hearing tests revealed no deafness. The speech tests were inconclusive and recommended that psychotherapy continue so that Kenny's "confidence would improve."

The birth of a baby sister triggered off intensive anxiety. Regressive play in the bathroom returned and once more ego boundaries seemed threatened. Kenny sat in the bathroom with the door opened which was unusual, as if oblivious to everything except the imminence of his own destruction. He held on to his penis looking forlorn and fragmented. He said pathetically, "My penie?" I named each body part and reassured him of his continuing ownership of all of these, including his penis. I tried to talk to him about the differences between himself and the new baby sister. He sat without a sign of response until I said, "When Mommy comes home she will want you to have your penis." At this his expression changed and once more he reintegrated. Again he was concerned with his badness and he asked me whether his loud or soft noises would be acceptable.

It was difficult to contact him at this time and he gradually subsided into silence, at times appearing robot-like. However, because of the strength of the therapeutic bond, he could reconstitute more quickly following the emergence of archaic rage. He felt that his own badness and loudness had triggered off the heightened anxieties at home. When I was able to help him to understand, he said, "Call me Kenny." He regressed briefly once more to infantile dependency but this did not satisfy his needs. After holding a baby bottle he decided, "I no baby, I Kenny."

Family circumstances again interfered with his life anl the progressive course of his treatment. The family moved to a new neighborhood which would, in effect, be a new start in life. The boys' jealousy and aggression grew to such a pitch of intensity that the parents talked of placement. After saying, "I be baby, no talk," Kenny for the next three months became a wild, silent physical expression of rage. He had been given a longed-for toy for his eighth birthday which his brother immediately destroyed. After this, Kenny's very silence vibrated with rage, but at first he could not offer a sound about this latest cruel injustice. I reminded him that babies could not talk, and that he had told me he was not a baby. His response to this was, "I wan' be hater." I wondered who he hated since he knew that his brother had destroyed his toy but he would not tell. I urged him to tell me, to say his brother's name. I pronounced the name very slowly and when I accented the sibilant first syllable, Kenny became frightened. He blew with his lips instead. He protested, "I no do da. I be dead."

Nevertheless he felt that I understood he had a right to express his angry feelings; still fearful of talking, he once more put them into action. He would bound into the Clinic, dash straight to the therapy room and once inside, would throw large building blocks at the window, door, light fixture and me. Interpretation of his feelings toward the therapist, who threatened the release of such dangerous thoughts and feelings, of his anxiety about losing his mother because of the new sibling, did not reach him. It wasn't until a few weeks later, when the move to his new home became imminent, that I fully understood. Kenny felt that he was going to be thrown away because all old broken things were abandoned like old homes and babies (himself). His actual fear was of being left behind in the old house and being replaced in the new by the new infant. It wasn't until this precise interpretation was given to him piecemeal and repeatedly that he was able to calm down.

Negative transference manifestations appeared more consistently and were expressed in body language. Instead of throwing things at me when he was angry, he would bend over and seemingly deliberately pass flatus, or spit. At times he filled the room with foul odors to indicate he felt bad, dirty, rejected and wanted me to feel it, too. Suddenly one day, he said to me after we had survived his unremitting aggressive hostility, "Why you like me for?" I gave him all the reasons and then reminded him of how he used to feel and that he used to say, "Boy do da." He then demonstrated, "I go like this," and assumed the old head down, withdrawn autistic posture. He had become more reality oriented, and past and present were now clearly separated in his experience. Memory was being restored.

He had begun to learn spelling and arithmetic at school, subjects he seemed able to grasp relatively well, after the initial resistance to and fear of new learning experiences were overcome. Numbers, like his developing speech, became organizing, cognitive principles, and he was preoccupied with them. He wanted to know why the clock had only twelve hours (does one die then) and asked, "Why so little numbers on the clock, why is it no got 13?" He kept testing me to see if I wanted him alive or safe. He was now using abstract concepts in an obsessive defensive way. He wanted to know if he could live to be 99 and would flip the calendar and would ask me on which day did I think that he or I would die. His preoccupation with living and dying finally led to his ability to tell the therapist that, "If I get real, real angry, I die."

In the fall of that year, in imitation of his brother, he wanted to join a boys' club. This imitation was not like the former fusion with the brother during which boundaries were confused. It was a true imitation of the activity of a separate person. At his initiation, he was able to go to the head of the room where his father and many other people listened as he responded to the initiation rites over a microphone. Even though his speech at this time was unintelligible, he played his part. He came to the Clinic afterwards flushed with pride over his performance and the acceptance by his family. He was transformed. He walked into the room with an erect posture, head up, eyes bright with his newest dream. He asked me, "What I do be club leader?" He revealed his fear of failure by asking the therapist, "What you do if I no make it?" I replied that perhaps we should think of the things that he needed to do. I reminded him that he was learning to read and write and do arithmetic at school; that he was going to speech class; that he came to the Clinic so that I could help him with his worries. Kenny thought this over very seriously and looking up at the therapist said, "I not afraid to live!" Kenny had declared his commitment to life. For the next few weeks he was busy trying to figure out the exact meaning of words. He would ask, "What means friendly; what means sad; what means hate; if a clock is fast does it mean it can go no farther?" Kenny now seemed to be preoccupied with the basic elements of life itself.

Obstacles to Kenny's development appeared very early in his life and the events of the separation-individuation phase resulted in psychotic fixation. Traumatic events and conditions continued to accompany him as he grew older. Treatment in the postautistic phase, therefore, continued for several years but in spite of his unhappy life experiences he continued to improve. When at the age of 14, Kenny graduated from the eighth grade, there were 3 A's and B's on his report card. Understandably he was very elated. Even though peer relationships were still fraught with unhappiness, he was encouraged by his mother to go to the school dance accompanied by his father. He was triumphant. When I complimented him on going even though he was afraid, I remarked that everyone in the family deserved credit for the mutual help they were giving each other. To which Kenny replied slowly and with effort, "Another person deserves credit, you helped me get my grades up." I reminded him that he had done the work and I wondered how he thought this change had come about. He replied, "It's like a light, a bulb. It went out, it went on and off. You helped me and the light went on." It was fascinating to observe the emergence of the meaning of this former ritualistic acting out now being revealed in Kenny's symbolically apt verbal statement. He exclaimed, "When I go to high school, I'll go to the school dances, this one woke me up!" This was a declaration of hope for the future and beyond his competence at that time. Nevertheless, the establishment of the self now helped him further to cathect the world of people.

To sum up, when Kenny began treatment, he seemed to be completely preoccupied with the struggle to make certain of his place in his chaotic world. He did this by alternating between psychotic incorporation of "the good mother" and ejection of the bad self as if this were the only way he could be defended against further fragmentation of his empty and disorganized self. The primitive form of his defenses and identities was revealed by the defective differentiation of self from animate or inanimate objects in his environment. Very early in infancy, Kenny's sensory and perceptive functions had become involved in avoidance mechanisms, so that he appeared not to look or listen. Preverbal elements of language as well as words became negatively associated with feelings of his own badness, in part, because of his harsh parental introject. The result was that language did not develop beyond its rudimentary elements, and all human contact was avoided.

When Kenny began to develop an attitude of trust and to form a secondary symbiotic relationship with the therapist, he was able to move out of the undifferentiated phase, and sensory-motor perceptual and cognitive functions were expanded. As each regressive phase was worked through, energies were released for further separation of the self and for gratifying experiences. Each step led to the expansion of the perceptual system, which could thus become more responsive to an increasing variety of stimuli.

The tenacity of his bad self-image prolonged the time in which this became the battleground for further individuation. It was not until he began to sort out inner and outer experiences that aggressive impulses and affects became available for the task of ego mastery.

His primitive defenses were highlighted in the choice of animate and inanimate objects around which he wove his conflict of survival. When self and non-self were undifferentiated, Kenny acted as if he literally became the object with which he identified. When the therapist entered Kenny's psychic orbit as a kind of magical auxiliary ego, Cluddy, a transitional identity, appeared. Now that he began to modulate feelings within himself, Kenny seemed to be changing the "shape" (13) of his self-awareness by becoming this non-existent imaginary child.

This permitted him to have affects, to feel and to be vocal about fear, to experience ego mastery and to sort out reality while gradually giving up autistic defenses.

Part identification with Cluddy was given up since it was limited in its usefulness and Kenny's ego was not integrated sufficiently to maintain synthesis and structure through a relationship with a fantasied object (6). The next short-lived choice in his quest for identity was that of Hal, his brother's friend. This identification, which might be characterized as a borrowed "ideal self," served as a defense against disapproval and loss of love since it appeared at a time when Kenny was faced with school failure. In the boys' club episode, when Kenny identified with his brother, he no longer fused with him but imitated and attempted to be like him. This process characterizes Kenny's attempts to incorporate every positive identity as a spur to progressive personality organization.

When Kenny had attained a unified self-representation he was able to exclaim, "Call me Kenny." His beginning tender feelings for the therapist made him wish to please her by taking on the identity of Kenny. This case, treated by psychoanalytic psychotherapy, illustrates the genesis and dynamics of the generation of a sense of human identity in a child who presented both autistic and symbiotic elements of infantile psychosis.

REFERENCES

1. ALPERT, AUGUSTA. "Reversibility of Pathological Fixations Associated with Maternal Deprivation in Infancy." *Psychoanalyt. Study of the Child*, 1959, 14:173.
2. BETTELHEIM, BRUNO. *The Empty Fortress*. N. Y.: Free Press, 1967, p. 36.
3. EKSTEIN, RUDOLF & FRIEDMAN, SEYMOUR. "On the Meaning of Play in Childhood Psychosis." In *Children of Time and Space, of Action and Impulse*, chap. 10. N. Y.: Appleton-Century-Crofts, 1966.
4. —— & MOTTO, ROCCO L. "The Borderline Child in the School Situation." In *Professional School Psychology*. M. G. and G. B. Gottsegen, eds. N. Y.: Grune & Stratton, 1960, p. 249.
5. ERIKSON, ERIK H. *Identity, Youth and Crisis*. N. Y.: Norton, 1968, p. 217.
6. GIOVACCHINI, PETER L. "Integrative Aspects of Object Relationships. *Psychoanalyt. Quart.*, 1963 3:403.
7. GOUIN-DECARIE, THERESE. *Intelligence and Affectivity*. N. Y.: Int'l. Univ. Press, 1966, p. 63.
8. JACOBSON, EDITH. *The Self and the Object World*. N. Y.: Int'l. Univ. Press, 1964, p. 48.
9. MAHLER, MARGARET S. "Thoughts about Development and Individuation." *Psychoanalyt. Study of the Child*, 1963, 18:307, 309.
10. —— & LA PERRIERE, K. "Mother-Child Interaction during Separation-Individuation." *Psychoanalyt. Quart.*, 1965, 34:4.

11. PELLER, LILI E. "Freud's Contribution to Language Development." *Psychoanalyt. Study of the Child*, 1966, 21:459.
12. RINSLEY, DONALD B. "Economic Aspects of Object Relations." *Int. J. Psychoanalys.*, 1968, 49:44.
13. SANDLER, JOSEPH, et. al. "The Ego Ideal and the Ideal Self." *Psychoanalyt. Study of the Child*, 1963, 18:152.
14. TYNAN, KENNETH. *Kenneth Tynan, Right and Left*. N. Y.: Atheneum, 1967 p. 112.

CHAPTER ELEVEN

Story of Robert and How He Got There: The Development of Object Relations in the Psychotherapeutic Process with a Borderline Psychotic Child*

The intention of this presentation is to follow a line in the ego development of a borderline psychotic boy from ages five and a half to thirteen and a half during eight years of intensive psychoanalytic treatment. Available to the child at first were the most fragmented, non-integrated, psychotic introjects that represented forerunners of self- and object representations, largely fused in a symbiotic position in which the child started treatment. Mahler has described this phase well (2).

For many months the first change involved a gradual differentiation of introjects of the self from introjects of the object, still within what Ekstein calls the symbiotic sac (1). Only very slowly did this psychological membrane melt away in the process of the differentiation of true self- and object representations as the capacity for identification emerged and began to lead to alteration and integration of the intro-

---

* Kenneth Rubin is the author of this chapter.

jects within the ego. The development of object constancy could then proceed.

It should be stressed that the progressive psychic movements were never constant, but always oscillated and gradually led from a position of a relatively lower level of ego functioning to one of a relatively higher level, from a preponderance of primary-process thinking to one of secondary-process thinking. And in the process the triggering of profound ego regressions was common.

Patient material to be featured concerns a progression of names he insisted on calling himself, against the background of a progression of characters he made up in stories he wrote. These invented characters dwelt in lands that started somewhere in Africa and gradually shifted to an Atlantis-like continent between South America and Africa, to Wyoming, to Oklahoma City and finally to Los Angeles, as the characters gradually became more like himself, his family and friends. The transference also offered a major window through which to view these changes. An attempt will be made to show the pertinent resistances operating at each stage and the typical interpretations that were made, at first within the metaphor, and very gradually with less distance.

Dick's parents, both college graduates, were relatively stable, cooperative, and helpful. Father was a small businessman, and mother, a housewife. A two-year younger sister seemed to develop normally in every way. Dick's oddness and inner directedness were noted from about age one and a half. The work-up at Reiss-Davis revealed a borderline psychotic child, with a major thought disorder characterized by a preponderance of primary-process thinking and poor reality testing. Psychological testing was rudimentary due to the inability of the child to cooperate. Environmental stress seemed not of the sort to affect a normally developing ego adversely. Dick seemingly was a child with faulty ego development due largely to constitutional and/or developmental or maturational malfunctioning. Of course, the impact of the environment interacted with the growing psychic apparatus as is always the case.

Dick began treatment, four times a week, as a very anxious, upset child. He seemed to be bright, to have well-developed speech and at times to be capable of using it for communication. He was brought for treatment usually by his mother, who had to remain in the waiting room during his sessions for over a year because he could not tolerate her absence. Dick was aware of the therapist, as treatment progressed, but ignored him at first and retreated to playing in a corner of the playroom with his back to the therapist. During most of the early hours he crouched in front of a blackboard he had unhooked from the wall and placed against the far corner of the room. He spoke as though

o himself, turning his eyes from side to side, glancing at the therapist
behind him out of the corner of his eye.

Though the treatment stages were not actually separate and distinct,
for writing clarity they will be organized into several phases.

The first phase of about fourteen months, concerned the struggle
that culminated in Dick's accepting the therapist into his inner, symbiotically based, world.

Dick began to introduce the therapist to his inner world quickly.
By the tenth hour he drew a stick figure and called it Leslie. Leslie
was a girl. Soon Leslie was he, and he insisted during his hours and at
home that he be called Leslie and that he was a girl. Leslie was also
a baby. By three months of treatment he said, "I'm not Dick. He's all
bad," and related over the next several hours how Dick hits and was
aggressive and no one liked him and we must not allow Dick in. Leslie
feared and hated Dick. During this period, Dick's mother noted that
he avoided looking into a mirror and told her, "I looked and no one
was there."

During this phase the therapist agreed in many ways that Dick
should not be let in if he were too bad; that perhaps he could never
be let in if he could not learn to control himself; but that maybe the
doctor and Leslie could learn to tame the bad parts so he could be let
in; but in the meantime Dick was sick and needed treatment.

Early in the treatment, Dick at times could speak to the therapist
directly, asking his name and how to spell it, but in the main, he
showed his need to avoid conflictual or personal material by writing
numbers endlessly and asking the therapist how to spell words. This
type of avoidance became characteristic and was used from time to time
throughout treatment.

Dick began spelling Leslie. At first it was spelled MBAIC; then
WAGOSY. He said, "Dick . . . Dick . . . is there a K in Leslie?" The
therapist replied, "Yes, a K for Dick." Leslie was spelled Lagernacky
and Kenny was spelled CANY. At another time during this period he
brought in a *Life* magazine picturing the christening of a Kennedy
child. "Is it Dr. Kennedy?" Dick asked. Thus he expressed the blending, yet fragmenting and isolating of parts of the self-object fusion,
Dick/Leslie/therapist (Dr. Kenneth).

Dick's essentially symbiotic position was reflected in these and other
ways. One hour Dick urinated and ordered the therapist to flush the
toilet, as though the therapist had urinated. In the same hour, the
therapist's stomach growled and Dick said it was *his* belly. He spent
hours drawing his and the therapist's houses and making them look
alike.

From six months on, drawing became Dick's chief activity during his hours and at home. He developed into a talented draughtsman during treatment.

At seven months of treatment, an event of great consequence occurred. Dick's younger sister had a tonsillectomy. Dick's mother reported that immediately after the surgery Dick took to his bed and like his sister, did not want to eat or talk. Then, a few days postoperatively, the sister hemorrhaged dramatically, with bloody vomiting and had to be rehospitalized, necessitating Dick's missing his hour that day. The hemorrhage was controlled and the sister was home again in two days.

The mother reported that as the sister was recuperating in bed painting with water colors, she asked Dick to change the rinse water. Dick refused. The sister angrily yelled that she would break him. Dick began to scream hysterically, tried to vomit, and was very upset, reacting to the threat in a concrete way. Concrete thinking often plagued Dick.

The next hour Dick became very irritable as the therapist hesitated in spelling words that Dick had not indicated clearly enough. The therapist began to interpret, "If Leslie (and Dick interrupted: 'I'm not Leslie, I'm Robbie!') could put the thoughts in his mind into words, they'd probably say: poor sister ('Yeah') . . . she had tonsil in her throat and they were taken out; but it seemed her throat got broken and she had to go to the hospital again. . . . Is she all right now? ('Yeah') Is she home?" ("Yeah)." Dick went on, "How do you spell bomber?"

The name change to Robbie became entrenched for a long time. The choice of Robbie signified the fusion of himself with the therapist Rubin. One of the main uses of this was to avoid the consequences of separateness from the therapist. This defensive use of fusion was interpreted in many ways. As though to hammer home the danger, the therapist became acutely ill a few days after the sister's troubles and missed two weeks of work. Coincident catastrophes had an uncanny way of happening during the course of Dick's treatment.

For many weeks after the sister's surgery, Dick, or Robbie, as he now insisted on being called, ordered the therapist to draw airplanes, copied from a book he brought, and then ever more fancy models. He especially favored the Constellation since at age three he had flown on this type during a family move and it represented all his feelings about any kind of change. At age four he lost a toy helicopter at the beach and had become anxious about helicopters and ceiling fans in stores. Having the therapist draw planes represented a constant finding of himself, the lost helicopter, as well as repeatedly establishing his body image. A change of schools at nine months of treatment, age six years four months, was reacted to by his feeling of fragmentation of the self,

xpressed by preoccupation with airplanes without tails and by pieces
of airplanes. This was pointed out to him by saying that when Robbie
alked about airplanes without tails, the therapist thought for a minute
Robbie was going to say how much in pieces it made him feel to change
chools. (It may be mentioned that for a few years this child required
pecial therapeutic schools. He never had problems with learning; in
act, he displayed a superior intellect. But he needed the smaller size
of the classes and the greater teacher-student ratio to buffer his social
levelopment that lagged woefully behind. For a long time Robbie was
ery passive and helpless with other children, afraid to play games,
und often the butt of aggression of the other children. Six changes of
chools were effected during the length of treatment as special inade-
quacies developed with each of the schools in turn.)

For many hours, Robbie asked questions endlessly, often seemingly
vithout any connection in context but apparently representing an at-
empt to use obsessive ego defenses to bind or give structure to primary-
process thought derivatives that continuously burst forth. The attempt
ailed at this stage because the ego was not nearly strong enough. This
naneuver was interpreted in many variations of the observation that
some boys wonder what a certain word means while others wonder how
you spell the word, which is less upsetting to think about. The endless
repetitious quality of many of these hours produced the first occurrence
of great sleepiness in the therapist, as he had to ward off unconscious
anger at the boy.

After a month's vacation, Robbie ushered in the next seemingly
endless, deadening play. He turned to the multiplication table and spent
hour after hour going over the 9's and the 12's, etc. At first he seemed
to mean by it his attempt to master the concept of time in relation to
the separation from the therapist, as in the number of days of his absence. But this maneuver, too, became a general way of getting distance
from feelings and an attempt to bind primary-process thought derivatives.

The crucial climax of this first phase of treatment now unfolded
over the next two months, beginning at one year of treatment, age
six and a half. Robbie introduced the idea one day: "When I am a
frog, where will you be?" The therapist replied, "A big frog, right by
your side." Robbie continued: "My daddy frog; no, my doctor frog."
Several hours later, he said, "Will you die before me?" "No, I will die
at the same time!" During this period Robbie vacillated between presenting his world in a more humanized form, introducing short-lived
characters, and dehumanizing the world as in reverting to playing with
numbers. The therapist said such things as, "Sometimes when you talk
about numbers it seems to mean how old is this person compared to

that one; but now it sounds just like numbers. How come?" His common rejoinder was, "Let's talk about that later."

Several hours after the one in which he had introduced the idea of himself as a frog, Robbie was questioning the therapist about how old the therapist would be when Robbie was this age, this age, and that age. The therapist replied, quietly, "I'll be here as long as you need me." With his back to the therapist and almost in a whisper, Robbie replied, "Will you be here a billion years?" "Yes, as long as it takes," the therapist answered.

One month later Robbie announced that he wanted to be a baby and told the therapist to paint a picture of a frog, a little one, and then a bigger one. "It's the daddy and the baby," he said. This marked the first time that he represented, even by having the therapist draw it, a family unit, albeit an animal one. Two hours later, he began animating the family. He had the therapist fashion a little frog out of clay. Robbie made some snakes. "Are snakes sad?" he asked, as though he were a visitor from a distant planet asking his guide to explain about the feelings of the human beings he was viewing. The next hour he made out of clay a mommy snake and a baby snake, all curled up, asleep. Then more to himself than to the therapist, he told a story about the "four snakes."

Three hours later Robbie told a story as he fashioned some animals. "Baby frog is a tadpole. This is the pond where the frogs live." He asked the therapist to put smiles on the frogs. "Do people cry?" he asked. "Yes, when they have a reason," the therapist said. "What's a reason? Do you frown when you cry?" he went on. Then he had the frogs leave their little pond (the table) and jump into the ocean (the floor). A whale tried to gobble them up and they escaped back to their own little pond. The therapist interjected, "I'm glad they have their own safe pond to go to when the big sea is too scary; but I hope they can learn to get along in the sea, little by little."

At this point, Robbie introduced the crucial addition. He had the frogs swimming around until they met a skindiver wearing a big face mask (the therapist wears glasses) and swim fins. Thus, by the simile of the frogman, Robbie accepted the therapist into his inner world. At this point it would be correct probably to describe this as evidence of a primitive form of separation of introjects of the self and object in Robbie's ego, *but within the symbiotic membrane.* As dramatic as this moment was, after fourteen months of therapy, it marked merly the beginning of the beginning of treatment.

After this, Robbie started, in his drawing pad, a story entitled "The Three Turtles." Over the next many hours, however, he was unable to stick to the story and spent most of his time numbering pages of the story that never got written. Though boys were introduced to take care of the turtles, at one point, in the midst of numbering pages, Robbie began drawing houses. Endless hours were spent drawing ever fancier, more modern houses. Robbie displayed real talent and became an excellent draughtsman. He drew his house and the therapist's house, (previously drawn by the therapist) stressing at times the similarities, the sameness, to avoid the consequences of separateness; but at other times he showed the differences as he tried to learn the differences between himself and the therapist.

At seventeen months of treatment, before the one-week Christmas vacation, Robbie prepared for the separation by drawing doors and door knobs as he dealt with the means of mastering the entrance to the place from which he would be excluded. The first hour after vacation he brought in a story he had written at home showing Popeye going on a space trip. In the story children wanted to accompany Popeye but Bluto, the villain (also representing the therapist) stuffed their heads in the gas tank, making them cry. "Draw them crying," Robbie ordered. The therapist said, "It's not what they *look* like that shows how they feel, it's what they're *thinking* about. I guess while Dr. Rubin was gone some kids wrote stories while other kids thought how sad they were that he was gone."

A few hours later, Robbie showed the expected outcome of symbiotic fusion via a story of a witch and a giant catching the children to cook them. But the children turn the tables by cooking and eating the witch and giant. Thus, if mother loves him, she eats him; if he loves mother, he eats her.

About this time he accepted coming to the office alone and meeting mother on the street after the hour.

The second phase of treatment, lasting about a year, began now, at about sixteen months, and consisted of his bringing in pieces of stories about a little boy whose name underwent a series of changes. He called these characters his "pretends." These stories represented brief, sporadic attempts to portray his inner world, mostly in terms of fragmented introjects of the self, each fragment of which had to be kept separate. The fusion of introjects of self and object resulted in the inability to sustain a story; he constantly put his features into the story about other characters, confusing the two. Nevertheless, in spite of the broad fluctuations in levels of ego organization, this phase reflected the capacity for a higher level of psychic organization and of presenting his inner world in a more human and recognizable form.

About this time Robbie, for the first time, could accept the therapeutic suggestion that he sit *opposite* the therapist at the table and tolerate this degree of physical separateness. During the hour he intro-

duced a brief story about a boy named Greg who was going to a new
school. Robbie's struggles with conceptualizing his self continued a few
hours later as he described his silly Pete Seeger record: "He thinks
animals are alive." Then he told about Pinocchio, the wooden puppet
who comes alive. A few hours later, as he approached the office Robbie
saw the therapist in the hall, wearing an overcoat (the therapist always
works in shirt sleeves). Robbie asked during that hour, "Are you Dr
Rubin, are you *really* Dr. Rubin?" as though seeing the therapist
dressed differently and out of the office meant he was a different person. This underlined the lack of a stable psychic representation of the
therapist as a whole object.

A somewhat related problem culminated during this period. For
many months Robbie often refused to urinate when obviously he was
suffering with a full bladder. The context in which it appeared pointed
to his inability to distinguish between a perception of bodily reality—
a full bladder—and an introject of external reality—a commanding
mother. This was interpreted to him in many variations of "Sometimes,
when a boy needs to pee, he can't tell if it's suggested by a full bladder
or if it seems mommy is inside him, ordering him to pee and he's
darned if he will."

Two weeks before his seventh birthday, Robbie's mother was hospitalized for two days for minor surgery. Robbie reacted by physically
leaning on the therapist more and by beginning endless stories about
Greg being sick with fantastic illnesses, as Robbie fused with his
mother's experience of being ailing and lonely.

Just after his seventh birthday Robbie drew pictures of Greg and
his "pretends." He depicted them by stick figures; the boys had long
heads and long noses in front, the girls, like the mirror image of the
boys, had long heads with pony tails in back. By this, Robbie showed
his confusion about the anatomical difference between the sexes that
matched his confusion between self and object. But, also, the images
were used defensively to deny the differences between people, to ward
off the consequences of separateness.

In a closely following hour, Robbie for the first time drew his house
and the therapist's house "as they really are," i.e., different. He was
able in this instant to tolerate the separation of self and object. By
the end of this hour, however, Robbie was very reluctant to part physically from the therapist.

Three hours later, Robbie attempted to write "The Life of Robbie,"
dropping for the first time the distance device of the "pretends." Nat-
urally, he could not maintain it and began making up outlandish names
for the characters in his stories as though he had conscious control over
this process. Actually, they were akin to neologisms.

A few hours later Greg's family and friends became "The Small Guys," and these "pretends" were to last a long time. They were like children.

Several hours later, Robbie drew Greg in pieces, his head, hands, feet, heart, brain, everything but the penis, as this part remained the most conflictual, non-assimilatable part of his body image. He had to keep the introjects of his self isolated because he could not deal with his whole self, including as it did the bad parts, any more than he could deal with introjects of a whole object.

A few hours later, via a story about a Useful Dragon, he permitted the idea for the first time that his fragmented, bad self-introjects could be beneficial. The therapist remarked, "I'm so glad. He thought he was so different. But now he found out he could be useful, in his own, dragonish way."

Soon Robbie became obsessed with the idea, via the story of Babar which he had read at home, of eating a bad mushroom and dying. This ushered in the theme of the old elephant king who dies and is replaced by the young elephant. At this stage Robbie's main fear seemed to be an archaic forerunner of separation anxiety, constantly strong in the boy, in which the loss of the symbiotic partner is feared, that is, the defusion of the introjected representations of self and object. In a subsequent hour Robbie said, "The reason the part about eating the bad mushrooms *hurts* is that I dream *I'm* a dead green elephant."

Now Robbie told the story of Babar quite factually. Then he introduced the character of a monkey, who was a famous doctor. This monkey-doctor (how like the original skindiver of months before, but representing a higher level of psychic organization) could protect Babar. Now the Babar theme took on the color of the boy being catapulted into the role of king without any preparation, meaning to Robbie at this stage the giving up of the symbiotic position.

Around this time the "pretend" Greg, became Craig, who was to have a long career. Robbie landed Craig momentarily in the United States. "He was born in Pennsylvania, Philadelphia," not far from his own birthplace. During this period Robbie talked at length about comparative heights ("How tall are you? How tall is so and so?") and measured himself against the therapist, all in the need to remain small and young and to be protected by a bigger, stronger person. It was a long time before any of the "pretends" reached Robbie's chronological age or he admitted to his own.

Via a story, Robbie indicated that Craig was skinny and fast, like a fence swift. The therapist interpreted the need to be able to run away from people and danger but hoped the fence swift could run to a safe place, peek out and learn what the people are like and how to get along with them safely. Being skinny and fast like a lizard became an important theme for Robbie. It seemed to match, in his drawings the thin-headed "pretends" which depiction lasted a long time.

About a month later the therapist announced an impending five week vacation, the second major break since the start of therapy a year and nine months before. Robbie began to ask quite openly where the therapist was going, then complaining that it did not take that long to get there (the therapist generally answered questions of this sort factually). A little later, while writing, Robbie said, "When a word isn't there, it's on vacation." He said he would write these words at home when the therapist was gone and that he would stay at home those days.

The next hour, Robbie played out Craig's being afraid of the monsters in the dark, but has the mother's voice reassure Craig. The following hour, he involved the therapist in play with "The Small Guys." Robbie made Craig be the teacher. Thus, Robbie stuck to the therapist to maintain the symbiotic relationship, but tries for the first time to identify with the lost object in a primitive way, having the "pretend" become a teacher—a most significant beginning capacity. Robbie then showed all the bad things that would happen to Craig as he played on the playground equipment at school. The therapist interpreted to him his concern with what would happen if the person Craig needs should go away. Then Robbie portrayed Craig lying down on the couch and sleeping, while all the school activity went on around him. The therapist said, "He hopes if he sleeps all the time, he won't feel so lonely and scared with the doctor being gone." Robbie said, "He doesn't cry. When he sleeps, there's a tear on the pillow."

In the next hour, regression was more marked under the impact of the impending vacation and the greater investment Robbie now had in the therapist. Robbie started out wanting to talk about his fear, not Craig's but his own. Then Robbie turned to play with "The Small Guys," whom he and the therapist had to feed. Then he announced that Craig speaks Kier, and did the therapist know Kier? The therapist replied that Craig invented a new language, which was safer, in case no one could understand him, but perhaps someone could learn the language and be able to help him. Robbie then asked "The Small Guys" what makes plants grow. They answered, "Corn, wheat, lima beans." Robbie laughed uproariously. Then he asked the therapist the answer, as a sensible person. "Water and sun," the therapist replied. Robbie was very pleased. Then he became the teacher and dictated words for the therapist to write. Robbie corrected them and gave the therapist an A. Then Robbie became both teacher and student as he dictated some words to himself. The day before vacation began, Robbie constructed a calendar with which he magically manipulated the time. Thus does the primitive ego organization struggle to cope with the problem of separation. The very indication of the anaclitic need showed the developing and growing capacity to separate the introjects of the self and object, still within the symbiosis, but perhaps less fragmented introjects.

In an hour shortly after vacation (the mother reported that Robbie openly missed the therapist and showed how sad he was), Robbie drew a baby turtle in an egg. It was only safe to come out if the momma were around. It turned out that Robbie's parents were going on a few days' vacation shortly. Robbie behaved in an anxious, listless manner. As fate would have it, Robbie's father became ill with mononucleosis and the vacation was cancelled. Subsequent hours revealed much fear that Robbie's wish that the parents not go away caused father to become ill. For instance, Robbie would ask a question seemingly out of context, "Is a bad cold pneumonia?" and indicate a belief in magic. In this hour he spent much time concocting a helicopter out of a pencil sharpener, presumably his old, fragmented, lost self. In a subsequent hour, he spoke of the "flock juice, the leftover crayon juice that gives red fever that turns the lungs red," and reported a dream of a gas chamber.

At two years of treatment, age seven and one-half, Robbie brought in a book about dinosaurs and became preoccupied with them. He continued drawing and writing titles of stories that never got written, including ones about dinosaurs. The therapist also likened it to the profile of "The Small Guys" with their long noses and their great speed so they could always flee to safety. In between, Robbie invented strange dinosaur species, complete with descriptions. The emphasis was on anatomical protection against being eaten. In this, Robbie seemingly struggled with the devouring aspect of the introjected object, if he gave in to the symbiotic pull and fused with the object, as well as trying to cope with the devouring, fragmented introjects of the self. Robbie introduced a dinosaur child friend of Craig named Rungaish.

About this time, a major change of therapy hours was instituted because of Robbie's school needs. The hour change, from early morning to late afternoon, triggered initially a sizeable ego regression. At first Robbie babbled about dinosaurs and spun a pair of scissors like the propeller of the lost helicopter or the airplane that moved him across country when he was three. He progressed to a feeling of utter chaos in introducing words that were apparent neologisms and throwing out thoughts that indicated his fear that his inner badness (fragmented self-introjects) had infected the therapist just as it had father.

But within two hours, he began to calm down. He played teacher again with the dinosaurs as students, thus consolidating his capacity to separate self from object and make use of forerunners of identification to identify with the therapist who might be able to help the sick dinosaurs. A few hours later, Robbie played by himself as a mixture of teacher and student or of students keeping to themselves. The therapist pointed out that sometimes the students/dinosaurs didn't want the teacher to know what they were playing because they are afraid he wouldn't like it or understand it. Soon Robbie became the teacher again. The next hour, Robbie attempted to finish with the dinosaurs, to act neither as teacher nor as dinosaurs, but as the one who *chronicled* them. With this budding observing ego, Robbie announced that he had finished the dinosaur book. All this was indicative of the increased strength of the ego at this time and the higher level of ego organization operative at times, all the more striking because it came about in the face of a change in his therapy appointments, a major adjustment which up until now would have triggered *only* a regressive type of ego functioning.

In subsequent hours Robbie reverted to a more regressed level as he seemed to cast about for a new mode in which to express his inner world. He started a story about Craig and Rungaish expressing fear of the bad mother who either would not understand or would cause the bad result in the first place. Robbie suddenly said, "Como se llamo usted?" (What is your name, in Spanish) as though to present the therapist with an impossible task to understand him. A little later, he said, "Sometimes I wonder if *you* understand me—you do."

The next hour Robbie brought in what the therapist thought of as Robbie's psychotic work book. It contained recent writings produced at home. While he played, the therapist read references to building houses, repairing houses, poisonous rattlesnakes around houses, and red fever. As the therapist read, Robbie in his play suddenly had a rocket blast off. The therapist remarked that the kids in the stories had important things to tell the teacher, but they wondered if the teacher had the patience to keep trying to understand, and whether they were too mixed up to learn anything.

Within a few hours, Robbie hit upon the idea of making a dictionary: "No, a *volume* of dictionaries," and he returned to the position of writing *about* writing but never fulfilling the promise. He talked about a "flanting cough" and composed a table of contents: one, Craig gets sick; two, Craig visits overnight at a new dinosaur's.

About this time another change in schools was made. The subsequent hours reflected Robbie's attempts to present and cope with the fragmented, bad self-introjects in the isolated way that he had to keep them. The therapeutic task at this time concerned trying to bring the isolated self-fragments together as preliminary to forming a psychic of the representation of a whole self. One hour, he showed, in attempting to play a baseball game with the therapist, that he could never learn to do things the way other kids did and could only do it his own way. The next hour he brought in a box with toy dinosaur figures. He questioned whether the therapist knew this one and that one. He questioned whether the therapist knew all the sicknesses which he named. The therapist replied that he did, and that for each illness the two of them could figure out a cure. Robbie then asked if the therapist knew Greek, and wrote his version of the Greek alphabet. The therapist opined he could if furnished with the key to the translation. As though the therapist had passed the test, Robbie superimposed the English aphabet upon the Greek one.

At this point, the therapist announced a Christmas vacation of one week. Robbie responded by making a map to Craig and Rungaish's house. Robbie interjected remarks about vomit, snot, BM, saliva, and spit, in the context that all were bad inner things that had to be gotten rid of to make one like other normal kids. The hour after vacation, the talk of disease took on a new meaning, and he actually slipped, fell, and incurred a bloody nose to show what could happen to him when the therapist was gone.

In a subsequent hour, Robbie said, "I have to go to the bathroom. You come. You have to see what I do." The therapist acquiesced, saying that Robbie wanted him to see all the parts of him. Later, Robbie looked at a picture of bugs in *Life* magazine. "Isn't it awful?" he asked. "Do you see him? I thought I was the only one to see him." In response to Robbie's concern of the fragmented, crazy parts of himself, the therapist suggested studying the bugs and classifying them and making sense and order and wholeness out of them. "How do you know who you are or what you are?" asked Robbie. "How does blood get into the body?"

A few hours later, Robbie asked, "Did you ever change your name?" The therapist replied, "No, but kids who are afraid of some parts of themselves do, to try to get rid of the bad parts." Robbie began to mix water colors in a glass of water calling them different names as he added colors: "Chocolate brown, unsavory mixture, blue crystal, diarrhea, vomit, BM, eh-eh." The therapist remarked that those kids who change their names are afraid there is such a mixture of bad parts inside them that they'd better keep them all separate or else it would result in an unsavory mixture, but that if we studied that unsavory mixture, we'd probably find much that wasn't bad at all.

Soon the therapist proposed writing a book, putting all the pretends together. Robbie immediately decided to draw a globe of the world, turning it so that only a part of a country showed at a time, such as

"ALIA" for Australia. He cautioned that it had to be turned carefully. "Yes, so all the parts of the country can get together," replied the therapist. This type of warding off the task of integrating his self- and object-introjects was typical of Robbie. If presented the task of writing a play, he built a stage instead. Nevertheless, the third phase of treatment was ushered in.

The third phase began at two-and-a-half years of therapy, age eight years one month. In this phase, a still higher level of ego organization functioned at times. The introjects of self and object became more humanlike, although the various parts of the self still tended to be kept isolated from each other. More importantly, Robbie began to superimpose his inner world onto the real world as he could not integrate the real world but only fuse with objects and external reality, but wide fluctuations of levels of ego functioning continued.

At this point, for a brief time Robbie briefly drew his characters looking more like real people, but quickly reverted to the "thin heads." The next hour he invented a country named Cairominia, where Craig was born, where gajrinylaslyi, the second most important mineral in the world, is. When the therapist hoped that the laws in this country would allow all the pretends to live safely together, Robbie dropped the theme. The next hour, the therapist sang, a la "How Are Things in Gloccomorra," "How are things in Cairominia? Is there room for Craig and Rungaish there? And room also for Dick there?" Robbie said that Dick lives far from Craig; Robbie is only three doors from Craig.

The next hour, Cairominia became Carominia, and the therapist finally understood that Robbie was referring to the land of Egypt where mummies are, because Robbie had recently expressed the fear that Mommy might turn into a mummy; that is, not only become dead, but change from a helper into a monster. For the next hour, Robbie brought a map of Cairominia with the size indicated, the location of chief minerals, and a high mountain plateau drawn in. The therapist expressed the hope that they had laws there that allowed emigration to California. The next hour, Robbie added to the map airports and planes going there. The following hour, the therapist asked Robbie about his weekend. For the first time, he replied with factual details about what he did. Then he made up strange names for the states of Cairominia and later in the hour gave these names to teachers in Craig's school. One of these names was Geranium Ghana. This name became more prominent and finally remained as the country where the "pretends" lived.

The next hour, Robbie went alone to the bathroom across the hall, almost for the first time. His mother, while not required to wait in the waiting room all the time, still had to remain there many hours, and Robbie checked on her presence every now and then in his great need to maintain the symbiosis. The hour after this, Robbie asked for the first time, "Do I *have* to come here? Could I *not*? I've been coming here a long time." In this way, he made a trial in thought of separating from the doctor/mother. But the thought was not yet capable of being the prelude to the act. At this point, Robbie got chicken pox and missed a week and a half of therapy. His mother reported that Robbie spent the time reading books on diseases, saying this was like being with Dr. Rubin.

A few hours later, Robbie asked why the therapist saw other kids, "Because if you spent time on imaginary things, you wouldn't be able to become smart?" The therapist replied that making use of an active imagination was no obstacle to becoming smart. In this hour Robbie mentioned Greg for the first time in a long time. When the therapist said, "Welcome back," Robbie replied that Greg had been sick. The next hour, Robbie again flirted with the thought of giving up the symbiotic position. "Can I come *different* hours and different days?" He announced he would go to the bathroom alone. Later he made clay figures. "No dinosaurs. This is Craig. This is Robbie (Last Name)— he's a pretend." The therapist replied, "Yes, he was Dick, who made up Robbie, who makes up all the pretends." Robbie rejoined, "Can't I stay here all the time?" Over the next hours the therapist spoke of actually doing things that one thinks about, referring it to Robbie's material.

Some hours later, the mother reported that Robbie had just read *Pinocchio*. She remarked that with his long nose, Pinocchio looked like the people Robbie drew. Robbie said that Pinocchio became a real boy. Later, Robbie developed a headache and said he did not want to go to his hour as one presumes he feared that the therapist would expect him to become a real (whole) boy before he was ready. When he arrived and the therapist interpreted this, Robbie began to ask questions about anatomy and diseases. In the context of the material over the next hours, it became clear that Robbie had to keep his introjects fragmented and isolated in order to avoid dealing with the *wholeness* of the self and object.

Over the next month, in the first indication of tentatively advancing to a new stage of ego development, separation-individuation (even though separation of self and object was by no means consolidated and the symbiotic position persisted most of the time), Robbie began a serious struggle at home to break Mommy's rules even at the risk of incurring her wrath and losing her love. Also, in this way, Robbie tested the limits of his inner psychotic world by his struggle with the external authority.

In his written stories he had Craig going to a school named Cold Pen Pens Valley School. The derivation of this interesting name took place over a number of hours. It started as Clearwater Canyon; then it became Coldwater Valley; finally it became Pen Pens Valley. Coldwater Canyon is the name of an actual street in Los Angeles which runs from the therapist's office to the Valley, where Robbie knew the therapist lived. He drew the Cold Pen Pens Valley School with features very like his current school. This was typical of Robbie's superimposition of his inner reality onto external reality. Then Robbie introjected the fused inner-outer reality. During this process his inner reality very gradually and spottily became modified to grow more like external reality as his capacity to integrate the isolated fragmented parts of his introjects of self and object grew.

Finally, the climax of the third phase occurred, again under conditions that in the past had triggered mainly ego regressions but now resulted in the opposite. This happened at two years ten months of therapy, age eight years five months. Robbie and his family were anticipating a vacation to the mountains and to the beach. For two consecutive hours Robbie wrote out his version of Dr. Seuss' story of "Gertrude McFuzz." In this story a doctor gives Gertrude pills in order that she grow two magnificent tails she had always wanted. The therapist interpreted Gertrude's wish to have her fairy tale come true just as Robbie wanted the therapist to make Robbie's make-believe come true, only because the real world seemed too different and scary. Following this, for the first time Robbie drew an elaborate realistic map showing all the correct landmarks and relationships of the cities and roads to and from the proposed vacation sites, worked out in detail. The next hour Robbie revealed the concrete thinking that made the real world such a perilous place for him. He drew a head with an arrow through it. Lake Arrowhead was one of the anticipated vacation spots.

When Robbie returned from his vacation, the therapist announced his four-week vacation to take place shortly. Robbie asked: "What happens if I get very sick?" The last hour before the therapist's vacation, Robbie started out by saying, "It's the start of the crash," and showed his fear that he would crash or that the therapist would crash.

In an hour shortly after vacation when therapy was resumed, Robbie announced: "Craig moves again to Jutko Hills." The therapist applauded and observed that perhaps this would be the place where the pretends could move in with the real people. Robbie replied, "Imaginary is real in the mind." He then asked, "Would you like to be Craig?" The therapist replied, "In many ways, except I'd like to be free to be a pretend some times and real other times." Robbie replied, "Well, he's just an *imaginary* person."

In a closely following hour, Robbie drew his first representational figure, a pretty mommy whose pretty dress, he said, causes a boy's penis to swell up. He went into the waiting room to show the drawing to his mother, telling the therapist he wouldn't *dare* tell Mommy what it is because she'd say it's *nonsense*.

The fourth phase of treatment, perhaps the beginning of the middle phase, began at three years of therapy, age eight years, seven months. During this stage lasting about a year, Robbie's invented stories became more autobiographical with a move toward emerging from the symbiotic state and toward a truer self- and object-representation, but still within the format of pretending. As part of the process, he changed his name for the last time and attempted to suppress his primary-process thinking completely.

This phase began with Robbie introducing stories about a new family, the Randoms, which were to undergo many changes. In between, in all these hours, he drew houses and garages incessantly, and asked disconnected, insistent questions as always.

A few hours later he said, "I wouldn't want to be naked in front of a pretty lady—it would *embarrass* me—who says embarrass?" The therapist replied, "A *little* boy who then doesn't have to wonder about a naked lady." Then Robbie sharpened a crayon in the pencil sharpener and said, "Put your head in the hole and sharpen your nose." The therapist added that this reminded him of the boy who wondered what would happen if he put his penis in the hole of a naked lady. Robbie laughed nervously and told how his teacher would not let him write the word vagina in a story. Here Robbie struggles on a pseudo-neurotic level of ego organization, although he is still without stable self- and object-representations, let alone progressed out of symbiosis to separation-individuation. Still, the level of psychic functioning is higher.

In a subsequent hour, Robbie brought in a book of *The Stories and Poems of Robbie* (Last Name). Then he drew a story of the Randoms moving with little Nardy, the first character to become established, who came up to the bottom of Mommy's skirt. Nardy cried that he didn't want to go to school. In the midst of this, Robbie said, "I love myself," and seemed to be rubbing his penis against the top of a chair. The therapist remarked that loving oneself was safer than loving someone else and having to worry about another person.

A significant change was noted in a few hours. Robbie was working quietly at the table. He said something under his breath. When asked what he had said, he replied that it was *nothing*. He asked if he *had* to tell the therapist. This was about the first time he showed the capacity to contain the usual breakthrough of derivatives of primary-process thinking.

Robbie questioned the therapist minutely, as he had done many times, about where he lived, how he traveled there, and especially what were the alternate routes. These relatively impersonal questions were answered in order to offer landmarks of external reality upon which Robbie could lay down his inner reality, then introject the fusion, a veritable bridge between him and his inner world and the therapist and his external reality. In a subsequent hour, Robbie demanded to know how many children the therapist had (not answered). He wanted the therapist to name the location of all the houses he had ever lived in since birth (answered). Robbie's parents were contemplating another house move at this time. Then Robbie felt his own cheeks and said his glands were swollen. The therapist observed that a guy wonders if he moves from place to place, can he keep in touch with the person he used to be, can he find his way back to that person, and can all the parts of the body come together and make a whole person. Robbie said, "Who was that boy in the waiting room?" (He had seen another patient.) The therapist replied that Robbie wondered whether he would come here some day and find someone else in his place. Robbie asked, "Is this my hour?" "Always," replied the therapist.

The drawing of cars, very fancy ones, executed with great skill and draughtsmanship, became the major preoccupation during these hours. In the Random family stories, Randy Random was introduced as Nardy's older brother and became the main character. During one hour he brought in a book of stories with a real story line for the first time, *The Randoms and Their Friends*, with chapters of Randy's adventures. This did not last, and the therapist began to put pressure on Robbie for the first time to stick to stories and follow them through, as a way of confronting him with the difference between thought and action. He was able to pursue this only very incompletely. In one of the hours he shifted to the Random daddy and announced that he was an architect. Robbie asked how much money architects make, as part of thinking about his own future.

In the midst of this progressive movement toward more separation of introjects of self and object came an hour of panic shortly before his ninth birthday. Robbie announced his presence in the office by pushing the button as usual. As the therapist was a little slow in responding, Robbie banged and kicked the door and screamed, "Open the door! Aren't you ever going to open it?" It turned out that it was a school holiday. He was brought by a family friend, and suddenly he was afraid that the therapist would not be there. Actually, this probably evidenced a breakdown from the higher stage of development of object relations of the separation-individuation stage, as the anaclitic object suddenly became essential. In a subsequent hour, Robbie was busy drawing cars; then he focused on license numbers. Then he asked the therapist the history of his cars. Then he asked the therapist for his car license numbers and wrote them down. The therapist said that now Robbie would really be able to keep track of where the therapist was at all times. Later that hour, he talked about twins and wished he had a twin, as he sought again the safety of the symbiotic position.

Around this time, a significant change occurred in Robbie's material. He went through many hours attempting to cover up his psychotic fantasies. There was no talk of the "pretend families." He was irritated in general with the therapist and spent his time drawing cars and making car noises of imaginary rides in cars. At home, he reportedly behaved similarly. In school, he was reportedly doing well and making friends for the first time. Robbie was apparently attempting to use obsessive defenses against the underlying primary-process surgings. That he was able to succeed even partially spoke for the growing power of his ego.

However, for the therapist this was a painful period. He well knew the work that lay ahead and the need to continue to uncover and understand the psychotic material. In addition, the hours became even more stereotyped and dull, and the therapist again had to struggle to keep awake in his unconscious anger at the boy. In one hour during this period, Robbie exclaimed that he came to see the therapist because he liked to. The therapist added, "And because we have work to do, like arranging to make it possible for all your pals to move here from Geranium Ghana." Robbie retorted, "I'm not making up any pretend countries any more." The therapist replied, "No wonder you stick to making car noises."

During this time Robbie's mother reported he wrote a letter to his maternal grandmother in which he said, "I can't write anything; I'm having a thought failure." This graphic phrase revealed the price Robbie was paying for attempting to suppress the breakthrough of primary-process modes of thinking. Unconsciously, actual repression was occurring. Any conscious use of imagination or fantasy became suspect as a vehicle for primary process and succumbed to repression. Of course, this also showed the growing strength of the ego. At his first opportunity, the therapist told Robbie that Randy had been troubled for a long time; he was afraid of his imagination; he was afraid people would think he was crazy; he was afraid of some of his thoughts, so he developed a thought failure which was no fun but at least seemed safe.

During this phase Robbie also seemed to be defending against masturbation fantasies. The frequent clutching at his penis seemed to take on a new meaning. Sometimes as he made car noises he grabbed his penis through his clothes and blurted out words like "fuck" and mentioned worrying about swollen glands. He was fascinated during this time by a photograph in a *Life* magazine of a young Negro woman with her head thrown back and an ecstatic look on her face.

In a similar vein, during one hour when the therapist pressed him to write a script instead of numbering the pages, Robbie wrote a story. "The boy goes to the house of the virgin. They get undressed and kiss." Then Robbie went to the bookcase and got down Rapaport's *Organization and Pathology of Thought* and the latest volume of the *Psychoanalytic Study of the Child* and "escaped" with a furious car ride. The car ride probably represented the impulse-defense on a nonverbal, non-thinking level.

However, the "thought failure" by no means interfered with important reshuffling of ego elements. The culmination of the fourth phase of treatment occurred in an hour in the midst of a period of quiet, anxious withdrawal. Robbie said, "Robert is a common name." The therapist remarked, "And Robbie is his nickname." "Yes," replied Robbie, "he used to be Dick." "Can you ever use Dick again?" asked the therapist. "No," replied Robbie, "no one would know me." This current integration of parts of the self-introjects on the way toward the development of representations of a whole self that was acceptable was of great significance. Robert gradually became the name he called himself from then on. The therapist had naively assumed that someday Dick would re-emerge by that name as all the formerly unacceptable fragmented parts of the self were welded together. Instead, a whole person was to re-emerge as Robert via the internal changes represented by changes Dick to Leslie to Robbie to Robert.

The name Robert had powerful determinants. Among other things it contained part of the therapist's surname and was the name of the street on which the therapist had once lived, which Robbie knew all about. The name offered itself as a convenient template in the process toward identification.

In the midst of all this, the parents decided to move again. A change in schools would also become necessary. The possibility that Robert might be ready for a public school was considered. Robert handled all this without too much trepidation at first. Robert moved into his new house while the therapist was away on a three-week vacation and dealt with it, the mother reported, by complaining about the doorknobs being the wrong kind. Doorknobs had been a much earlier preoccupation in the days before Robert could tolerate animating the world around him.

The fifth phase of treatment, lasting about two years and featuring

urther consolidation of ego gains, began as work was resumed after
vacation. Four years of therapy had passed and Robert was nine years
even months. The use of maps to pin down reality became a prominent
levice. A more reality-oriented Randy Random emerged.

Under the impact of the significant changes in his external life,
Robert—for now I shall call him this, as he did—went through a period
of great shifts in the level of his ego organization. In the course of the
next several hours, he verbalized in a way that graphically exhibited
his reaction as though each new change was completely new without
any past experience at all to draw upon. It was as though Robert were
saying: If I don't see it right now, I have no idea what it looks like (he
could not draw a picture of his new house); if I don't see you right
now, you don't exist; if something is happening right now that is exactly like something I've experienced before, the gap in time renders
it completely new and unpredictable." Most of this emerged as he
talked about the new house and the new school in terms of the names
of new streets. All this was interpreted to him.

Robert started in a new school, a public school for the first time.
In an hour in which he did not want to talk about the new school,
Robert suddenly asked the therapist if he would like to see his penis,
and in the same breath pulled it out, complaining about how soft it
was. Thus, in the context of his fear of being swept away by the changes,
Robert reverted to checking the intactness of a valued part of his body
which probably represented a primitive separation anxiety resulting
from fear of the loss of the self.

In another hour, as though suddenly overcome by all the changes
and perhaps also triggered by the parents' plan to go away the coming
weekend, Robert began to babble in a chaotic manner with great pres-
ure of speech about a flood that he had heard happened elsewhere in
he country. The flood had devastated a wide area, washing away houses
and killing a number of people. Before that, Robert had read about
tidal waves and had used tidal waves as a metaphor to express intervening fears of being swept away by external or internal forces. The therapist interpreted Randy's fears that in a new situation where he didn't
know the streets or the people he was afraid he could just be swept
away. Robert shrieked and whistled to drown out the words.

The next hour Robert tried to draw a map of the country involved
in the flood as a way of making himself knowledgeable about the external reality and so mastering the anxieties stirred up internally as a
consequence. This means of learning about and internalizing external
reality as a method of mastering anxiety about internal forces was used
more often. In the past, Robert had tended to use maps as a means
of laying down his chaotic inner world onto the external world, as

in drawing Geranium Ghana, the land of "the pretends," as a continent off the east coast of South America. For Robert, drawing a map
also was like touching his penis, to make sure everything was in place
and intact.

A few hours later, Robert turned to a map of Los Angeles in the
telephone book. He began indicating by dots where Randy and his
friends lived. The therapist remarked how glad he was that Randy and
his friends finally moved to Los Angeles: that he'd always thought
they'd like it here. In another hour Robert brought in a gas station map
of Los Angeles, and in high excitement went over it. He outlined dis-
tricts. He called himself "nuts" when he outlined a border incorrectly.
The therapist interjected that it wasn't nuts, that it was important to
know exactly where everything was so that even disasters such as floods
could be dealt with.

A therapy hour was changed with Robert to allow him, at his
request, to participate in an after-school program of learning sports.
This reflected Robert's shift at school towards giving up the position
of being the crazy one and becoming like the others. He reacted to
the hour change as though all his landmarks were gone. He asked the
therapist to list all the places he had lived all his life, and spent the
hour concentrating on maps. For the next few hours, Robert worked
on maps of Los Angeles and especially the Valley, where the therapist
lived. He asked for the therapist's home and office telephone numbers.
He worked on a book about the Randoms that never got written.

The Christmas break of a week revealed more true separation anxiety than ever before, evidence of the consolidation of separation of
psychic representatives of the self and object and the dissolving of the
symbiotic membrane. The mother reported frank expression of missing
the therapist. Robert ushered in the post-vacation hours by bringing in
a transistor radio and showing a great interest in rock and roll songs,
especially those with a theme of love. The toleration of the idea of
self and object separateness and of love for an external object was quite
remarkable.

Soon Robert brought in four gas station maps of Los Angeles. He
pored over them, asking endless questions. "I don't trust maps!" he
exclaimed. The therapist agreed, not unless they have in addition to
real places all the places one has made up in one's mind. He urged
Robert to work with the therapist to construct such a map so that they
could always be able to find their way. Robert drew maps for several
hours, but working alone without much contact with the therapist. A
period of avoiding bringing up his thoughts followed, mainly by playing
rock and roll records in the service of this resistance.

Finally, Robert started a new story of Randy, the surname now being spelled Randomme, the form that persisted until the end. This story was written on index cards. For the first time, problems with teachers and school became the theme of the story. There was a bad substitute teacher who was angry with the children and had a cold stare.

The therapist announced his impending five-weeks' summer vacation. Robert reacted by talking about different kinds of watches and asking if it were all right if he yelled "shit!" in here. The therapist replied that if one could *think* about it, one would probably say, "I don't *like* it when Dr. R. takes time off and goes away on vacation. It makes me *mad*. But instead, one wonders about watches and if one can yell 'Shit!' ". In subsequent hours, Robert tried to establish a continuity with the past and future by questioning the therapist about where he lived all his life. Then he asked directly where the therapist was going on his vacation and who would stay with his children. During this period the mother reported that Robert was taking long solo bike rides with much pleasure. In this way, Robert tested out the idea of separateness, on the one hand, and on the other hand checked out map routes so that he could always find his home and the therapist's home and the way to get to each.

The first hour after summer vacation, Robert brought in a long typewritten story about "Rocket to the Moon." In this way he dealt with his feelings about distance the therapist had traveled from him. A few hours later Robert engaged in very reality-oriented talking about new cars. In the midst of this, he drew a picture of the Randomme house and told about a TV commercial in which the cartoon character came to life. Robert asked, "If I use flesh color in drawing Randy, would he be real?" The therapist replied that he'd always thought that Randy had lots of good qualities.

More and more, Robert brought in material about school. He reported that he had told the kids that he goes to a psychiatrist, and they called him crazy. Robert skipped a grade and was very upset by that. He wrote a story about Randy Randomme at school in which Randy was abused by another boy and turned to the teacher for help. The teacher helped him but Randy could only relax when the bully was not in school. The bully gave Randy a bloody nose and called him "spaz" and creep." Another treatment hour change was reacted to by Robert's saying that the clock was weird. The therapist replied that it pointed to the new meeting time instead of to the former time. Robert rubbed his penis as though checking if it were there. He began a story of the Randommes in which they drove up to friends', rang the doorbell, and the whole house collapsed; they fled in terror.

One hour, Robert came in with stories about the Randommes covering many pages. He discovered that several pages were missing. He hunted frantically for them. Robert got very upset and said, "I might die." The therapist sympathized that any gap or lack of connection seemed to be permanent. Robert cursed and screamed and calmed down with difficulty.

From time to time, Robert revealed his thoughts more directly via the stories, (once, he told a story about a greedy, awful boy, thereby introducing an aspect of his own feelings) but, in the main, for many hours, Robert again retreated to a position of withholding or avoiding his thoughts. He spent hours playing the card game War with the therapist. Robert's focus in the game was to do anything to avoid losing his high cards. The feeling he gave about this was that the high cards represented powerful internal protectors, the loss of which would reduce him to a feeling of being little and helpless. Nevertheless, the sameness of the hours caused the therapist to react by becoming very sleepy again. Later on, Robert showed his fear that the therapist was mad at him or had left him when the therapist became very sleepy. Robert told the Peanuts story in which Charlie Brown went to substitute psychiatrist, Snoopy, who fell asleep, and then went to psychiatrist, Lucy, who also fell asleep. Robert showed much primitive identification with miserable Charlie Brown.

Robert's concrete thinking persisted as one of the chief contaminants of primary-process thinking. The therapist's vacation in Yosemite was misheard as "cemetery," which conjured up images of death due to parting. Before school started, Robert reported that his mother quizzed him about history, and he was afraid he had lost his mind: if the recall was lost at that moment, it seemed gone forever—knowledge being equated with mind.

The concrete thinking was especially strong in the area of aggression. In an hour during this period, Robert asked, "Would you like me if I had a crazy sense of humor?" "Sure," replied the therapist, "or if you had a crazy sense of anything." Robert then told about an actual occurrence. There was a bully in school, and two of them were not strong enough to hold him off. Robert went on, "I told the other guy I'd hit him (the bully), but I might *explode* and I was too tired to explode—is that humorous (anxiously)?" The therapist replied that it wasn't a question of humor: that he must have thought, as boys do, that if one *felt* mad enough to explode, one might *actually* explode, and who would want to do that? "It's just an expression," Robert said quickly. "But sometimes one fears that they are literally true," added the therapist.

After five and a half years of treatment, when Robert was just eleven, the therapist reduced the number of weekly therapy sessions to three.

It seemed possible to do so without diminishing the continuity necessary to drive the process, and this was borne out. Robert responded by arriving a half-hour late for the next hour and telling a story about the Randomme's moving, asking if they would like it. The therapist replied that no one likes changes.

The bulk of the hours during this time, as was the case most of the time, was spent by Robert drawing, usually cars, and mainly keeping his thoughts to himself. In the condensation resulting from reducing eight years of material to a few pages, the impression is given of rich and abundant material. Actually, the dominant impression of the treatment process was that it tended to unfold in an exceedingly slow-moving and tedious manner. And so the work with Robert went on. The therapist attempted to use leverage to open up into Robert's thoughts, to get at and resolve his thought disorder, to allow conversion of more and more primitive thought processes into secondary process modes. Robert resisted as much as he could, more successfully as his ego structures became more prominent.

The next spurt of material came into the open as Robert began to struggle with the idea of going to a summer camp and living away from home for the first time in his life. "Camp (Name) has *girls*," announced Robert one hour. The therapist questioned Robert about what he anticipated at the camp. He expected there would be baseball; there was a train ride up to the camp, and what if he got sick? Fear of vomiting had always been prominent with Robert ever since his sister's tonsillectomy. Robert then drew a picture of a girl swinging a bat and hitting Randy on the head, graphically showing how dangerous it was to play with girls.

The next hour Robert brought in an 88-page typewritten story about Randy Randomme in which he anticipated and pretested in story form situations current and future that were upsetting to him. Though this was not yet a level of thinking directly about conflict situations, it represented a higher level of ego functioning than one that reacted to changes by babbling about a flood. The second chapter described Randy going to camp on a train, involving a very perilous journey; the third described Randy as a Little League baseball hero. In subsequent hours the story writing lost the capacity of thought as anticipation, as Robert was momentarily overcome by his fears. Randy was reported falling down a cliff, bitten by a black widow spider, taken to a hospital where he vomited. The fear of the thought disorder returned in another hour, as Randy met a new friend in the new neighborhood and was afraid it was going to be a crazy neighborhood. A few hours later, Randy was playing baseball in Little League. He kept dropping the ball and making a joke of it but he was really *sick* (mentally).

A few hours later Robert invited the therapist into his real life by asking him to attend an open house at his school. He said the therapist could eat with him and ride with the family and that Robert would introduce him as his uncle. The covering over of the thought disorder continued as Robert made cartoons of his Randomme family in which he borrowed events from the cartoon Peanuts. The therapist remarked that Robert had a wonderful imagination but seemed to fear it might run away with him. Robert responded by asking questions about the war and killing and leaving home. "I'd probably cry if I were away from home," he said. Robert began coming late for every hour as he practised separateness and independence. The therapist complimented him on his growing independence and his wish during his hours to "cut out the crazy stuff."

The fifth phase ended as summer came and Robert departed for camp for four weeks. When Robert returned, the therapist's summer vacation of three weeks was imminent. The therapist prepared Robert for psychological testing to see what this modality would reveal about the state of Robert's ego. Robert responded to the idea of testing by saying things that showed he feared either he would fail the test and be ruined or pass the test too easily and be kicked out of treatment.

A battery of psychological tests was administered by Elaine Caruth, Ph.D., an experienced member of the Reiss-Davis Childhood Psychosis Project. Robert was eleven and a half at this time. The results confirmed the clinical impression to a surprising degree, showing a verbal IQ of 130: performance 99: overall 117. There was minimum evidence of a thought disorder. Mainly, Robert was seen functioning as a schizoid, affectless boy. Neurotic defense mechanisms were developing; there was a consolidation of identifications. At this point, the therapist had a conference with the parents, reporting his beliefs that more could be accomplished and urging that treatment continue. The parents consented.

The sixth phase of treatment began when the therapist returned from vacation. Six years of therapy had elapsed; Robert was eleven years seven months old. This phase corresponded roughly with the seventh year of treatment. During this phase there was a further advance of psychic functioning. Despite fluctuations, the symbiotic position was over. There was a fairly well established separation of the psychic representations of self and object. Separation-individuation was strengthened. The oedipal theme, presented sporadically in primitive form before, emerged in clear focus. All of this was shown by the more direct way Robert presented his thoughts. The schizoid, affectless boy began to change slowly. "The thought failure" vanished.

Robert greeted the therapist upon his return from vacation with an open recital over the next few hours of Robert's scary experiences at camp during his own vacation. He did not use the Randomme family or any gross distance devices but spoke directly of the train ride, the thirst, the constant fear that someone would vomit, which was awful because he could see it and *hear* it, his fear at first of sleeping in camp, his largely refusing food the first few days until he began to relax and eat with gusto.

Soon Robert introduced "Archie Comics," a regularly published comic book that was to assume great importance for him. This comic featured endless stories of Archie and his girl friends in a high school, innocuous, innocent, largely asexual boy-girl setting. Gentle jealousies and rivalries were shown. In the hour in which Robert first brought in this comic book he asked, "How do you meet a girl: how do you open a door for her?" a question from a much higher level of ego organization than the one that pertained when Robert asked a similar question about what people were like years earlier, "Do snakes smile?"

A few hours later Robert brought in a lengthy Randomme family story, typewritten on regular size typewriter paper. Robert told of his plan to actually have the story *published*, and discussed this with the therapist. The story now had a new beginning. The family moved from the cold climate of Montana to Oklahoma City. Randy was frankly depressed by the prospect of moving. In a dramatic moment he was left behind inadvertently as he went from room to room in the old house saying goodbye. Randy hopped on his old bike which he had elected to leave behind and, riding frantically, caught up with the departing family car. They arrived at the new location. Randy inspected the much more modern, nicer new house and decided all he needed was one new friend.

Two weeks later, Robert introduced the oedipal theme in a clear way for the first time, age 11 years 8 months. He reported a *dream* (dreaming had been reported occasionally throughout treatment). He went into *Archie Comics*: he and Archie, Betty, and Veronica, the main characters of the comics, went off to war: he and Archie were practising with swords. Suddenly Archie disappeared and there was blood on Robert's sword. He was at his desk in the school; a schoolmate shook the desk and he woke up. "Boy, am I glad it was just a dream!" The father was displaced by a peer in the oedipal rivalry.

Later in the same hour, Robert related a story of the Randomme family in which the mother had a baby and later built for the growing child a display case for his rock collection, even though Randy had a rock collection of his own. Then the family went on a vacation during which Randy fell down a waterfall and was almost killed collecting rocks, and cut all his fingers. The oedipal material triggered a regression to a position of sibling rivalry. The therapist remarked that he thought Randy could let himself *react* to what happened to him and think directly: Mother, if you had a baby, I would feel like dying.

The next hour Robert continued with the oedipal theme. He related the story from *Archie Comics* in which Archie was afraid of a bigger boy because he liked the girl that the bigger boy also liked. Robert then began talking about girls. "Did you ever dream of going to school in the nude?" "Sometimes I wish I were a girl." The therapist asked why. "Girls don't have to go to war." The therapist replied it was no wonder a guy wished sometimes he were a girl to avoid the fighting that boys seem to have to do, even fighting over girls.

Two weeks later, Robert actually mailed the whole Randomme family typewritten manuscript to a well-known publisher. This represented the farthest advance Robert had yet made toward putting thoughts into action, which is one of the hardest tasks for a borderline psychotic individual. Usually, action is confined interminably to the realm of promises, which indeed was the case with Robert for years. Robert waited impatiently for a reply, even a rejection, which unfortunately never came. Robert started a new story, bringing in the first forty pages including a chapter about Randy going to camp on a train. Robert said, "It's funny, Randy's adventures are just like things that have happened to me."

And so treatment went on for the next few months. Robert began to struggle with breaking away from his dependency on the therapist. In one hour, Robert complained bitterly about his Friday hours. He threatened that he would not come on Friday any more and let slip that he did not want to come any more at all. The therapist acknowledged Robert's concern with being stuck in the vulnerable position of *needing* the therapist. Robert went on reading from a *Highlights Magazine* in the office. He made fun of a story for being such "a baby story." The therapist agreed that no one wanted to be stuck in the position of being a needy baby. Robert continued by asking, "What's the real name for bellybutton?" The therapist replied, "Umbilicus, and what it means is that at first the baby is very attached to its mother, then less and less so, until finally, by age 12 or 13, he doesn't want to be reminded of needing mother at all." Robert broke in irritably, "okay, okay!" Then he began talking about slums. He had expressed a fear of slums and being poor and needing money for a long time. He had even begun stealing change that his parents had left around. Being poor meant being in a position of being needy and thus exposed to all the consequences of having to depend on someone. This theme continued sporadically for many months.

As the next summer approached, Robert faced the prospect of starting junior high school. He reacted by regressing to writing a story in which a new character, 12-year-old Charles Chydell, awakened on a boat, forgetting he was starting a vacation boat trip and thinking that a tidal wave must have carried off his house while he slept. Then Charles had a dream about impossible tasks and a terrible, punitive teacher.

The seventh and final phase of treatment began after the summer break. Robert was twelve and a half. During this eighth year of treatment, Robert gradually emerged as a neurotic boy, a very odd boy, but one who functioned mainly on a neurotic level. Psychological testing was repeated and treatment was terminated.

In the first hour after vacation Robert revealed his intermittent problem in going to sleep as a fear of sexual thoughts. He made a slip of the tongue while reporting some events of the summer. "I didn't like sleeping with girls—I mean, in a *house* with girls," he said.

Two weeks later Robert wanted to talk again about his fear of vomiting. He approached this in a very straightforward manner as a problem that he would like to get rid of and understood that the way to do this was to discuss his thoughts about it. He now traced the whole history of the vomiting. At age four he had been sick and vomited often. At his age 6 his sister had the post-operative throat hemorrhage and vomited blood. Later, some boys vomited at camp and he was afraid to sleep. He was afraid of the sound of it and that it might get on him. All this Robert volunteered. The therapist pointed out the progression of fears: he might die; the reminder, sister might die or he would, if it got on him.

By the middle of that year, when Robert was almost 13, the therapist gradually became aware of being vaguely uneasy, as though something were happening that he could not pin down. As the therapist thought about this, he realized what seemed wrong. Robert had been presenting himself as a neurotic boy. The therapist was talking to Robert as he did to neurotic youngsters.

For example, in one hour during this period, Robert was talking about school. He asked, "Do you know who Danny has a crush on? Cindy Doran." The therapist remembered that Robert recently had confessed painfully that he liked this girl. "Too bad," the therapist said, "the one you liked." "Oh, no, who wants to like girls!" replied Robert. Then he asked the therapist to remove his glasses to see what he looked like. "Cindy has *round* glasses now," Robert observed. The therapist asked Robert to describe her. "It's impossible to do," he said. "Oh, fuck, I mean fuzz." The hour continued. Robert asked the therapist what kind of piano he had and did it have a sustaining pedal that hung down; *his* broke off; he hoped he didn't have to pay for it. All the time he spoke, he was fiddling with a pen that he said had belonged to a girl and which he had broken and kept. He said he hated to hear guys in college talk about degrees and classes and grades. The therapist said that it seemed as though a guy was expected, right now, at age twelve or thirteen, to know how to do everything, like how to handle girls; and a guy is afraid he might hurt a girl if he's the kind of guy who tends to break things. Robert replied, "I like dirty jokes." He told some. "One guy asked another how babies are made. The other replied, intercourse. Idiot, said the first, they're found under a cabbage leaf." (Incidentally, the cessation of concrete thinking and the development of real humor were among the last things to develop with Robert.) Robert went on, "Want to hear an old Archie Comic?" He told the story of Archie and Betty and Pug and Veronica waiting at the pier for the arrival of an Italian boy and a French girl who were exchange students. The Americans joshed and argued about who would win the newcomers as boy and girl friends. When the boat arrived they learned to their chagrin that the foreign students had already met and become boy and girl friend.

And so the final six months went. The decision was made to terminate treatment. Robert responded with understandable trepidation but with some pleasure and no significant ego regression.

The therapist proposed psychological testing again, as a point of comparison. It was made clear to Robert that termination was decided and did not depend on the testing. Nevertheless, the psychologist, the same one who had tested Robert two years previously, reported that Robert was exceedingly anxious and upset the first day of testing, age thirteen and a half. In spite of this, the testing revealed dramatic progress to a now essentially non-psychotic level of functioning. There was no evidence of a thought disorder. There was a firm allegiance to the secondary process and to reality. There was a marked improvement in body image. Sexual identification was established, though weak. There was security in his identification as a truly animate member of the human race. The people around him were seen as real flesh-and-blood creatures. He was able to integrate emotionality to some degree into his life so that he was no longer the schizoid, affectless child of two years before.

REFERENCES

1. EKSTEIN, RUDOLF & FRIEDMAN, SEYMOUR. Prolegomenon to a Psychoanalytic Technique in the Treatment of Childhood Schizophrenia. *Reiss-Davis Clin. Bull.*, 1968, 2:107.
2. MAHLER, MARGARET S. *On Human Symbiosis and the Vicissitudes of Individuation.* N. Y.: Int. Univ. Press, Inc., 1968.

Part Three
THE DYING AND LIVING OF
TERESA ESPERANZA

We start again from the split of our experience into what seems to be two worlds, inner and outer.

The normal state of affairs is that we know little of either and are alienated from both, but that we know perhaps a little more of the outer than the inner. However, the very fact that it is necessary to speak of outer and inner at all implies that an historically conditioned split has occurred, so that the inner is already as bereft of substance as the outer is bereft of meaning.

We need not be unaware of the "inner" world. We do not realize its existence most of the time. But many people enter it—unfortunately without guides, confusing outer with inner realities, and inner with outer—and generally lose their capacity to function competently in ordinary relations.

This need not be so. The process of entering into the other world from this world, and returning to this world from the other world, is as natural as death and giving birth or being born. But in our present world, which is both so terrified and so unconscious of the other world, it is not surprising that when "reality," the fabric of this world, bursts, and a person enters the other world, he is completely lost and terrified and meets only incomprehension in others.

R. D. Laing

CHAPTER TWELVE

Teresa

Teresa Esperanza became my patient in the fall of 1960, when she was fifteen years old. One day the following spring, she brought with her to my office a hand puppet that she had made at school. The puppet was an Easter bunny named Lizzie, after Elizabeth Taylor. For most of the hour, Lizzie and I talked while Teresa listened.

I asked the puppet whether Teresa would like to be a puppeteer when she grew up, and Lizzie answered, "Well, that would be wonderful. But, you know, Doctor, this is something I want to tell you. She wishes she could become many things, not only that, she wishes she could become a movie star, a nun, a nurse, a doctor, a lady that sells in a toy store, that sells toys for the children or that sells nice things, jewelry or perfume or, you know, things for the ladies that they use, you know, or also . . . that she would make cakes herself . . . and she would sell them and have her own sweet store, you know like in Mexico those stores."

Teresa's wish to "become many things" is one common to most adolescents, and, like Teresa, most adolescents are self-absorbed and live at times in a world of their own. They experiment—in fantasy and in outward behavior—with a variety of actions and feelings. They seem to believe that they can reach any goal they choose, but for the time being they commit themselves to none.

The normal adolescent sooner or later begins to establish firm goals and to acquire the skills he needs to achieve them. As he moves toward adulthood, his abilities, his goals, and his daily behavior bear an increasingly close and consistent relation to one another. With the psychotic adolescent, this does not happen. His illness frustrates all his attempts to formulate and to move toward the goals of an adult.

In her late teens, one of Teresa's most pressing practical problems was to be able to leave the school shower room in time to meet the volunteer worker who brought her to the clinic, instead of remaining there, lost in fantasy, for hours and hours. At 20, she reported as a major achievement—which, indeed, it was—that she had taken a bus by herself. She could not execute whatever larger plans she was capable of developing; they seemed to remain forever part of her infantile and primitive fantasy world.

Teresa's difficulty in achieving even the smallest, most short-term practical goals indicates that her investment in the world of reality was minute. If her energies were not directed at realistic goals, then where were they going, and why?

In order to answer these questions, it was necessary to find some way to communicate with Teresa. With psychotic patients, this task is difficult at best. Sometimes any contact with the therapist is too threatening for the patient to stand. At other times, contact can be maintained only briefly.

Thus the therapist must take advantage of any avenues of communication the patient can open up. In Teresa's case, one of her first attempts to communicate took the form of violent and irrational behavior. Later, she spoke through a third party, the puppet Lizzie. Throughout her treatment, she used "borrowed fantasies"—incidents from television shows and movies that she transformed into allegories and metaphors of her own problems.

Through these media, Teresa was able to show that her actual goal was simply to stay alive.

When Teresa began treatment at the age of 15, she was hardly reachable at all. At best, she behaved like a nine-year-old child. She constantly demanded gifts, food, and love; she thought that life should consist of Christmas and Easter, of valentines and birthdays. She was diagnosed as suffering from a schizophrenic reaction, childhood type, with a massive hysterical facade.

Teresa openly stated that she hated growing up, which to her meant temptation that she could not cope with. Growing up made her "nervous," and when she was "nervous" she was prey to delusions and hallucinations. She could not differentiate between past and present, outside and inside, object and subject. Her uncontrollable anxiety, and the rage and murderous impulses that accompanied it, could be kept down only if she returned to the relatively safe base of childhood.

During her first encounter with me, Teresa described herself as a good girl who was possessed by a demon. During the course of treatment, the demon continued to represent Teresa's illness: he was a "monster" who was attempting to possess her mind. As such, however, the monster came also to represent the therapist, whose efforts to propel Teresa toward reality were as threatening as the demon's attempts to drive her toward open psychosis.

Teresa revealed the dual nature of her monster in an early session. There was the sound of furniture breaking in the waiting room. When I came out of my office and asked Teresa what had happened, she said that she had broken a lamp "carelessly." I said that she looked angry, and she admitted that she was, attributing the feeling to something that "bothered me in my mind, that I imagined."

"I don't know what thought it was," she said. "It was just a strange thought that bothered me, that got me in a bad mood and got me so angry that I felt like breaking anything so I ruined the lamp and I had to break that, that . . .

"You know, it is sort of something like an imagination. You can imagine yourself, that you lead yourself, you know what you do and what you're not supposed to do and what you're supposed to do. But then suddenly you can imagine another person that, well, thinks that he is more greater than you and that person would think that, that he can do . . . that he's more stronger and he can do better than you and then he will tell you, 'Look! I'm stronger, so I'm going to lead. Not you, you're weak. You do what I say.' So then he, he makes me do what he says and that's what gets me in bad mood, that he thinks he's more stronger and more smart than I am . . .

"And then that, that person when he does . . . suddenly he gets me in such a bad mood that my imagination, and he's scolding me in my imagination, he's punishing me, he's getting angry at me, and then that is what gets me angry. That's what gets me in a bad mood. Then I grab something I feel like grabbing and just breaking it . . ."

I suggested that she wanted to show me she was stronger than I, that she feared I was strong enough to make her well, to take the lead away from her. Our conversation went like this:

P.: That's imagination, it's something like that. It isn't that. It isn't that another person thinks he's more stronger than me. It's something like that. It's a creature, funny.
T.: That's right. But I'm the creature in your mind.
P.: No, you're not that creature.
T.: Teresa, you told me through your act. You told me, see.
P. (screaming extremely loudly): You're not that creature, you're not that creature . . . You're not that creature!

But Teresa had told me through her act. Parenthetically, it should be mentioned that acting out is behavior that classic analytic theory considers undersirable. Some patients, however, have no real choice available. They cannot replace acts with words; indeed, they cannot distinguish between the two, just as they cannot distinguish fantasy from reality. In psychotic patients, acting out can be a step forward rather than a defensive maneuver. Teresa was in closer touch with reality when she broke my furniture than she was, for example, when she sat on the floor of my office and literally turned her back to me.

Many psychotic children live with monsters. They are terrified of them and beg to be rid of them. They say to the therapist, in essence, "Let's love each other but hate my monster."

The therapist does well to refuse this invitation. The child uses the monster as a repository of his own "bad" impulses; by personifying them, he tries to establish distance between himself and them and to deny that they are his. If the therapist accepts the monster as a part of the child, he paves the way for the child to do so as well.

Since the monster represents not only what the child hates in himself but also what the child hates in the therapist, it is doubly important that the monster be brought into the analytic hour, where it is available for the same kind of interpretive work as is accorded the patient. The therapist can treat the monster as a common property and, when appropriate, engage in a dialogue with it. In this way, the monster becomes someone with whom both therapist and patient can negotiate, and both can try to influence the monster toward less punitive and less destructive ways of controlling the child's behavior.

Eventually, Teresa could say of her monster: "I haven't been trying to just get him out of the way or just get him out of my mind or by other means get him out of me . . . remember before how hard I would try? . . . Now I just try to ignore him, that's the best . . . before I would want to get angry at the creature, he's the one who would get me angry, nobody else, he started it and I would want to finish what he started and instead I would wind up doing it to someone else . . . but I found out that's not the best thing to do to tame him . . . the creature bothers me now with a reason."

Despite this rapprochement, Teresa continued to fear that the creature might reassert itself and destroy her. She therefore allowed herself, from time to time, to act as if she were the creature. As a defense against the notion that the monster was real, this behavior was a step toward the mastery of psychosis, toward a recognition that her psychotic thoughts were her own and had to be integrated with the rest of her personality.

TERESA AS PUPPET

It was not long after the lamp-breaking incident that Teresa brought the puppet, Lizzie, to my office. During the hour, a transformation sim-

ilar to the one that I have described in the monster occurred in the
puppet. At first, the puppet was primarily a spokesman for Teresa's
aunt, who was taking care of her at the time. The aunt constantly tried
to keep Teresa's behavior within limits by telling her what she should
and should not do. Thus the puppet reported to me, for example, that
Teresa had been overeating: "She's still been stuffing herself . . . she's
still harming herself by doing it, it's not healthy for her body, it's
unhealthy."

As the interview progressed, the forbidding puppet who spoke of
limits became a reflecting puppet. It tried to explain Teresa's behavior
and to create a rationale for her difficulties. At one point Teresa said,
in her own voice, that she wished Lizzie could really talk, so that
Teresa would not have to speak for her. She went on: "But if I wish
that she would talk instead of me making her talk, that really gets me
more sick than what I am, Doctor."

T.: You mean if you would really think that that thing's alive.
P.: Umhmm, that's right, that would get me worse than what I am,
     and I might really see it, and I don't want to see it, I would be
     frightened, and that's why I shouldn't even think of it. It's some-
     thing to see even a cartoon, you know, funnies, talking cartoons,
     like Donald Duck, you know—at least I can make her move as if
     she were alive, she seems to be alive, see.
        (Reverting to puppet's voice:) Well, so she felt uncomfortable
     to sleep without a pillow because all her curlers were bothering her
     and were aching her head and she couldn't just sleep well, so she
     asked her aunt if she could let her sleep with a pillow, so she slept
     with a pillow in the night and she slept comfortably and every-
     thing and next morning she, well, well, she fixed her hair nice and
     everything and now she has this nice hair-do—what do you think
     of it?
T.: Very nice hair-do—grown-up girl hair-do.
P.: Thank you. Yeah, that's what I think. But, you know, the poor
     thing she always feels she's a child, you know, and . . .
T.: Suddenly she has a big girl's hair-do.
P.: Well, you know, she's mixed up, she's in between the two, this is
     something hard to explain, but I'll explain it to you at one time.
     She acts both ways—sometimes she acts like a grown-up and some-
     times like a child, and she doesn't know which to choose, which of
     the two, she's mixed up, you know—it's something like if, let's say,
     you go to a store, and you see two dresses, let's see—this girl sees
     a very pretty dress, and she sees a beautiful dress, and they're both
     so pretty she doesn't know which one to choose, she gets mixed up,
     you know, it's the same way with her. You understand what I mean,
     Doctor?

T.: Yes, I understand that very well. I just wonder why she doesn't want to choose the one or the other, Lizzie.

P.: Well, it's—that's a part of her sickness, don't you understand? 'Cause if she were cured, she would choose one of the two dresses.

T.: She sure would.

P.: Of course. But the reason why she doesn't is she gets mixed up about it and starts saying, "Well, I want this one or this one." She goes for the two but she doesn't know which one, she gets mixed up, confused, it's in her sickness, you should know that, I'm sure you know it, don't you?

T.: Sure. But tell me, what would be the trouble if she were to choose one part, just leave out the other?

P.: Well, um, uh, let's see, let's see.

T.: Oh, Lizzie, you gotta do a lot of thinking.

P. (giggling): I know what you're saying.

T.: Yes, well, if you can think that out, you've got a good thought.

P.: Well, what do you think would be the best thing? Which of the two dresses would you choose? (Lizzie addresses Teresa here, who answers, "Well, I think I would choose if I were cured, I would choose the beautiful more than the pretty one.") See? She would choose the beautiful one.

T.: She'd rather be the grown-up woman.

P.: That's right. Well, that would be both for a grown-up woman and girls, you know, but she would choose the beautiful one, you know what I mean? You understand me, don't you?

T.: Yes, she would want to be the beautiful woman.

P.: Yes, that's right. See? You like my voice, isn't it sweet?

T.: It's sort of like a bunny's voice.

P. (giggling): Oh. Thank you. You're very nice.

The image of the therapist had largely replaced the image of the forbidding aunt. However, the use of the puppet kept both figures at a safe distance. Part of Teresa, speaking through the puppet, could collaborate with the therapist, but that part of her was still, as it were, a puppet in the hands of her illness.

TERESA AS EURYDICE

Teresa's use of "borrowed fantasies" began with her first interview, when she described a television show about Martian invaders. Among them, she said, was "a girl that came from another planet . . . a devil girl, I mean, she was horrible." Some five years later, at about the time she reported her new ability to take the bus by herself, she used the screenplay, Black Orpheus, to describe the powerful inner struggle that lay beneath her reality-oriented attempts to master small tasks.

Teresa had been speaking of such realistic goals as keeping appointments and learning a simple trade. She complained that she was tired of even the slightest criticism from the Sisters at the Catholic home where she lived. Later, she began to play with the idea of being like the Sisters, a fantasy role that was opposed to her desire for a romantic involvement. When I remarked that Teresa did not seem to know whether to become a nun or get married, she disrupted the conversation, lost contact with me, and tried to remember a movie she had seen. Like an attempt to recall a dream, her tortured attempt to recall the picture was an effort to return to the conflict that had been the subject of our discussion.

As the fragments of *Black Orpheus* emerged, it became clear that Teresa saw herself as Eurydice, killed by the hateful and jealous Aristaeus, the Snake-Man. Orpheus was both her savior and, when he turned to listen to her pleas for rescue, her murderer. Eurydice's death by snake-bite reminded Teresa of Cleopatra and the asp, and of her own fantasied attempt to poison herself.

P.: I took poison. But I didn't take a little. I took plenty. But you don't believe me yet, do you?

T.: I believe that.

P.: No, you don't have to believe me, if this sounds like a make-believe story, sounds as if I'm making it up. But I'm not. I wish I could tell the whole world that it's true. But nobody could believe me. It's hard. Mysteries do exist.

T.: You have no idea how much I do believe you.

P.: I have no idea. Maybe one day I'll notice it because I really can't see it. I really think that, ah, that you're just being, you want to be sweet to believe me, you're pretending to.

T.: You still don't know . . .

P.: 'Cause if you wouldn't really believe me you would hurt my feelings and you'd say, "Poor Teresa." I don't want . . .

T.: Teresa, I don't mind hurting your feelings if it helps us. I don't mind hurting your feelings. You know, you're a big girl, you can stand a little hurting. It's like when you go . . .

P. (*shouting*): But nobody knows.

T.: When you go to the dentist can't you stand a little pain? When the dentist works on your teeth?

P.: You start talking about these stories and I mention a story and I start thinking about myself and I'm so scared that I don't know (*sobbing*) I don't know who I am. I don't know what I'm doing in the world, why I keep walking around. I don't know why I'm alive. I'm supposed to be dead. Why am I alive if I'm supposed to be dead?

T.: Because I want to make you completely alive.

P.: It's just like if the devil came and he killed me. Well, I know the devil and I killed myself. I don't know why. I didn't know what I was doing. I just didn't know.

T.: Do you know the story of Eurydice?

P.: Well, somebody killed her. But she really died. But in my case I really didn't die. I died and I lived and I came back to life. Both things at the same time.

Teresa is dead and at the same time miraculously alive. Like Eurydice, she moves backward and forward between life and death. She does not look for goals that make life meaningful; rather, she struggles for existence itself.

Her fantasies of great achievements—of becoming a movie star, a famous singer—are not really goals. They are self-promises that, for the moment, transform utter helplessness into omnipotence and defend Teresa against her terror of dying. Like the promises of a child, they are things to be made, not to be kept. A child makes promises in order to secure his parents' love; Teresa made them, in the form of fantasied plans and achievements, in order to keep her self-hate from becoming great enough to destroy her.

Teresa's "promises" changed from day to day. Indeed, change could be said to typify her life, as it does the lives of most psychotics. They cannot maintain a constant image of any object, mental or physical. This means there is always a danger that the self will be lost—that it will "die."

The normal infant learns very early that his own body is a discrete entity, separate from the rest of the world. Then he learns that the rest of the world includes different people and different things, which can be distinguished from one another and which remain essentially the same from day to day. The child may be angry with his parents one day and not the next—his feelings and his thoughts may change—but his parents themselves remain intact.

For the psychotic, all things change: they flow together and become one another. During therapeutic treatment, the psychotic patient cannot keep himself and the therapist separate. Merging means loss of self, and the patient must at times retreat farther into fantasy in order to preserve his own existence.

To one patient, a boy of about 20, I sometimes appear to be a movie of a therapist rather than a real person. I have no life; I am merely a celluloid strip in black and white. When he wants to find out whether I am more than a movie, he must come toward me and touch me.

In fantasy, this boy sees himself as a powerful genius, a potential world leader, a great pianist. In reality, he is now attending an acting class, but at times the class presents insuperable difficulties. The drama coach once asked him to perform a pantomime of a man rolling a bowling ball down an alley. When he began to imagine the bowling ball, it suddenly lost its shape, became weightless, and started to look like a sheet of plastic.

As long as the objects in the phychotic's world are unstable, he must devote most of his energy merely to maintaining his own existence. The more stable they become, the more energy can be released for permanent and realistic goals.

The process of change is long and gradual, and the outcome is always in doubt. Some patients make excellent recoveries, others do not; most at least improve. At 15, Teresa would sit on the floor of my office playing with tiny toys like a five-year-old child, delusional and unable to talk. At 17, she could not read the time or change a dollar. Now, at 21, she lives on home relief. She can keep within her budget and arrive for appointments on time. She tries taking a course occasionally, and she recently held a job as a cafeteria helper for a few weeks. She could not keep up the pace and lost the job, which discouraged her for three or four months, but perhaps some day soon she will try something again. Once she acted out so violently that she had to be institutionalized. That is over. Teresa will probably never be a normal adult, but she has come a long way from where she began. And she has put away her puppets.

CHAPTER THIRTEEN

The Orpheus and Eurydice Theme in Psychotherapy

Most of the versions that came down to us from Greek mythology stress the deep commitment of Orpheus to Eurydice, who was taken from him, having been killed through a snake bite. His beautiful poetry and the power of his songs persuaded Persephone and Pluto to release Eurydice from Hades, to return with him to the upper world. But as they are on their way he yields to Eurydice's appeal and turns around, forgetting Pluto's injunction, and thus he loses her forever.

Current versions of this myth read like a cautionary fairy tale and are to remind the Eurydices of our time that forbidden love will be punished; and they are to warn the modern Orpheus that he who yields to plea and helpless passion rather than creating conditions of mature love must fail. Other versions of this myth tell us that the death of Eurydice was caused by the jealous Aristaeus, who reappears then as the killing serpent. Much generic psychological truth in this myth has made it survive even though its specific reinterpretation in modern civilization hints at culture's costly price, that is, the increasing repression of the original struggle, as Freud (1) has elaborated in *Civilization and Its Discontents*.

I wish once more to revive this old tale, but this time as seen through the eyes of a psychotic adolescent girl and her therapist and against the background of a specific transference paradigm.

Teresa Esperanza, who owes this fictitious name to the expression of hope that better treatment techniques can be developed in order to help children and adolescents suffering from schizophrenic disorders and related conditions, is now 20 years of age. She has been in treat-nent with us since the age of 15 as one of the cases of the Project on Childhood Psychosis (2). She is seen in intensive analytic treatment nd the illustrations to be used, excerpts from the tape recordings, are rom the 455th treatment hour. Earlier published communications dealt vith the opening gambit (3); her use of puppet play (4); the nature of the psychotic acting out (5); and her particular use of the delusional reature (6). Work has also been published concerning our contact with he responsible relative and the supporting agencies (7) (Ch. 20, this ol.). Diagnostic studies, based on test material, as well as theoretical onsiderations concerning her notions of inner and outer reality, have lso been part of our research activities (Chapters 2 and 4, this vol.).

Much of her struggle consisted of an attempt to suppress psychotic naterial. The failure of repression expressed itself in her use of avoid-nce, denial, and suppression of the psychotic thought, leading at times o catatoniclike states, to a total inability to meet the tasks of everyday ife. Reconstitutional activities led to childlike behavior, reminding one of an eight-year-old child rather than of a late adolescent.

The attempt to help her create a continuity between the acceptable nd the unacceptable is described in a paper (6) discussing techniques nd suggestions concerning a working alliance, a therapeutic alliance vith the monster—that delusional creature which expresses both disso-iated parts of herself as well as dangerous and forbidden notions about he psychotherapist. While in years past she tried to deal with that reature by urging the therapist to destroy the creature, to not remind ler of him, she has now come to a point of development in the thera-eutic process which permits her to consider the creature a "past hal-ucination," a "crazy thought," which does not really exist, and which s gone forever. But in order to make sure that this thought, that there s a creature outside of her who can persecute and destroy her and kill ler or can force her into forbidden actions and thoughts against her eliefs, can be banned from her mind, she allows herself, from time to ime, to act as if she herself were the creature. This thought, the psy-hotic version of the identification with the aggressor, though a temp-ation for her new-found strength, serving primarily as a defense against he notion that the creature may really exist, is a beginning mastery ver the psychotic content, a step toward the idea that these psychotic houghts are her own and must be integrated with the rest of her ersonality. However, it is not only in the service of adaptation but, at he same time, leads frequently to new regressions, and reminds one f the parental injunction that he who plays with fire is in danger of eing burned. This capacity to cathect the observing function of the go, for her a newly gained acquisition, is like a weak plant. It grows a the hothouse of therapy and undergoes the constant risk of being exposed to the rest of the world where there is no maintenance of tha[t] artificial emotional climate which is necessary to the survival of thi[s] new but still labile function.

Much of this struggle expresses itself in the vicissitudes of the wildl[y] fluctuating psychotic transferences which allow her to see the therapist at times, as the benevolent helper and rescuer who is to bring her bac[k] to the upper world of reality, and, at other times, as the jealous, th[e] destructive and archaic monster, that forerunner of the superego, th[e] creature guided by the talion principle but without reliable capacity t[o] distinguish between self and the world of objects, between inner an[d] outer reality.

A telescoped account of this hour will permit us to revive the ful[l] emotional impact of the encounter and, at the same time, to benefi[t] from this illustration which is to give us insight, in a magnified for[m] indeed, into tactical and strategic problems of analytic work with schizo[-]phrenic adolescents. Their particular struggle, although as human a[s] the struggle of any other patient, because of its tragic enormity, its pow[-]erful exaggerations, will lend itself well to serve as a kind of X-ra[y] view by means of which the hidden anatomy of the therapeutic proces[s] becomes visible to the naked eye.

At the beginning of the hour, Teresa enters the consulting room[,] hardly aware of the therapist, seemingly looking straight through him[.] She struggles to reestablish contact. Her first comments are feeble an[d] unskilled moves by which she tries to pretend to act as if things wer[e] normal and her life were a going and well-controlled concern. Actually she had not been doing more than—to use her own words—"movin[g] around a little bit," "helping the sisters a bit" in the Catholic hom[e] where she is residing now as a boarder, with no work or school pro[-]gram except some token gestures. When it seems that these first fe[w] comments about the realities of her life might become too self-con[-]fronting, she continues as follows:

Patient: Umm, let's see. Let's start talking about something nice, eh.
Therapist: Oh, anything you want. Now remember, you're here to ge[t] well. We don't just have to be pleasant with each other.
P.: Yah.
T.: You tell me anything that is of concern to you, anything you're in[-]terested in.
P.: Well, I feel I'm improving these days. The Creature still bother[s] me, but he bothers me now in a strange way—with a reason. No[t] in a strange way, but with a reason.
T.: I wish he would have reasons because it's much easier to deal wit[h] the Creature when there are reasons.

>.: Now, now it seems he has a reason when he does it. Before he just . . .

C.: What is he telling you?

>.: Well, that if I stop imagining these things and I get these thoughts out of my mind and I just relax and be like anybody else, so, this will all end. It's up to me . . .

C.: That's what he said?

>.: And if I keep on with this being tense, and yes—he doesn't say it, but somehow he, he lets me know. And, but, if I keep getting myself tense and that I don't want to pay attention to what he says 'cause he's telling me the right thing to do, then he'll keep bringing up these things. It's not so bad now.

C.: I think if we can look at the thoughts of the Creature—

>.: It's going away because I keep doing these things and the more I do them, they're vanishing now.

C.: But I think if we can look at the thoughts of the Creature we can then check whether they are good thoughts or bad thoughts. Maybe some are good, maybe some are bad.

>.: Well, you know I have explained to you, um, when I, ah, kind of, um, when the Creature isn't around I want to take his place. Something like that, you know. And other foolish things, other ideas I get of doing things when he's not around. But still he's around and I know it. He says, "Oh, I caught you. If you keep on with that, poor you, I'll keep digging you in. So you better stop that and then I'll leave you alone."

.: You mean—

.: And he'll be mean to me if I'm mean to myself. If I'm nice to myself . . .

.: He tries to be someone who always stops you?

.: He's trying to help me. He's trying to stop me being mean to myself. Because he knows I'm mean to myself.

.: You know, that's nice of him. Except one thing I want to ask you about Teresa.

.: Yeah.

.: You know it's nice that he tries to stop you from being mean to yourself. But I'm worried about one thing.

.: Yeah?

.: Suppose he stops you so much that he stops you from all things you do. You know, if he doesn't know where to draw the line . . .

.: Well, he says, ah, he talks to me not in words but he, he tells me, "You're the one who's trying to stop yourself from everything, from doing everything. But I won't let you do it." And he's trying to do this kind of thing, that pains me and hurts me very much so that I get all these things of wanting to do, you know.

.: You know what I would like to teach the Creature?

.: What?

T.: To know where the line should be drawn. You know, what shoul‹ be stopped and what should not be stopped.

P.: Well, maybe he's just trying to help me and maybe he thinks h‹ draws the right line.

T.: Well, sure, except if he draws the wrong line then he doesn't hel‹ you too well.

P.: Yeah.

T.: Let's say if you are angry with a situation and you say, "Oh, ‹ could really say nasty things to you," that's one thing. But if i‹ your anger you smash a door, that's another thing. And I think i‹ the Creature stops you from smashing a door the Creature woul‹ help you. But if he stops you even from expressing that you a‹ annoyed about something, then he would be wrong. Don't you see‹ There's a line between the two.

P.: I see.

T.: And I'd like to help you and the Creature to find what the lin‹ ought to be.

P.: What if he's trying to help me and he thinks that he's helping m‹ the right way but he's not. I told you that . . .

T.: Yes, but that's where you and I have to force the Creature to le‹ us in on what the line is so we can slowly help him to establish th‹ right line, instead of the wrong line.

That creature, shifting as he does from being a fused figure of threa‹ ening parental introjects and infantile precursors of superego element‹ to one representing more current objects and awareness of expression‹ of self, has recently acquired more up-to-date methods and, at times, ‹ considered a helper, albeit an unreliable ally in the struggle for sel‹ control and self-guidance. Can he be taught to draw the line betwee‹ thought and act, between inner and outer reality? Can Teresa mai‹ tain a stable contact with the therapist? Can she identify sufficientl‹ with his therapeutic efforts, that is, primarily his interpretive work, s‹ that she may acquire stable ego functions? Can he become a stable intr‹ ject leading to her capacity for identification on a higher level instea‹ of having available only primitive mechanisms of incorporation an‹ introjection? The more advanced ego functions are necessary to replac‹ archaic psychotic mechanisms with stable representations of self an‹ object. These new ego functions must take the place of primitive ps‹ chic positions which are but part object and part self-representatio‹ ruling tyrannically a chaotic inner world of uncontrolled impulses an‹ catatoniclike inhibitions.

Teresa seems to ask that question as she ponders the therapist‹ quandary as to whether one can help the creature maintain a line ‹ clear differentiation between a violent act and an angry thought. Sh‹ then returns to considerations of realistic tasks such as keeping certai‹

nterviews with people who might help her, taking an academic school
ourse or learning a simple trade. She complains about being tired of
earing even the slightest criticism from the Sisters, with negative
houghts about one of them particularly, a faint warning to the thera-
ist lest he put too many demands on her. Then therapist and patient
eview together her earlier hospitalization following her aunt's angry
nsistence that she leave the home because of her wild and destructive
exual acting out (5), comparing this with her current ability to main-
ain herself without serious new blowups in the Catholic home for
;irls. In the following dialogue, she plays with the idea of being like
he Sisters, a fantasy role that is opposed to her desires for a romantic
nvolvement. She also sees the Sisters, themselves, as being opposed to
his kind of involvement. Only recently she had been engaged in an
bortive attempt at a sexual relationship with a young colored man who
rightened her immensely, as do intruding fantasies about the therapist.
he was forced to use the Sisters as protectors while, at the same time,
he also saw them as standing in the way of her wish toward her pro-
essed desire for this young man and for the transference wishes he
epresents. The following interchange alludes to it and could be under-
tood as the day residue giving rise to the later development of the
naterial just as the day residue creates the raw material for the dream.

T.: After you got out of the hospital, and after you left the home of
your aunt, I wondered whether you were going to last very long
in that Catholic home.
P.: Yeah, I wondered, too.
T.: Didn't you wonder, too?
P.: Umhmm.
T.: I wondered whether you can behave so we could keep you there or
whether there was going to be a new blowup.
P.: No, no, no.
T.: But I guess you think that you're going to make it.
P.: Yeah, yeah, heh, year. No, it's not so bad.
T.: I was thinking the other day about it, you know, because we had
no, we really have no move left after that. But you made it, and I
think you had a few incidents at the home, isn't that true? It got a
little upsetting, but nothing too serious.
P.: Ahhum. No.
T.: So Sister E. and you—you think she's a little too fat.
P.: Little too fat. (*Giggles*)
T.: And it looks like you are afraid for her so she loses a little weight.
P.: Nah.
T.: No?
P.: No. I can't do nothing with that.
T.: But I guess she's a nice person essentially.

P.: Umhum. Umhum.

T.: Even though she makes you angry sometimes.

P.: Why do you say sexually?

T.: I said "essentially." I didn't think of it "sexually."

P.: Oh, essentially.

T.: I couldn't quite imagine . . .

P.: Oh, pardon me.

T.: I said essentially.

P.: Pardon me. (Giggles)

T.: What would sex have to do with a Sister?

P. (Giggles): Let's not . . .

T.: Let's not mention it. It's enough it has to do with you. These Sisters have many prayers so they won't have to think of that.

P.: Oah. (Yawns) And if they weren't Sisters and then they would get married and it would be all right to dream about it.

T.: Right. But the way Sisters live now they are not supposed to get married.

P.: The way they live now they're not supposed to get married?

T.: I mean, Sisters, nuns, are not supposed to get married.

P.: No, of course not. If I would become a nun . . .

T.: So they better not think of sex.

P.: When I used to dream being a nun—that wasn't the only thing, I was dreaming of being other things, too. I was, but I noticed that if . . .

T.: If you are a nun you can never allow a man to touch you.

P.: That's right. But if I would become a nun I would just . . .

T.: You would have to accept that.

P.: Yeah.

T.: Sort of forget about sex. Or just think about it.

P.: Yah, but I don't know if I want to get married either. I don't know.

T.: Well, when you would be a happy healthy girl you might want to get married. Some girls do.

P.: I don't know. Yeah. Maybe later I'll decide.

T.: You've got plenty of time.

P.: Ahhum.

T.: Because if you got married right now it would be like in one of these movies that you told me about. It wouldn't be a very good marriage. Probably blow, blow, blow. But you don't know what's going to blow.

P.: I wouldn't be blowing all the time. (Giggles)

T.: Well, or a blow on the head. Well, here's Teresa, who doesn't know if she should become a Sister or get married.

P.: Well . . .I'm trying to think about something. There's a movie remember, I was going to talk to you about.

At this moment she disrupts the conversation, loses contact with the therapist, changes the subject and tries to remember a movie. This

ortured attempt to recall the picture is like an attempt to recall a
ream, an attempt to return to her inner conflict. The screen play
erves as a borrowed fantasy which seems to fit the inner dilemma. The
orgetting of that fantasy is a defense against awareness of that unre-
olved internal civil war. It is actually a description of her awareness
f the lack of object and self-constancy, her self-observation of loss of
elf and objects and her struggle against reconstitution. The therapist
ad not seen this particular movie, and perhaps fortunately so, since
hus we may observe his own struggle, as well, as he tries to regain
ontact with the patient and to enter her inner world without knowing
he play's plot which is to allude to the patient's current inner battle.
et us see how she recaptures the memory of the movie which turns
ut to be her quasi dream, her living nightmare. Her first attempt to
ecall the story's hero makes her think of Little Black Sambo, who
as afraid that he would be eaten by the tigers, only to eat them him-
elf after they melted into butter, having been turned into harmless
nd tamed creatures which could be incorporated without danger.

.: Well . . . I'm trying to think about something. There's a movie,
   remember, I was going to talk to you about.

.: A movie you saw?

.: Yah. I want to talk about it. Remember I said so?

.: Yes, you did mention a movie, but you know, you're an old movie
   goer. You see so many movies I never know which you have in
   mind. What has that movie to do with?

. (Long pause): With going to heaven. Something like that. At the
   end the two angels fly to heaven because before they came down
   to earth they were angels and then God decided, well, from angels
   they'll become human beings. And when they die they'll become
   angels again and then come back to heaven where they were before.
   So in the meantime, because I believe, I used to believe these things
   and imagine them, I think, before a human being would come to
   the world while he would be in heaven, that he would be maybe
   air, that he would be an angel. When he would come to the world
   he would be a human being either or he would be an animal or a
   plant, or, you know. And then the human being would go, he
   would be an angel again. So now . . . yeah, I told you about this
   movie I was going to talk to you about. But, you see, I have it
   written on my list too. And I think it's a kind of a movie may be
   you saw. It's about, ah, it takes place in, ah ummm.

.: Where does it take place?

.: . . . in Rio de Janeiro.

.: In South America.

.: Yes.

.: That's a beautiful city, Rio de Janeiro.

P.: Yah. That's where it took place. You know, I was surprised. Th
first time I saw that movie it was one night, the girls were in th
TV room and this movie starts and they start playing this strang
music with drums and the women were walking around and kin
of wiggling and dancing and carrying things on their heads.
thought it was, how they live in the jungle, or in Africa, that's wha
I thought it was about. And later I walk in, when the movie kin
of started, or a little after it started, it keeps on, and I walk in.
was curious to see what it was about, you know. And then, I hadn'
noticed that it took place in Rio de Janeiro, but the second tim
when I saw the movie I saw it when it started again. That was
movie they had shown for over a week. And then the girls tell m
at the end, while I was watching it, it took place there. And I wa
surprised, I didn't know. And, um, it was kind of sad, you know
Starts kind of happy.

T.: Starts happy, like a nightclub or something, isn't that it? Dancin
women.

P.: Kind of . . . like a nightclub (*laughs*). More than a nightclub.

T.: Well, there are women dancing and wiggling.

P. (*Giggles*): Yeah. Well, they used to sing and fly. They used to
they thought they were in heaven and they could be free and fl
through the sky and the clouds. Of course, they were free. Bu
they weren't in heaven either, you know. They were happy ever
day. Every day they had a carnival.

T.: They could have nothing but carnivals and enjoy each other. Hov
did it turn out?

P.: They had carnivals every day, they had parties every day. Every da
they roamed around the streets getting together and singing an
dancing and laughing. Every day they seemed to be happy.

T.: Sounds like one big party.

P.: And there was a little stream up in the mountains, in the hill
where a bunch of poor people lived, poor people, you know, anc
um, when I mention the movie it makes me feel terrible.

T.: Really?

P.: Well, not exactly, but ah . . .

T.: Something bad must have happened in the movie.

P.: Oh. Of course.

T.: Would you like to tell me?

P.: So that word, ah, maybe you've heard of the movie, um, means lik
Little Black Sambo, you know, but it isn't Little Black Sambo. I
was like Big Black Sambo. Not Big Black Sambo though, no
Mambo, Mambo was . . .

T.: Maybe Big Black Sambo Little.

P.: Um, no.

T.: Must have gotten after a girl.

P.: This wasn't Sambo, this was, um, what was his name? I forget hi
name now. Black Cavern, something like Black Cavern, or . . .

T.: What did he do? Did he go after a girl?

P.: Ummm . . . Black Orpheus.

T.: Black Orpheus. Now, I have heard about that.

P.: Ah, I thought you had. Did you see the movie?

T.: No, but I've heard about it. I would have some idea of what there was in it.

P.: Yeah. Did you hear that it was sad though?

T.: Yes, it was a sad story.

P.: See, they were showing it in a theater near where I live and I kept passing by and they kept showing it and the title "Black Orpheus," I didn't know what it meant. I thought Orpheus meant a bunch of people, black color, black skin.

T.: No, Orpheus is an old name. It's a name from a Greek myth, an old Greek story.

P.: A Greek story.

T.: The Greeks had a story that was called "Orpheus and Eurydice."

P.: Then who were they, the . . .

T.: Well, Orpheus was a happy fellow who found a nymph once, whose name was Eurydice. He found her in the woods, a lovely girl.

P.: He found her in the woods?

T.: Yes. That's the old story, it goes that way. And they danced around and they had many happy days. Except that one day a snake bit her. She died and she came into the underworld. But what did that make Orpheus do in your story?

P.: No, the girls told me, Stella, you know, she said there did exist long ago a queen, I think she told me, a queen, and her name was Eurydice. She was a queen. That's all. She didn't tell me the rest.

T.: Is that the story that took place in that town in the south? You just spoke of Rio de Janeiro.

P.: Yeah.

T.: That's where Black Orpheus took place.

P.: Yeah, but this other Orpheus and Eurydice—was he black, and she was black, too?

T.: No, not in the Greek story. They were Greeks, they were . . .

P.: No.

T.: . . . light-skinned people.

P.: Yah. She was white, she was white, and they both were white.

T.: But what happened in your movie with Eurydice?

P.: But you said she went in the forest and the snake bit her.

T.: They were in the forest and they were engaged in love play. They loved each other very much.

P.: And they used to roam around in the forest.

T.: They used to roam around in the forest and the snake bit her and she died.

P.: But what did the snake . . . That's what happened to Cleopatra!! She killed herself at the end. She was beautiful, too.

T.: Yes.

P.: She took this snake because they wanted to kill her, all the bad soldiers, they wanted to kill Anthony, Marc Anthony. And he killed himself also, with a knife, and she killed herself, she . . .

T.: That's true.

P.: . . . took a snake that she kept in a basket and she let it bite her. But you know snakes have poison in them, it's the . . .

T.: Yes.

P.: . . . the most disgusting thing. That's what I did to myself. Remember? Long ago. Remember?

T.: What did you do?

P.: Well, don't you know?

T.: What?

P.: I told you.

T.: You did, but I forgot.

P.: Well, I took poison. I took poison. But I didn't take a little. I took plenty. But you don't believe me yet, do you?

T.: I believe that.

P.: No, you don't have to believe me, if this sounds like a make-believe story, sounds as if I'm making it up. But I'm not. I wish I could tell the whole world that it's true. But nobody could believe me. It's hard. Mysteries do exist.

T.: You have no idea how much I do believe you.

P.: I have no idea. Maybe one day I'll notice it because I really can't see it. I really think that, ah, that you're just being, you want to be sweet to believe me, you're pretending to.

T.: You still don't know . . .

P.: 'Cause if you wouldn't really believe me you would hurt my feelings and you'd say, "Poor Teresa." I don't want . . .

T.: Teresa, I don't mind hurting your feelings if it helps us. I don't mind hurting your feelings. You know, you're a big girl, you can stand a little hurting. It's like when you go . . .

P. (Shouting): But nobody knows . . .

T.: When you go to the dentist, can't you stand a little pain? When the dentist works on your teeth?

P.: You start talking about these stories and I mention a story and I start thinking about myself and I'm so scared that I don't know. (Sobbing) I don't know who I am. I don't know what I'm doing in the world, why I keep walking around. I don't know why I'm alive. I'm supposed to be dead. Why am I alive if I'm supposed to be dead?

T.: Because I want to make you completely alive.

P.: It's just like if the devil came and he killed me. Well, I know the devil and I killed myself. I don't know why. I didn't know what I was doing. I just didn't know.

T.: Do you know the story of Eurydice?

P.: Well, somebody killed her. But she really died. But in my case I really didn't die. I died and I lived and I came back to life. Both things at the same time.

`.: But that's what happened to Eurydice.

`.: Wha-a-t?

`.: In the Greek story.

`.: Oh, tell me, tell me.

`.: I wanted to tell you.

`.: Go on. And then I'll tell you . . .

`.: Do you know that Eurydice in the Greek story . . .

`.: That's why I'm lost, because . . .

`.: . . . goes into the underworld . . .

.: After the snake, right?

`.: . . . where the dead people are. And Orpheus is grief-stricken because he loves her very much. And he was also known because he could play an instrument, a lyre.

.: A guitar.

`.: What would be like a guitar, but a Greek, a Greek lyre, you know. He went down and he sang to the god of the underworld.

`.: What's the god of the underworld?

`.: There was a god in the underworld, in Hades, you know. He sang to him and he told him please, let me take Eurydice back to the world, because she was a good girl. It was just a tough break she had with that snake, you know. She went around barefoot instead of wearing something. In those days the girls went around barefoot.

`.: Well, those snakes. I could have twisted its neck off before it bit her.

`.: Well, you know what the god said, he said you can take Eurydice back to life.

`.: The god said . . .

`.: He said that, yes. "But you must learn one thing."

.: Well, of course.

`.: He said, "You must learn . . .

.: But then he would have to die one day, too, so don't worry, dear.

`.: No, he said . . .

`.: He said, "You will all have to die. You think she's the only one who will have to die. One day the whole world will end and that's when everybody floated away." No.

`.: But that's not what the god said to Orpheus.

`. (Laughs): No, but if he could have said that Orpheus would have understood better.

The screen play, *Black Orpheus*, leads her to a core conflict. The observer of the movie cannot maintain the position of a distant spectator and the account of the plot becomes a powerful autobiography, albeit one in which the biographer reexperiences rather than recounts. She is reminded of Cleopatra who kills herself and drives Anthony to suicide; she becomes Eurydice who is lost and dead, who pleads and begs for

rescue and who sees the rescuer as the helpless Orpheus who must yiel
to temptation which will destroy him as well; and she sees him also a
the hateful and jealous Aristaeus, the snake man, who must kill th
woman who spurned him in an everlasting nightmarish pursuit.

Teresa describes the violent transference struggle in which the d
fense against dangerous transference love and hate, the discovery o
sexual wishes as well as homicidal impulses toward the therapist,
psychic death, the closing of the sluices of motility, the draining o
affect, the catatoniclike withdrawal, the lack of contact, the inability t
use insights toward mastery of actuality. This psychic death is th
equivalent of suicidal and homicidal impulses fused in a schizophreni
world destruction fantasy.

While in this particular account Teresa sees death as a psychologica
inability to move, to experience herself, she has previously repeatedl
played out and acted out, and seriously so, homicidal and suicidal im
pulses. The delusional fantasy of self-poisoning and the actual sel
destructive events described elsewhere (5), were frequently almo
undifferentiated.

What are the technical problems of the therapist? He sees Teresa
like Eurydice, gravitating between the position in the upper world an
the one in Hades, the underworld. As she slowly recathects reality, th
positive aspects of the transference, he helps her move toward a mo
mature position. He is not Orpheus who is driven to rescue the gir
but he knows he is so in the mind of the patient. He knows that suc
patients must go through an endless repetition, as part of the workin
through process, of going to and from the two positions; the back an
forth between Pluto and Orpheus; the demands of the Thanatos an
the Eros principles. The fluctuations of the psychotic process provok
overoptimism as well as hate in the countertransference. Can he avoi
repeating the mistakes of Orpheus? Let us follow Teresa and her docto
once more and see whether he can or should; whether the disappointe
love of Orpheus must be paralleled by the therapist's technical failui
or helplessness.

T.: In the Greek story, now, what the god said to Orpheus was that
    you do not turn around, meaning if you are patient and if you ca
    wait and if you're not hasty, and you go step by step and you hav
    lots of patience, then you can make her alive. That was the stor
    So Orpheus . . .
P.: That's what I'm doing. Look what God did to me, he did the sam
    thing. He brought me to life, because I did the right thing.
T.: That's right.
P.: Because I'm innocent. I didn't do nothing wrong.
T.: You know what I learned . . .

°.: I didn't mean to kill myself, and well, he knows me, he knows me.

°.: You know what . . .

°.: See, nobody else knows me but him, nobody. I know what he has in mind, anyway, about me.

°.: But Teresa, you know what I learned about that story?

°.: I follow him.

°.: . . . what I learned from that story?

°.: What? What?

°.: I learned this—that you must learn something, I must learn something from Orpheus.

°.: Did she come back to life anyway?

°.: Well, let me tell you. I learned something from Orpheus.

°.: Ahhuh.

°.: And that is, if I want to be a good doctor to people who are dead . . .

°.: Umhum.

°.: . . . but could be alive, then I have to lead the way and I shouldn't lose patience, and I shouldn't turn around, and I shouldn't become bossy, and I shouldn't be impatient, and if I can go straight on regardless of what I hear, regardless of what these patients tell me, like Eurydice, you know, whether they cry or complain or holler or laugh or sing—I should be willing to listen to everything—but not turn around. And if I don't turn around I can bring them back to life and those who are dead people . . .

°.: That's me, let me not turn around.

°.: I won't turn around.

°. (Sobbing): You know, I don't want to be half-dead and half-alive. It scares me. I feel like a ghost. And one day if everybody notices that I'm a ghost, they're gonna faint. They're going to come in and ask me. "What are you doing here? Why aren't you under the ground and dead in the grave?" What am I going to answer?

°.: You know what I . . .

°.: I want to be completely alive again, live in the world. Oh . . .

°.: You know what you . . .

°.: . . . boy. Well, a person like that has to be lost in his life. Before I was lost, when I was a child, but now I'm more lost than I was before, because of that.

°.: You know what you could answer?

°.: Nobody knows I'm dead. Nobody knows. That priest didn't believe me. I tried to tell him it's true. He said, "Oh, that's impossible. What are you talking about, child? Of course, mysteries exist, but not that kind of a mystery. God would never create that kind of a mystery. That you are alive—the moment you die you become alive again? Immediately? And, then you are both dead and alive." "Well," he said, "my child, I can see you're alive. I don't see you're dead. You breathe, you talk, you move. What's dead about you?" And I asked him, "Well, don't you think I smell like a dead person?" "Of course not. I think you smell all right." You know, I tried to give him a lot of explanations but he didn't agree. He kept saying no, he thought I was, he kept saying it's all in my mind, I'm imagining it. Nope. I'm not. It's true.

T.: But Teresa, if I had been you, I would have said to the priest. "You have forgotten to believe in miracles. But I am a doctor who knows the story of Orpheus, and who has learned from Orpheus that the only way to make Eurydice alive is to not turn around. If you believe in her . . .

P.: That's what happened in this movie. That God-damned Orpheus. He heard Eurydice's voice and one day he, let me tell you this part, one day, after he had lost her, he went looking everywhere for her and he asked everybody. And he went through an old building and he asked a man where she could be. And he said, I have no idea but let me take you to a place where there are people who —ah, spirits of the dead people come into them and they react in such a way, you know what I mean, these kind of places?

T.: Yes.

P.: He went there, and there, at the end, he heard this woman talking and she had the voice of Eurydice. And Eurydice was in her, her spirit, you know, like someone possessed by the dead one? That's a horrible movie I saw long ago, possessed by the dead. Ughh. I don't want to talk about that though. Well, Eurydice started telling him, you know, he didn't even notice, he just heard her voice first then she kept telling him; "Orpheus," she started yelling to him, and, "Come to me," and, "I'm here." And she said, "If you turn back you'll never see me again. So don't look back." And he asked "Why shouldn't I look back?" "Because you'll lose me forever." "No, don't go." And she says, "Oh, but you will lose me forever my butterfly boy, if you turn back." (Laughs) So, then, finally later he does turn back while he was there, he turns back.

T.: You know what the trouble with Orpheus was? He was so eager to touch her, he wanted the girl, he turned around, and the girl who was not yet fully alive . . .

P.: Yeah, but this Eurydice in the story, she was so pretty.

T.: Yes, I know. But if he had not turned around, he would have gotten her and the way to do that is . . .

P.: She was as innocent as me. And as sweet as me. That's for sure.

T.: But Teresa, if someone is half-dead, you don't touch them.

P. (Shouts): Well, I'm half-dead. So don't touch me. If not, I'll die altogether and you'll faint.

T.: I'm not going to touch you.

P.: Oh, I'm afraid I'll die altogether. Either I'll die or I want to come back to life altogether.

T.: I'm not going to turn around. I'm going to listen.

P.: Well, call for Orpheus and maybe he'll bring me back to life.

T.: I am Orpheus. I am Dr. Orpheus.

P.: No you're not Orpheus.

.: I'm not that Orpheus.
.: You're not Dr. Orpheus. You're Dr. Rudolf Ekstein.
.: That's right, that's . . .
.: Okay.
.: I'm not going to turn around.
.: If you were Orpheus I would want to see you black because I like Black Orpheus. He was good looking and he was black, too. He was a blue prince.
.: I am the white Dr. Orpheus.
.: Okay, so you're not him.
.: Can't we talk about that next time a little more?

The therapist must realize that in analytic work with patients, neurotic or psychotic, transferences cannot and must not be manipulated. Transferences are but the patient's as yet dim vision, via the psychic mamentarium he has available, of earlier unconscious situations recreated in the present and projected onto the therapist. This vision in the case of a psychotic patient is experienced more like a religious visitation, a kind of reexperiencing with a minimum of maintained reflection. Teresa not only experiences endless self-torture, psychic death and then the slow and painful reconstituting of more advanced psychic organization, but she reexperiences the splitting of self as well as the splitting of object. The therapist is seen not only as Orpheus but also as Pluto. He is the powerful representative of life and love, the hapless and impatient lover who does not heed Pluto; and he is also the jealous, vengeful Aristaeus, and he cannot, and actually should not, prevent it. As Teresa moves back and forth between Pluto and Orpheus, the therapist must understand that he is assigned both roles, and often simultaneously so, in the vicissitudes of this transference battle. A part of the patient's chance for recovery lies in the therapist's capacity to accept both assigned roles—the twin expressions of overt ambivalence. Saint George was challenged to kill the dragon. Eurydice pleads with Orpheus to kill the snake man; and Teresa begs the therapist to kill the Creature, to forget him, not to mention him. But there is no psychic growth without the full working-through of the unconscious conflict. Saint George needs his dragon. Orpheus needs Pluto. Eurydice needs both Orpheus and Pluto as she does Persephone and Demeter. Teresa needs her Creature. The therapist needs to accept his double role if he is to sustain the process. Neither of the great protagonists can be destroyed. They can only change as the work toward a synthesis—the emergence of new ego functions which allow new conflict solutions—proceeds. Interpretations, on whatever level the patient can use them, are the main tools of the therapist in this seemingly endless, and frequently experienced as hopeless, struggle toward higher integration.

We may raise the question as to whether Teresa will ever be abl to harness and to synthesize the forces of love and hate, of Eros an Thanatos, of life and death. This question is presently beyond ou predictive capacity. The blending of a firm therapeutic commitment an a deep scientific interest creates the will, guided by some insights int the transference and resistance struggles of Teresa, but not as yet th certainty of therapeutic success.

As I reflect wistfully on this long-range endeavor, I am guided bac to Freud who ended his volume, *Civilization and Its Discontents* (1) with this comment on mankind's struggle:

"The fateful question for the human species seems to me to b whether and to what extent their cultural development will succee in mastering the disturbance of their communal life by the huma instinct of aggression and self-destruction. It may be that in thi respect precisely the present time deserves a special interest. Me have gained control over the forces of nature to such an extent tha with their help they would have no difficulty in exterminating on another to the last man. They know this, and hence comes a larg part of their current unrest, their unhappiness and their mood c anxiety. And now it is to be expected that the other of the tw 'Heavenly Powers,' eternal Eros, will make an effort to assert hin self in the struggle with his equally immortal adversary. But wh can foresee with what success and with what result?"

REFERENCES

1. FREUD, SIGMUND (1930). Civilization and Its Discontents. *Standard Editio* 21:64-145, 1961.
2. MEYER, MORTIMER & CARUTH, ELAINE, eds. Project on Childhood Psychosis *Reiss-Davis Clin. Bull.* 1:54-106, 1964.
3. EKSTEIN, RUDOLF. The Opening Gambit in Psychotherapeutic Work with Se verely Disturbed Adolescents. *Amer. J. Orthopsychiat.* 33:862-871, 1963.
4. ————. Puppet Play of a Psychotic Adolescent Girl within the Psychothera peutic Process. *Psa. Study of the Child* 20:441-480, 1965.
5. —— & CARUTH, ELAINE. Royal Road or Primrose Path: Psychotic Acting Ou In *Children of Time and Space, of Action and Impulse,* Rudolf Ekstein, ed New York: Appleton-Century-Crofts, 1966.
6. —— & ——. The Working Alliance with the Monster. *Bull. Menninger Clin* 29:189-197, 1965.
7. ————. Discussion of "Psychological Effects on the Child Raised by a Older Sibling" by Milton Rosenbaum. *Amer. J. Orthopsychiat.* 33:518-520 1963.

CHAPTER FOURTEEN

Object Constancy and Psychotic Reconstruction*

There is a tide in the affairs of men,
Which, taken at the flood, leads on to fortune;
Omitted, all the voyage of their life
Is bound in shallows and in miseries.

SHAKESPEARE

When Teresa Esperanza, our patient, was a little girl less than ten years of age, she lived with her maiden aunt in a swank apartment on the Paseo de la Reforma in Mexico City, near the Statue of Independence. She loved that monument and its golden angel on top which had been shattered into many pieces during one of the violent earthquakes but was now completely restored and as good as new, at least on its shiny and glittering surface.

That was between 1956 and 1958, years before she started treatment at the Reiss-Davis Child Study Center. Later, when psychotherapy became a desperate necessity, her aunt gave a vivid description, a condensed account of the child's life at that time. The aunt had given the child a charming little poodle which they owned for about two years. Teresa gave the dog the name Trampa, the Spanish equivalent of Tramp, the Disney character in the movie *The Lady and the Tramp*. The dog had been bought originally because Teresa had wanted

---

* Seymour Friedman is the co-author of this chapter.

179

a dog, but soon, without anybody knowing why, the animal became attached to the aunt. Recently Teresa told her aunt how she had threatened the dog by making motions to throw him out of the ten-story apartment window right on the Paseo de la Reforma and had dashed the animal's body against the tile floor; that she got on the floor and devoured his food; and when this had become uncomfortable, she had deprived the dog of his raw meat, taken it to the table, and eaten it like a dog. All these observations helped Teresa's aunt to real-ize how ill the child had been. The aunt found herself devoted to the little animal and she recounts how, some two years later, this dog died in Ecuador, having caught a fish hook in its throat when he was on a boat as they were out fishing with Teresa and her little cousins. He was rushed, not to a veterinarian, but to regular doctors because every-one was so devoted to him. It was Sunday and the animal was hospi-talized in a regular hospital, where he died from the effects of anes-thesia after the surgeon had removed the hook.

At the time of this interview, the social worker* had felt that the aunt's awareness of the child's deepening illness was covered with a deep distrust of doctors who cannot help.

For our present purposes, though, we want to take these observa-tions as a quasi-independent account of an adult observer who thus describes to us the strange love-hate relationship that Teresa developed toward the little animal. We are thus in possession of an observed fact, an actual episode of that phase of the child's life, a piece of personal history, a fragment of a continuum in the life of an individual who struggles with the problem of *acquiring constant self and object repre-sentation*, of restoring some continuity in her life by means of restitu-tive processes, the *psychotic patient's equivalent of reconstructive activity* (2).

In this paper we shall follow Teresa and her therapist through two sessions, treatment hours 578 and 580, to observe the specific psychic work she must accomplish in order to re-establish her relationship with him each hour, to restore the continuity of her life by gaining access to memories until then unavailable and dreaded, to make these memo-ries serve the selective purpose of restoring object and self constancy, and of regaining the capacity to function in her current situation.

If we were to analyze a dream, we would try to move from the manifest content of the dream to its latent meaning. In this specific example, we have put the latent meaning ahead when we described the murderous situation between her and the dog. We now return to the actual psychotherapeutic material in order to show how this psychotic

---

* We are grateful to Mrs. Beatrice Cooper for the use of her records.

girl's mind works its way from the current psychotic life situation to the restoration of appropriate memory, and how we attempted to bring this process about.

Teresa came to the 578th interview* about half an hour late. She had canceled her two preceding appointments by telephone. The patient started the hour acting apologetic. She feared that she had disappointed the therapist, referred to the weather and complained of the heat and mugginess. Her manner was that of a petulant, frightened, reluctant girl on a date, deeply involved in a silent love relationship, with a passionate yearning for the lover to whom she cannot and dare not openly confess her need, but to whom she can only make protests, irritated excuses, and complaints of discomfort, and finally end up with the impulse to escape and postpone the contact for another day. She can remain committed to therapy only if she dictates its structure and has the freedom and power not to turn the relationship into therapy, but to make a safe situation for therapy. Although the patient sought to convey that this contact was more like a casual chance meeting in the street that began with chit-chat and irritated complaints about the heat and muggy weather, she inwardly yearned, as well as feared, to restore the love relationship with the therapist and to confess that she loved him, yet could not see what he looked like and what he really was.

The therapist endeavored to convert this brief encounter into a therapeutic session by reacting to her comments about the weather as a metaphoric expression of her inner and outer psychological and emotional climate, and by attempting to re-establish the severed contact from the last therapy session. He reminded her of her intent at the end of the last hour to relate something important to him in the next session. This led Teresa to her customary borrowed fantasy from a TV show, her characteristic mode of reconstituting the transference by love-hate relationships, and her defensive and adaptive establishment of optimum distance to withstand maximum closeness.

Teresa related her fantasy version borrowed from a film depicting the destruction of Pompeii by volcanic eruption and devastating earthquakes. Her account revealed her confusion and vagueness regarding details, facts, and persons involved, reflecting her tremendous inner anxiety and lowered intellectual functioning, as well as communicating the subordinate relevance of the content of the fantasy to its transference meaning and purpose. As if in a hypnotic trance, she essentially gave this account to the therapist.

Somewhere in a park in the vicinity of what she identifies as a plane-

* Previous accounts of our work with Teresa appear in Ekstein (2), and Chapter 13, this volume.

tarium in Los Angeles (actually her misinterpretation of the TV show —a misconception in the service of recollection of aspects of her own life and the transference position), a street sweeper, cleaning up a mess rummaging in the sand for trash, comes upon a stone hand which turns out to be part of a statue of a Roman soldier dating back to the ruins of Pompeii, buried under volcanic lava. As the statue is removed via truck to a museum it comes to life, becomes violently destructive and murderous, and has to be restrained and confined. The therapist's interventive comment during the patient's account of the story, that this story impressed him so much in demonstrating that there was no protection against danger in being a lifeless statue, since it became alive and angry and could do great harm, brought from the patient the retort that it was a ghost from the past, and that after the orgy of killing either to comply with or to escape from the vengeful, destructive wrath of the people, it walked into the ocean and slowly began to vanish and disappear, as it seemed to melt into the water. The therapist's repeated attempts to focus her attention on his interpretation of its meaning and relevance for her identification with the immobile, lifeless statue and her fear of her own anger, destructiveness, and consequent self-destruction are countered by her own need to control the interpersonal process and the therapist's participation by her repeated interruptions.

She continued by enumerating a variety of factual details, in this way warding off the therapist's interpretative intervention and explanation of the fantasy and its relatedness to her life because she herself had experienced a catastrophe, like an earthquake. After again interrupting his attempts to explain her need to be lifeless and immobilized, she remembered having been in a terrifying earthquake in Mexico, followed by an agonizing nightmare in which she desperately but unsuccessfully tried to awaken the aunt in order to be comforted and protected. The nightmare had ended in the death of the aunt, the dog, and herself, as well as the destruction and collapse of the building.

The therapist successfully continued his effort to explain her need to be a lifeless, immobile statute, paralyzed for work, school, and other normal activities, out of fear that, alive and active, she could become destructive and harmful and make other people angry with her, wanting to destroy her in their vengeful wrath. As a lifeless statue, paralyzed and harmless, she remains safe and at peace, a good girl who is not angry and who is even enshrined eternally in a museum. She appeared to accept the interpretation, as well as the therapist's reaffirmation of his wish to help her so that her mind and body can be safeguarded from both outside and inside earthquakes, but she ended by wanting to re-

ate a spooky love story which she promised to tell from the beginning
in the next session. The love story ended with the danger that the girl
would vanish into the sea together with the restored lover from the
past, but she is saved by the police as the deadly lover disappears.

Teresa's fantasy communicates her explanation, justification, and
rationalization of her inability to come to this hour on time and to
enter actively and openly into its therapeutic purpose and goals, just
as her whole life has been confined to a paralytic stalemate of active-
passive ego inactivity and expectant waiting (3). In the fantasy she
inadvertently reveals her theory regarding her *lack of object and self
constancy*: that it is the consequence of a violent and catastrophic blow
from the outside, as if she had been trapped in a vise by an accident of
fate and of nature—a grandiose and omnipotent rationale to restore
self-esteem in the infantile experience of complete helplessness and impotence, loss of control and of self-esteem. The patient's theory and rationale, however, succeed no more in restoring her self-esteem than the
interpretative activity of the therapist, who attempts, via interpretation*
to establish or re-establish the effective functioning of the mind and
with it object constancy as well as constancy of the therapeutic process
and of the therapist as the object.

Via the metaphor of digging in the ruins and cleaning up the mess,
the patient permits re-establishment of the therapeutic situation, re-
constitutes the object, restores the past and its reservoir of old objects,
presumably dead, lifeless, and buried. Thus, in her varied and apparently distant, irrelevant, and trivial communications, equivalent to the
fragments, stones, and trash of the fantasy, the patient provides us with
her imagery that becomes the psychoanalytic tool for reconstitution of
objects, past and current, and furnishes the deceptive façade concealing
the past and its relationship to the live and lived-out process in the
current relationship with the therapist.

The themes of identity formation and object constancy run through
and are dealt with in the patient's material. The therapist is regarded
as a god of Roman antiquity who creates the weather, to whom the

---

* Psychotherapy can become addicted to the explanatory function of the interpretation which unsuccessfully attempts and only deceptively appears to restore self-
esteem and object constancy. For purposes of productive research and incentive, we
must resolve to give up *explanation constancy* as a condition both of research and
therapeutic activity, with the conviction that the objective of psychotherapy and of
our research is not to explain but to understand the working of the mind and of
the therapeutic process. Interpretation facilitates contact, process, and object relationships, and therefore creates object constancy; explanation provides quasi-mastery,
disrupts contact in process, and fosters object separation rather than constancy, establishes the omnipotence of the therapist, and may, in the total process, impede the
formation of mutuality.

patient responds by bringing her irritated, depressed complaints of dis
comfort and fear. The reconstitution of the object of the therapis
permits the emergence of archaic shadowy memories and affective ex
periences out of which the therapy relationship arises. Rather than
recalling, talking about, and reflecting upon the theme, the patient live:
out the problem of object constancy with the therapist in the present
For psychotic and borderline patients, object constancy is externall:
represented by their content in whatever form of ideation, whether o
love, politics, films, trash or weather, that serves to maintain the contac
with the therapist. Contact between patient and therapist constitute
the agent of both inner and outer negotiation and interaction, out o
which emerges the psychological construct of object constancy. And
just as the agent for contact can be represented by any communication
each of equal value, so can the object remain constant yet be repre
sented by the opposite images of the warrior hero of Roman imperia
grandeur with a sword in his hand, or by the clean-up man who gather
up the trash with a broom and shovel in his hand.

In a normal or less disturbed personality development, founded o:
more stable and reliable object constancy, object and self are in mu
tually accepting relationship to each other, surviving changes in role:
and adapting to each other in whatever role each may appear. I:
psychotic and borderline patients the relationship between object and
self remains not mutual but antithetical and reciprocal, in which botl
together form a unit and can survive in a united relationship only i
a rigid equilibrium is maintained in which the net change is zero, and
the equilibrium of the combined forces remains static and immutable
As on a teetertotter or seesaw, the equilibrium of the closed system mus
remain unchanged so that, if one goes down, the other must go up. I:
one member is active and alive, the other must remain inactive and
lifeless. If one is omnipotent, the other must remain impotent. If one
becomes too much alive, the other must die; if one is active, the
other must remain passive. In the archaic reciprocal autistic-symbiotic
relationship, the equilibrium can be maintained only by following the
dictum, "You do what I tell you, no more and no less." So it is witl
the internal equilibrium reached by the various roles comprising the
object. The world as extension of self and as object responds to the
psychotic patient as he manipulates its roles. If the world as objec:
becomes alive, it becomes dangerous and has to be returned to the
world of the dead via the omnipotent, delusional power of the psychotic
ego to perceive in a manner that serves its needs for survival, or the
self must become dead. To remain constant and to retain self and ob
ject in equilibrium, one of them must be dead. In the therapeutic
struggle the therapeutic goal is lost in the battle of quasi-self-constancy

which can be achieved only by wiping out the object. Yet, conversely, the only means of keeping the therapeutic relationship and process alive is by maintaining this equilibrium between live and dead partners, active and passive participants.

The problem of object constancy in the psychotic and borderline patient lies in this closed struggle between motion and stagnancy. We usually attribute the disturbance to the psychotic patient feeling threatened by the omnipresent, persistent, and fluctuating loss of object, the ever-present threat of loss of object constancy. What we begin to see, however, as a *core problem* is the rigid persistence and implacable constancy of the destructive, dangerous object (having grown out of negative introjects), which by its danger to the ego and patient and world must constantly be destroyed lest it destroy. Life destroys and must in turn be destroyed. Only in psychic death and lifelessness can object constancy be maintained.

Object constancy is not to be understood in terms of the fixed, permanent position of the object in time or space as external fixtures that can be identified in a person, thing, place or time dimension, but rather as an internal psychological ego process which in the normal situation remains vital, dynamic, and in flux, and permits the object to assume and to consist of many varied roles, images, and attitudes. By contrast, the psychotic ego is rigidly rooted in the past, stagnated in a position of constant adherence to and recognition of only one role, image, and attitude, that of inevitable, terrifying destruction, and permitting no modification, changing imagery, or additional role increments to the object in the course of time and in the present.

The fantasy related by Teresa via the destruction of Pompeii perhaps illustrates the familiar etiological theme of the original trauma, the volcanic and earth-destroying upheaval that originally destroyed the psychic life of the patient—and coincidentally the world—not as a completed event but as an enfeeblement of the ego's vitality and capacity for continued development and maturation, leaving it in a paralyzed state of shock, petrified into stone and impotent rage, overwhelming her psychic apparatus into passivity, stagnation, and suspended deanimation, a form of psychic death. As if to justify her attitude of interminable, inert waiting to be rediscovered by future events, fortune or therapy, she acts as though she borrows from the legend of the Dybbuk to explain her passive waiting to be released, as if by exorcism, from its stultifying imprisonment of her life energies in order to free her psychic apparatus to complete its life task of actively conquering its rage or giving vent to its murderous destructiveness, to seek safety in the mother ocean which was denied in the original trauma, and to complete its life cycle by achieving its progressive life goal at the same time it returns to its peaceful intrauterine reunion with the mother. As an idealized statue she can gain entry into a museum; as a live human she can only become an agent of the dead and must return to the dead, which paradoxically also saves her life.

In Teresa's psychotic illness we see the problem of object constancy manifested in her inability to perceive and meaningfully to appreciate as a reality the emerging new roles of the object as they become manifest in the course of time. Rather, she can perceive and react to, as reality, only the object's rigid roles of the past in the form of destruction, catastrophe, terror, panic, and death. In Teresa, as in other psychotic patients, rigidity maintains constancy; constancy is equated with psychic death. Stagnation, paralysis, and immobility guarantee safety and survival. The object is permitted to exist and has the power to exist only if it remains rigidly unchanged in terms of past perceived reality. Imminent perception of the object's new roles, even, or particularly, of a positive, health-identified nature in terms of love, reliability, trustworthiness, commitment, etc., immediately leads to the ego's flight from, denial of, and wiping out of the object, or overwhelming it under a barrage of irrelevance and triviality, or violently destroying it in fantasy, thus guaranteeing the *status quo* of the original traumatic object, and in effect experiencing the loss of the new object. The object is allowed to be only that which the psychotic ego prescribes its role to be—i.e., an echo—and if the object attempts to change, it must be destroyed. The psychotic ego cannot accept or realistically perceive the new object, but permits it to exist only as a mirror of reflection of the object of the past that is seen only in terms of hate, fear, and death. The psychotic patient cannot accept the new object as it is. Instead, the new object has to be to the psychotic patient what it is not, and therefore cannot in reality exist. A dilemma thus arises: although the patient is in constant threat of losing the real object as it is because the object has to be what it is not, that is, a copy of the real introject, he can maintain object constancy only by maintaining the object, not as it is in reality, but as it was in the past. The conception of the past object also need not have corresponded to reality, but may have been shaped by fantasy and delusion. The situation is comparable to the task of having to erect a building on a foundation of quicksand.

In the normal object representation, the ego can perceive the object in its manifold roles, has the capacity to accommodate them to each other, to accept each of the many roles on its own integrity and merit, and to synthesize them into a consistent entity. This capacity is absent in the psychotic ego which, to maintain constancy, has to maintain rigid and unchanging image representations of the object and to turn all roles and images into the devil, the witch, the creature or some delusional destroyer.

Object constancy depends upon the capacity to accept changing object images and representation as they emerge in the external reality of the patient's life. Object constancy depends on the synthesis between the enforced imposition of the image and the real person with the capacity to determine in reality what the object really is. In normal object constancy the ego has the capacity to perceive equally the two sides of the coin—buffalo and Indian head—as together constituting the coin. In the psychotic ego, object constancy depends on perceiving and accepting only one side of the coin and on vigorously excluding the other side. The function of normal object constancy makes possible the integration and synthesis of present objects seen in totality and reality with the memory of past objects and object representations. It can be likened to the two-headed Janus who simultaneously looks to the past and the present, *integrating and synthesizing memory and perceptions into one effective object entity.* In the psychotic process, only the powerful, raw, past images predominate and the present perceptions are rigidly cloaked in past images.

Object constancy therefore must be understood not in terms of external realities of space and time, in such external objects as mother, bottle, feeding schedule, place of existence, and other external events— although these are necessary external conditions that mirror the internal process—but as an inner reality in psychic function, the achievement of the ego's capacity for synthesis of permanent, fixed images of the past with impressions and perceptions of the present in the service of creating realistic object representations for optimal ego functioning.

The therapeutic task in childhood psychosis is thus to transform the psychotic concept of constancy that is equated with stagnation and death to the realistic view of constancy as a dynamic *synthetic function* that makes possible an active fulfillment of life. Object constancy is thus seen not as an agent of cure of the psychotic illness as provided by mother, therapist, appointment time or therapeutic commitment, but as the achievement of the ego created by the cure for which the agent, techniques, methods, and psychological tools of the therapeutic process still remain a largely unexplained mystery and provide us with the goals of our research interests, efforts, and reasons for collaborating in a research project.

Much of what we have been presenting here was the result of discussions that took place in our research group. As we realized that Teresa was struggling with the restoration of that time described at the beginning of the paper, we were acquainted by the social worker with her version of what the aunt had told us about this phase. The social worker was certain, and all of us agreed with her and thought the same, that Teresa, standing on the balcony of that apartment house on the Paseo de la Reforma, had taken the little French poodle in sudden anger and had thrown him down to the pavement. We were convinced that she struggled with the recollection, that painful memory, repressed, distorted, and under the dominance of the primary process, of the murder of the dog. It is indeed a curious thing that a whole group of people, including the therapist, must unquestionably accept the distorted account of the murderous fantasy, the memory of the fusion of object and self, in such a way that it appears to be secondary process memory, an actual fact outside, thus for a moment shifting our analyzing attention from the internal process to an external traumatic event. Our invention of quasi-fact was a kind of metaphoric representation on a secondary process level of a psychotic state of mind. We were nevertheless able to use that quasi-fact, expressed in our language and within the framework of our logic, in order to enter the mind of the child and to reconstruct what must have happened within that mind. The invention of outer reality, then, becomes the metaphor which permits us to guess inner reality. In this case, the progression which forced us to introduce our kind of reality testing actually forged the inner facts, but was nevertheless in the service of the therapeutic ego, the reconstructive ego which permitted us to understand the psychic work of the reconstituting ego, that psychotic substitute for reconstruction.

As we were preparing the final draft of this paper, our scientific conscience suggested that we check the established memory against the recorded data. For a moment we identified with the feeling that Freud must have had when he discovered that his assumption of sexual etiology in the neurosis of hysterics was related to fantasy, to inner reality, rather than to an external fact. This peculiar error, in our case a distortion of our own memory and not the patient's, rather than standing in the way of understanding the material, was our way of coping with the attempt to understand the patient, such as her strange way of "remembering" via the fantasy material, borrowed and delusional, which helped her to get back to the past, to separate past and present, and to create continuum out of chaos.

We follow therapist and patient and enter the consulting room in the midst of the 580th hour, in order to see how the patient completes the reconstructive work with the therapist.

Treatment Hour 580

T.: You sleepy? You're yawning.
P.: Umm. Yeah. I'm always tired.
T.: Did you get enough sleep these days?

P.: No, I still go to bed late.

T.: Oh, well, no wonder.

P.: But I decided that one day I'm going to start going to bed early. I don't know why I—

T.: Well, how many hours of sleep do you like to have?

P.: A lot! Why can't I just be like—I mean, want to be like—I just feel like if I—am an animal.

T.: You are like a little kid.

P.: Yah, I know. Sometimes I feel like a little child. Other times I feel like an infant all born again—

T.: Teresa, even children sleep enough, and animals—

P.: And I also feel like an animal, and sometimes I feel like a—like a ghost—like I'm an old woman. The woman who never was—a ghost! I feel like all different persons.

T.: That's right, but the animals sleep. Maybe ghosts don't sleep, but animals sleep enough. You ever had an animal at home?

P.: The last animal I had was this little baby poodle dog.

T.: Oh, yah? Did he sleep a lot?

P.: But I didn't care for him. He died. He got killed, because of me. I feel that I'll always still blame me for it.

T.: Oh, really.

P.: Yeah. He died.

T.: Did you feed him enough? What did you do wrong?

P.: Well. . . . You see, he was supposed to be my dog. My aunt gave me that dog to be for me. I always wanted one, but the kind of dog I always wished for was a collie or a German shepherd. You know, those big dogs? The only thing is that they cause a lot of problems in taking care of them. Then, one thing my aunt keeps mentioning, mostly when we talk about these dogs, she says one of the worst things that I found about these dogs is that they shit in the house. They shit everywhere (laughing). They shit all the time. They never stop shitting. You have to give them a pound to eat of food, a pound of food, not the (inaudible).

T.: Those big dogs. . . .

P.: And when they shit (laughing) they shit (inaudible) (laughing). And that's true. But, at that time that's the kind of dog I wished for, and she really knew the right thing and she never really. . . . And she tried to tell me the problem in having one of those dogs. She tried to show me. And she really insisted on knowing. She never really wanted to get me one. She never did. So she got me this little poodle dog, see, because I like poodles also. And she got me this cute little baby poodle. And right after I had seen The Lady and the Tramp, that Walt Disney picture; you know, the Tramp.

T.: Yes, I remember it very well.

P.: That male dog? Well, I haven't even (inaudible) like the Tramp in the Walt Disney (laughs). I haven't even tramped a single (in-

audible) in Spanish because I like them when they're sorta cute (*inaudible*) a little Tramp. When he was a baby dog, though, he was the cutest thing, Trampa was. So it was when he grew bigger that I didn't care for him anymore, because I thought he wasn't so cute. I don't know, I didn't like his looks (*inaudible*).

T.: Well, that was the time when you didn't—

P.: (*loudly*) That's the time when I didn't care for him anymore when he grew bigger. I didn't go for it anymore, and somehow it wasn't like it took my place and kept on with it. And I used to be mean to him many times, and I also used to wish to kill him, and I used to wish that he was dead. I couldn't stand him like this. I hated him. But I was a very sick child at that time. I was a child, and I was sick. Something was wrong with my head, and nobody knew. Everybody thought I was normal as can be (*inaudible*) normal when I was a two-year-old or three or four. No. Maybe. I was normal, but as I kept growing from there is when I started to get rocks in my head. As I kept growing that's when I started to get rocks in my head.

T.: That's why you got afraid to grow up, because—

P.: Then finally the day came I had to kill myself, which I find wholly a mystery. And I still can't believe that if I'm dead, how can I be alive. I never heard of such a mystery, did you?

T.: Yes, that was the black Teresa.

P.: Well, it's not my mind that's dead.

T.: I know, but the white Teresa doesn't want to do it. It's only the black Teresa.

P.: That's why I live such a rotten life, because I'm dead. I'm just a dead corpse. I—I—I'm—I'm a ghost. I happen to be a ghost, but one of those kind of strange ghosts that really never existed and then finally it does, it came to, and it does exist.

T.: Yes.

P.: I'm a new kind of ghost, I guess.

T.: But we want to make that Teresa ghost alive again and the white ghost—

P.: Because ghosts are usually invisible and transparent, they can just pass through one wall and another, but not me. I'm the kind of ghost who can't. Because I'm made out of flesh and bones and blood. I bleed when I cut myself like any human being does, when I hit myself it hurts, and I yell with pain, and I yell.

T.: So. . . .

P.: So, I'm a very strange ghost. I'm a human one, which means I'm a flesh and blood and bone human ghost.

T.: That's right. You're the kind of ghost that can. . . .

P.: Isn't that strange?

T.: . . . come to realize this.

P.: Though I know it's true, I still can't believe it, it's hard to believe especially when it happens to you and not to someone else. You find out that someone else . . . and you try to make them believe it, which is different than. . . . He doesn't have the problem that you have. And when you have it, that's when it's really hard to believe that it's true. Because you're in it already. But if mysteries exist, especially the biggest one, because this isn't a little mystery. This isn't the tiny baby one. It's one of the hugest, most enormousest mysteries that could ever exist in life. . . . One of the biggest, in fact maybe. . . . I don't think it's possible, but it's one of the hugest. It's a gigantic giant.

T.: Except that you and I will make out of this whole—

P.: It's a fact of life totally. It grows out of the world. It's a fact of life.

T.: But you and I will make out of that, these three ghosts, a real person again.

P.: And that's why I am like this?

T.: That's right, but you also want to be a new person. Where the white Teresa will be stronger than the black Teresa and the purple Teresa and all the other Teresas. And I guess that's hard to believe, too, isn't it?

P.: (long pause) Well . . . I think I'll—

T.: You think you'll keep on fighting with me so that we can get you to be as fully and thoroughly forever and ever the complete Teresa rather than the Teresa ghost.

P.: (long pause) Well, that little poodle dog that I had which was supposed to be mine. . . . Why when he died, why didn't he fall in the same case I fell in? (crying) Why . . . when he died, he didn't remain at the same time alive? If that would have been— Now this is another example I want to give. If that would have happened to him first before it happened to me, then I could see as an example. Well, that is a very strange mystery. Golly! You know what I mean. And then I would never know what happened to me. Suddenly, but then let's say a while after it happened to him, it happened to me suddenly, and then I would understand better, you know what I mean? Because I, I, I would have seen it before . . . happening to someone else, a little animal . . . or a human being. And that would make it easier. Then I wouldn't have such difficulty in believing it . . . in believing that it's true . . . and taking it hard.

T.: You took it hard that you lost the dog forever?

P.: I would . . . you know—

T.: You reproached yourself because you hated the dog, you know. You really also loved the dog. You reproached—

P.: No, I didn't hate the dog.

T.: Well, you said sometimes you hated him.

P.: Well, I really didn't. It's my illness that hated him.

T.: It was really your illness that hated him, but you loved him. The ghost of you hated him, but the real Teresa loved him.

P.: Yeah, yeah.

T.: And I think it was a terrible thing—

P.: So, that's what I'm saying. To give you an example, if I really would have seen this same mystery that happened to me. If I really would have seen it at first in him, happening to someone else . . . after that, then it happened to me, I would understand better, and I would take it easier to believing it.

T.: You would have taken it easier—

P.: But, it never happened to nobody, never. Only to me. So that's why I—I—I . . . It's hard to me to take. That's why.

T.: It's harder to understand—

P.: And if I would have seen it on someone else before.

T.: It's harder to understand.

P.: I—I also believe that the mystery of Juan Diego, this little Mexican Indian of Mexico, that had gotten into this strangeness, the mystery that happened to him of the Virgin of Guadalupe appearing, which was a mystery. Yes.

T.: Yes. I think—

P.: And I think . . . I also find it a great mystery when she, she put her image in this beautiful cloth mantle that she showed to everybody. That's the only way they would believe it.

T.: But he won out.

P.: He won.

T.: He won, and you will win, too, like him.

P.: Then they finally believed him.

T.: That's right—

P.: That was a big mystery too. I believe it was.

T.: And the ghost became real.

P.: That was a. . . . No, let me tell you. I do believe that that was some . . . thing of a mystery, and I believe that it was a big mystery—But I also believe that it wasn't the big mystery as mine. I still believe that. Though his mystery was quite strange and big, I still believe that mine is even twice bigger than his.

T.: Could be, but maybe that you and I—

P.: Twice bigger, it is!

T.: Teresa, but it just means that you and I have twice as big a task. But then, we're two people. He was only one (pause).

P.: Now, he somehow got help then in, in with the mystery—

T.: Well, but we want to get other things—

P.: And I really haven't reached up there—

T.: Teresa, may I remind you next Tuesday about what we talked about, so that we can continue it?

P.: Sure.

T.: Would you like me to? Good. Now we know a little better what it means to carry a burden. Bye-bye, Teresa.

Freud (5) speaks of the *technical activity of reconstruction* in the following terms: "When one lays before the subject of the analysis a piece of his early history that he has forgotten. . . ." He also refers to the process of working through, which permits us to help the patient restore continuity between the past and present as well as the future.

To what degree are such patients as Teresa, who suffer from the lack of object constancy which characterizes their peculiar psychotic transference manifestations, capable of restoring this continuum?

Rather than answering this question and commit ourselves to undue therapeutic optimism or nihilistic therapeutic pessimism, we want to suggest that our material poses a scientific question, the answer to which lies in the careful study of long-term analytic treatment of patients such as Teresa by committed therapists, a study which must allow for the objective evaluation and analysis of records by the therapist, supplemented by the taped research data, by psychological retesting, through the participating team, and independent research observers.

The question concerning the individual capacity of a person for object constancy and reconstruction, a study really in ego psychology, has been anticipated by Freud. As we followed Teresa's attempts to establish a kind of archaeology of her mind, we recall Freud's frequent comparison of the work of the psychoanalyst with the work of the archaeologist. One of these comparisons, an analogy which allows us to formulate new questions, may help us in rediscovering that *reconstruction* implies restoring the patient's access not only to past events but also to the *then available ego organization* which "wrote" that personal history. Freud (4) suggests in *Civilization and Its Discontents*:

> . . . that everything survives in some way or other, and is capable under certain conditions of being brought to light again, as, for instance, when regression extends back far enough. One might try to picture to oneself what this assumption signifies by a comparison taken from another field. Let us choose the history of the Eternal City as an example. Historians tell us that the oldest Rome of all was the *Roma quadrata*, a fenced settlement on the Palatine. Then followed the phase of the Septimontium, when the colonies on the different hills united together; then the town which was bounded by the Servian wall; and later still, after all the transformations in the periods of the republic and the early Caesars, the city which the Emperor Aurelian enclosed by his walls. . . .
>
> Now let us make the fantastic supposition that Rome were not a human dwelling-place, but a mental entity with just as long and varied a past history: that is, in which nothing once constructed had perished, and all the earlier stages of development had survived alongside the latest. This would mean that in Rome the palaces of the Caesars were still standing on the Palatine and . . . the beautiful statues were still standing in the colonnade of the

Castle of St. Angelo, as they were up to its siege by the Goths, . . . the observer would need merely to shift the focus of his eyes, perhaps, or change his position, in order to call up a view of either the one or the other. . . .

There is one objection, though, to which we must pay attention. It questions our choosing in particular the past history of a city to liken to the past of the mind. Even for mental life our assumption that everything past is preserved holds good only on condition that the organ of the mind remains intact and its structure has not been injured by traumas or inflammation. Destructive influences comparable to these morbid agencies are never lacking in the history of any town, even if it has had a less chequered past than Rome, even if, like London, it has hardly ever been pillaged by an enemy. Demolitions and the erection of new buildings in the place of old occur in cities which have had the most peaceful existence; therefore a town is from the outset unsuited for the comparison I have made of it with a mental organism. . . . The fact is that a survival of all the early stages alongside the final form is only possible in the mind, and that it is impossible for us to represent a phenomenon of this kind in visual terms.

REFERENCES

1. EKSTEIN, R. (1959). Thoughts Concerning the Nature of the Interpretive Process. In: *Readings in Psychoanalytic Psychology*, ed. M. Levitt. New York: Appleton-Century-Crofts, pp. 221-247.
2. ———. *Children of Time and Space, of Action and Impulse: Clinical Studies on the Psychoanalytic Treatment of Severely Disturbed Children*. New York: Appleton-Century-Crofts, 1966.
3. ——— & CARUTH, E. (1966). Activity-Passivity Issues in the Treatment of Childhood Psychosis. In: Panel on Activity-Passivity, rep. P. Gray. *J. Amer. Psa. Assn.*, 15:709-728.
4. FREUD, S. (1930). *Civilization and Its Discontents*. London: Hogarth Press, 1946.
5. ——— (1937). Constructions in Analysis. *Standard Edition*, 23:255-269. London: Hogarth Press, 1964.

CHAPTER FIFTEEN

The Working Alliance with Angels, Good Spirits and Deities

> What is destructible
> Is but a parable;
> What fails ineluctably,
> The undeclarable,
> Here it was seen,
> Here it was action;
> The eternal-feminine
> Lures to perfection.
>
> JOHANN WOLFGANG VON GOETHE

A collaborator and I have suggested that in therapeutic work we start with the acceptance of the delusional monster and try to bring about a working alliance with that part of the patient's personality (7). We expected that later in the process we would have helped the patient to accept and synthesize his "monster" parts, as well as his persecutory and destructive feelings about the therapist. We summed up our interpretive strategy as "the taming of the monster," and suggested that where unstable introjects rule, capacity for object relations could develop.

These suggestions for additional technical improvements were expanded from earlier insights derived from clinical investigations of therapeutic work with borderline and schizophrenic children. The notion of "interpreting within the metaphor" (5) (Ch. 13, this vol.) had followed the expression of a technical attitude described in Coleridge's terms as "suspended disbelief" (4). These technical assumptions attempted to meet the distance devices of the patients—their ego regressions and fluctuations in the service of defense—with appropriate methods of establishing workable contact.

In some cases, the technical innovations brought about enduring recoveries and remarkable improvements in our patients. In other situations, our early insights did not bring about lasting successes, and we felt at times as if our work had led us into a dead-end street.

The case that I am now utilizing to present some of our present investigations seems to exhibit a number of questions which must be answered in order to improve our technical armamentarium. These questions are partly technical and partly theoretical. The case itself was used in the communication on the working alliance with the monster. It was also used in my discussion of the Orpheus and Eurydice theme in psychotherapy (Chapter 13, this vol.), as well as in a communication by Friedman and myself on "Object Constancy and Psychotic Reconstruction" (Chapter 14, this vol.).

The patient is Teresa Esperanza, who, during the past several years, has been the therapeutic concern of, and has provided much of the basic data for, my research group at the Reiss-Davis Child Study Center. Teresa's treatment started in the fall of 1960 when she was approximately fifteen-and-one-half years old. A bilingual, Spanish-Mexican Catholic, she was diagnosed at that time as suffering from a "schizophrenic reaction, childhood type, with hysterical personality features." She is still in treatment, so we are now dealing with a late adolescent or young adult rather than a child. But that often is the fate of psychotherapeutic work with such children. These later phases are of vital concern, and, for some form of successful closure, I have come to think in terms of a decade (2, 3, 6). We should not be surprised if more and more treatment reports appear in the literature wistfully describing time commitments of this sort (Chapter 12, this vol.).

There is no question in my mind that the clinical team's next reappraisal of this patient will again come to the independent conclusion that we are dealing with a schizophrenic person. But I am also committed to the notion that psychotherapy brought about significant changes in this patient. For a number of years Teresa has lived apart from her relatives, and has made a fair adjustment in a Catholic Home for girls with South American backgrounds. The Home is run by Spanish-speaking nuns who have been very understanding and cooperative, and as supportive of treatment as can be expected in an outpatient arrangement.

Teresa receives a welfare allowance, budgets herself, takes care of her room, finds her way around town by bus—no mean achievement in Los Angeles—comes to the Clinic, and keeps all of her appointments quite well. I see her regularly, and she is also seen by the social worker, who discusses such social issues with her as her varied attempts at working or rehabilitation. Teresa once held a cafeteria job for three weeks, and now occasionally sells articles for a cosmetics firm. She maintains some contact with relatives, and has distant associations with the girls at the Home. Her essentially isolated way of life must be measured against the fact that during the first few years of treatment she could not come alone to the Clinic, could not take a bus, could hardly count money, could not shop, or take care of her room, and had many moments of submergence in her delusional world in which she was violent or completely inaccesible. In the other clinical papers we described her homicidal and suicidal outbreaks; her gorging herself with essentially inedible foods when unsupervised and when trying to restore the lost object; a time when she went to sleep with a can opener—that uncanny substitute for a teddy bear; a representation of transitory fusion of self and object, of the inaccessible breast and the violent teeth.

According to the conclusions of the communication on the alliance with the monster, we would have to assume that Teresa should now be able to accept the creature which dominated her life as part of herself, instead of as an alien and dangerous enemy. She should now be demonstrating a re-integration, a new synthesis of good and bad, to guarantee the developing of increased capacity for ego functioning on an adaptive level.

The following material may indicate to what degree this prediction can be substantiated, to what degree it was perhaps no more than a self-fulfilling prophecy, and to what degree the technique failed; or, in an optimistic outlook, whether it points towards a positive reassessment which may suggest different and additional technical maneuvers.

The phase of treatment under discussion covered a number of months between spring and fall of 1968. Teresa had been seen for more than 700 hours (not counting many other contacts with the social worker, volunteers, or other professional and semi-professional personnel). She had always been quite faithful to her therapeutic program and missed very few hours. During certain phases of treatment she was sometimes late, but she usually telephoned, or at least resumed contact some time within the hour. The phase started with a kind of therapy fatigue. It is difficult to say whether it was solely the patient's or whether it was also the therapist's "battle fatigue"—which Winnicott might refer to as an expression of sublimated hate in the countertransference.

After having missed two previous sessions, Teresa came very late to the 716th hour. The therapist interpreted her lateness as a way of avoiding a discussion on the possibility of ending. For several month she had been expressing a wish to end treatment by the end of 1967 then had revised this date to the first part of 1968. These comment were usually utilized by her and the therapist in the conventional sense and she had easily accepted the desirability of making the best possible use of therapy time until it was ended. This time, she eagerly responded to the explanation of her tardiness. The therapist also suggested that this year the Clinic might again wish to re-assess her situation (she had been retested approximately every 18 months in the past). He suggested that the assessment might indicate whether she had come to the point where she was satisfied with her achievement and no longer needed help. She responded extremely positively and suggested a bizarre way of assessing her reality to prove that the therapist was correct: namely, that she came late (i.e., could not function) *because* she was ready to end. She suggested during this 716th hour that perhaps she was losing job after job, and giving up plan after plan, because she was now so used to the Clinic as a baby sitter, that she saw herself as a "queen who has to be served by the Clinic." But if she stopped coming to the Clinic, she would no longer be a queen, would no longer be served. Perhaps then she could make herself into a real person who could deal with life. The ending of treatment would prove that she was well.

A few seconds later she started to laugh in a bizarre way, and suggested that she laughed this way because sometimes when she looked in a mirror, she saw herself in a peculiar way. When she had no mirror, she went on, she saw these aspects of herself in other people, as, for example, in the therapist. Just now, he had become strange and funny, and his voice had changed into that of a crazy, perhaps a dangerous, man.

One can see how this material was suddenly dominated by psychotic projection and reversal. Her wish to avoid the therapist or the task was acted out. The fantasy that she will be well as soon as she can end— a reversal of the facts of reality—was eagerly projected into the therapist, whose suggestion for re-evaluation quickly became the proof she needed. The tests were no longer a task confronting her, but were seen as a fulfilled promise, and one does not know whether that promise originated in the tester or the testee. Schlesinger's contributions on the nature of primary and secondary promising (10) are pertinent here. In addition, however, I hope to show that in Teresa's case one must see beyond her attempt to regain love through the act of promising, and also understand it as an attempt to regain the loss of psychotic self by forging and altering reality so that it agrees with impulse and fantasied wish-fulfillment. Inasmuch as this kind of promising includes a special arrangement between self and object, between internal self- and object-representation, I would like to refer to it as *fusion promising*.

Thus, the phase of treatment described took place during a time of special stress: the re-assessment of the therapeutic situation. This could be considered a decisive issue in assessing the problems encountered, but I do not wish to overemphasize it, since similar situations had arisen before during the years of treatment. As a matter of fact, this constant threat to the therapeutic situation—the recurring question as to whether one may continue or not, the possibility of losing or being dismissed by the patient, the feeling that the case is hopeless—is characteristic of this kind of case. This problem is directly related to the issue of object- and self-constancy and the transference paradigm that it creates.

During this same period, the social worker* attempted to review with Teresa the way in which she filled her time with unrealistic programs. For example, she took high-school courses in art, typing and French, but only made a pretense of doing the work which was beyond her capabilities. She also avoided any of the realistic rehabilitation programs offered her. In other words, she maintained a fictitious type of activity, a kind of psychotic action-promise, like Mr. K's job as surveyor in Kafka's *The Castle*. As she described, with her powerful psychotic obsessionalism, all the steps she would have to take in order to prepare for "action," it became clear that all the delay was an effort to ward off anxiety as well as reality. All Teresa's actions were in the service of the ego's passivity. They allowed her to maintain the degree of equilibrium which sustained her kind of optimum self- and object-constancy: a teetertotter activity between self- and object-representation, between good and evil, between fusion and defusion.

I am referring to a psychotic system of checks and balances, a complex system of delay mechanisms that permitted her to function from time to time on a pseudo reality-principle level. This system, however, lacked the capacity for utilizing thinking as trial action which is necessary for secondary-process, goal-oriented activity. One might suggest that Teresa gave token allegiance to the reality principle so that she would never have to translate it into the actuality principle.

Freud (9) suggested that "judging is the intellectual action which decides the choice of motor action, which puts an end to the postponement due to thought and which leads over from thinking to acting." The particular difficulty of this and similar patients is that they can-

---

* Beatrice Cooper, M.S., contributed the casework material.

not judge, plan and act on a secondary-process level; they cannot test reality. This occurs because of their inability to maintain either sufficient object-constancy or differentiation between self and object, between inner and outer reality. Their precarious remnants of self- and object-constancy can only be maintained by means of *suspension of the act*. They cannot alter reality for fear of destroying it and being destroyed by it.

Such psychotic patients cannot integrate new perceptions with memories of earlier, archaic introjects that were the former perceptions of the object: the devils, witches and monsters they need to maintain.

As Teresa continued in treatment, she permitted herself the integration of new perceptions with memories of earlier object representations, through the introjection of the therapist—that precursor mechanism of identification. Consequently, there evolved secondary-process-like object and self-representations, capacity for reality testing, self-observation, differentiation between dream and waking, and the like. But all these identifications with the therapist—still mainly on the level of introjection—ended in a kind of pseudo-identification, with capacity occasionally to think and observe like him, but not to act like him. A good example of this is the attitude, mentioned earlier, towards psychological tests. She did not expect the tests to reveal something about her; instead, the tests would make decisions, so to speak, that she was well and could stop treatment. The psychological test procedure turned into a kind of positive influencing machine, rather than an assessment for new plans which would have to be acted upon. The test itself was seen as an act, curing her rather than indicating her state of health.

This pseudo-allegiance to the secondary process, to the words of the therapist—an allegiance which leads to the thought but never to the act, to the promise but never to its fulfillment—showed that something in her working alliance with us had changed. We might compare her with a political candidate who tries to bring about an impossible alliance between opposing factions with entirely conflicting interests and attitudes, but who, under certain ideal conditions, can be persuaded to follow and elect him, thereby becoming instruments for political power.

Teresa's introjects, with their divergent interests and conflicting demands (replicas, as they are, of past and present outer pressures), had to be welded together by her into such an alliance to permit the functioning of an active ego with available synthetic function.

In "The Working Alliance with the Monster" (7), I suggested that the therapist, rather than requiring the suppression of the monster or attacking its evil nature, make it serve his patient. I suggested, too, that this alliance is particularly necessary when there are no other available forces with which to ally. But as the patient becomes capable of allowng the inclusion of thoughts and demands which previously had been projected into the monster or devil, and can see them both in herself and also in the therapist, she brings other forces into play which complicate our strategical problems.

I should like to quote from my summary of the 719th therapeutic session in order to introduce a new struggle: a power battle between devil and God, the evil and good spirits, the fallen and the celestial angels.

Teresa expressed her fear about going out and selling toilet articles in the neighborhood lest someone attack or murder her, and mentioned that she preferred a job as saleswoman in an elegant record shop (this latter the unrealistic suggestion from her aunt, who thinks of Teresa as much too ill to live with, but dreams she can adjust to a complex job situation). She then tried to avoid a discussion of her reality situation by telling me she had meant to tell me about a dream she had. As I was pressing her for the content of the dream, she could not really express the content of the dream, but all of a sudden all of life became a dream. It was a miracle of God that she had not really killed herself some years ago and was now dead, but the actual truth was that God had made her dream these things. The interesting thing was that not only did she dream about it, but I, too, was really just dreaming. There was not much chance for me to wake her up and get her out of this dream to face life because I, myself, lived in a dream world. While I could not directly ascribe to a particular school of philosophy this point of view, it indeed reminded me of Leibnitz. In his Monadic theory, he proposed that all of us have a private world of our own very much like a dream, and that there was really no contact between people except that they sort of dreamed about others; it was just by chance that these dreams ran parallel, etc.

I was now confronted with the fact that I had no place outside, and I could see exactly what this kind of psychotic obsessional struggle meant. It was a new defensive device, albeit psychotic, to ward off any return to actuality, to the tasks at hand. If I were to suggest that God meant us to wake up, and if I were to ask how both of us could help Him so that both of us could wake up and face the world, she would carry things a step further. She would say that, of course, God would wake us up in due time, but we would then wake up in paradise. Her wish to return to a dream world, to a world of her own choice, and not to go out and face the real world, was limited by the fact that sooner or later God would wake her up. Some people He would wake up and send to hell, and other people He would awaken and send to paradise. When she woke up, she would be in paradise. Of course, we knew that in paradise the same rules existed as in her dream world:

primary-process rules, instant-satisfaction rules, and no tasks to be
met.

I tried to battle within that psychotic metaphor. I suggested
that since God would indeed decide whether we wake up in hell
or in heaven, He had at least given us the privilege of helping him
make that decision. He allowed us to see what we could do now,
what we could prepare, what we could begin in this dream in
order to wake up in the right place. Would He punish or reward
us? This led her to a kind of concession that at least within the
dream she should try to get a job, and she wasn't meant to get
a job in the record shop anyway; but of course I knew that the
search for the job would be carried out in dreamlike fashion.

It was interesting to see how I could carry the struggle to her
within this fantastic elaboration. The mental struggle brought her
immense emotional strain. She started to perspire; she had to close
her eyes. I suggested that there was no reason for her, in the dream
that God gave her, to close her eyes to escape from the dream; she
might as well open her eyes. She opened them and again was with
me, but within the dream structure. This went on all through the
hour. Unfortunately, the dictated word cannot quite reproduce
the power with which she maintained these constructions, and the
effort it took for me to enter them and maintain some kind of
contact. One is tempted to place the stress on the grammar, on
logic or her lack of logic. One might say that her psychotic illusions are dressed up in a perfectly logical system, a kind of philosophical position for which, in our day, unfortunately, Teresa will
not get a chair as a professor of religious philosophy. Instead, she
will have to suffer the passivity, the inactivity, the paralysis of a
person who defends herself against impulse and external demands
by maintaining life through a philosophy that insists that *all of
life is but a dream.* The poets, after all, always knew about that.

The therapist was very much in the position of the prince who
tried to cut through the thorn hedge in order to get to the Sleeping
Beauty. Teresa went on dreaming and waited for the miracle. In the
past, she had seen herself as a kind of devil, and spoke of having killed
herself, of being sentenced now to be "dead and yet alive." She revised
this notion to one where the idea that she had killed herself was merely
the content of a dream, and it was up to God, that Prince of Heaven,
to wake her up. Surely He would put her in paradise rather than in the
therapist's vale of tears—which required reality testing and an active
life.

During this phase, her internal life was not dominated by the
monster but by a new construction—that powerful God who pulled
the strings, but from outside. He had become the personification of
megalomanic power which she had been used to project at least par-

ially onto the therapist, from whom she now removed it in order to make him, too, an ineffective, helpless, inmate of her mental prison. Part of her dream, fused with her in inactivity, the therapist was, nevertheless, with her, so that they could talk to each other in the dreamlike fashion which permitted contact but required no fulfillment of promise. The promise would be fulfilled by God. The monster had been replaced by God. Her life was dominated by God's timeless miracle.

The capacity to dream and to remember a dream, to observe it, report it, and analyze it, is a psychological achievement. In this case, the early differentiation gave way to fusion. As she reported the dream, she seemed to surrender to the dream world—the psychotic construction which warded off rage, anger, aggression, sexual acting-out, the victory of the monster. The price she had to pay was the inactivity of a paralyzed ego which must watch in horror, and only rarely in delight, what God permitted her when He induced her into dream states. Such were the fantastic promises of heaven that she expected from the therapist, active gifts which required her only to wait for his capacity to "make miracles."

We now had a working alliance with God. Less upsetting and disturbing, perhaps, than the one we had with the devil, it was much more difficult since He is so much more powerful, and kept her asleep and inaccessible.

In the 720th hour, Teresa continued the earlier theme. Again I quote from my notes of that hour:

> God is the one who had given her the dream; and all the earlier thoughts, namely, that she was killed by God and had killed herself, were but parts of the dream that He gave her. She was now living in a dream world in which the bad thoughts were abolished "once and for all." If they were to come up, they would only come up in dreams, and there was a way to remedy that. There was a bad dream that she had, and as I pressed her to tell it to me, I learned that it had to do with a vampire, somebody who looked like a man. This man was making love to her by seemingly kissing her neck and her throat, but he was actually sucking the blood out of her. This was turning her into a vampire who, if she were to make love to a man, would suck the blood out of him, and the result would be that she would become the mother of vampires. She somehow described the sexual intercourse as mutual murder, with the creation of dried-up babies. Fortunately, the dream did not quite end that way, because while she had the thought that this would happen, the dream actually ended sort of positively because God wanted her to end it positively. Thus she described the struggle against evil thoughts. Her attempt to conquer them

was simply to deny them by making them into dream thoughts and to claim that only the good thoughts were real.

God tested her with all of this, and I tried slowly to bring this test of God to the tests she was to have at the Clinic. She in turn, wanted to make this into a test for me. While she got lost as she tried to formulate the question that she had in mind, after considerable pressure on my part, she finally came to the question. She asked me whether I thought the good thoughts of the dream were truer than the bad thoughts. I said that they were, and she recognized that the bad thoughts came from the devil who did not really exist, but the good thoughts came from God, who really did exist. I said I understood now why she had such problems which would forbid her to wake up and live in heaven, and really get to work: she constantly tried to maintain the good thoughts and had to use all her energy in order to make the bad thoughts irrelevant, untrue, and non-existing. But if once and for all she could help God with the good thoughts and put them into good works, something would happen.

She struggled against that with the obsessional psychotic mechanisms that have been so often described, although she did want to make her concession towards turning the good thoughts into good works. First of all, she spoke to Sister Elena (the nun in charge of the Home for girls) and she had some good news to tell me. Sister Elena was still waiting to get some news from the other sisters about a job that Teresa could do for the nuns. So far, she had heard nothing. She had told Sister Elena about her discussion with the social worker concerning the possibility that she might find someone who would go with her and together they would look for work, perhaps even that weekend. This, of course, was her way of turning the good thought into good works.

She ended the hour with a description of another attempt really to turn good thoughts into good works. All of this, of course, was in response to my comments concerning thought and act. She described how she went to church weekly to pray and how she attended the service, and how she always gave some money when the basket was passed around. It is interesting, incidentally, that she stressed that the church is very near the psychiatric day treatment center she once attended. (Catastrophic sexual acting-out at that center with a young schizophrenic patient led to her being thrown out of her original home.) But she reproached herself for giving so little money, though sometimes she'd like to give an enormous amount, perhaps ten dollars. Did I think that was too much? I said it was too much now since she had only welfare money, but I felt it would be wonderful and beautiful if she could turn those good thoughts into good works that could come out of her salary. She agreed with all this, but as she left she said she found it very difficult because of all the nervous tension that was in her.

She felt she had some kind of body symptoms, summer pains perhaps. It was, of course, her way of saying that the pressure I put
her under with my talk about the ideal of turning good thoughts
into good works was about the limit of what she could bear. It
was on that note that the hour ended.

It is apparent that during the psychotic regression the internal war
between good and evil—between murderous act and repressive goodness
—was projected out into the heavens. God was responsible for the
creation of the devil, for the creation of evil thoughts in bad dreams,
for her turning into the evil woman who could murder in the love act
and produce evil children. But God is also responsible for this being
only a dream, and for His capacity to make her good thoughts into
something much stronger and more real than the bad thoughts. This
miracle of God which saved her was perhaps a useful metaphoric description of her capacity for self-observation. Its price was an arrangement by means of which she reduced certain self-awareness by projection, mastered forbidden impulses by repression, and maintained the
therapeutic relationship by displacement onto borrowed fantasies, which
stemmed from science fiction and mythology, as well as her religious
background. The synthetic and integrating functions were somehow
put into God, who maintained her in a psychotic balance, and permitted her to share her dreams, her inner world, with me. Thus she
permitted me—by saying to her, via her God, whatever was interpretable on this level—a kind of object relationship within a dream, that
protective garment which allowed us to talk to each other and to remain differentiated even though we were fused within it.

One might say that Teresa, in permitting her inner world of introjects to be populated by figures of good as well as evil, was thus able
to observe with me that powerful Armageddon of the mind.

In the 723rd hour:

Observing her "little problems" at the Home (where she was
criticized for talking to herself, behaving strangely, etc.), she
wanted to stress that these conversations were not with herself but
with the devil. At certain moments she recognized these as dialogues and as fantasies, and at other moments the devil was seen
as real. I tried to assess with her what the devil was doing to her
in this dialogue. It turned out that he was not exactly a seducer,
or one who did all kinds of mean things, possibly who talked her
into masturbating, etc.; rather, at one moment he even said to
her that she should talk nicely to him. She answered in anger,
screamed at him, and he screamed back, and thus it went back
and forth. After a while it became clear to me and to her that

the struggle between her and the devil was exactly the struggle we had discussed in the past; namely, her struggle to be good, to live up to the requirements that the world sets for her, while the devil tries to get her away from these requirements. When the struggle became too powerful, she tried to save herself by saying that it was all a dream, and that within that dream the devil really did not exist. She thus tried to devaluate the devil, downgrade him; she referred to his having been thrown out of paradise, and to his origins as an angel. When I called to her attention that the devil wanted her to be good and to talk nicely, she suggested he did that because she talked that way to him and told him to stop swearing. It seemed that the dialogue between the two consisted of both good and bad elements. I wondered whether perhaps the devil wanted to learn from her, wanted to become better, because he wanted to go back to paradise. This she could not accept. But it became clear that the dialogues she had with the devil were the kind of dialogues that she had with me. They were carried on in such a way that certain ugly notions that she projected into me reappeared there; sometimes, positive notions were projected as well. The material is a classical illustration of psychotic mechanisms of projective identification and identificatory projection.

It became clear that this internal struggle was a strange reflection of the dialogue that took place between her and the adult world around her, the people who made "demands" on her. She was constantly beset by the problem that she could not clearly differentiate what came from the outside or the inside. One can even observe that within herself the notion of good and evil, the notion of God and the devil, constantly fused and differentiated back and forth. This is, of course, exactly her dilemma. I suggested at one moment that the reason she was so angry with the devil had to do with the fact that she thought I believed the devil's predictions that she would never have a husband and was condemned to stay the way she is. She started to scream at me because she said that I was siding with the devil. I said that I really did not believe the devil, but she did. I said, for example, that if I were to tell her that the walls in this room and the couch were made of golden damask, would she get angry, and would she believe me? She said she wouldn't get angry. I said that here we saw the problem: it was obvious that whenever she got angry it was because she actually believed what was said and worried that I— that the devil—might be right, because she herself questioned whether she would ever get well.

She then said that if I said these things often enough to her, she might have to scream at me, because I might force her to believe that nonsense. This, in many ways, was a significant insight because it indicated that she was aware that she might not be able to maintain her own judgment, and felt her mind could be overrun.

This is exactly what takes place in her, and therefore she has that terrible anger against herself whenever there is a voice of doubt. Slowly, as this doubt dissolved, the situation between us became friendly again. When I suggested later that the only way to fight the devil was not by screaming at him, because screaming at him meant that she became the devil, but by action, by working and doing something, she said that she did that, too. It turned out that by action, she meant "praying," and the devil sometimes made fun of her. She got angry when he said to her: "Holy, holy, holy!" in a mocking and derogatory way.

In the next hour, the 724th:

She described the problem that she had with the devil, who tried to get her away from prayer and away from God and thinking about God. And then she said that she had brainwashed him. As a matter of fact, she had called the devil by a peculiar name: "Brainyak," which she said referred to being brainwashed. I thought to myself that perhaps this also had to do with her idea that I was so brainy. In any case, she tried constantly to counter his evil suggestions and his evil thoughts. Then I decided to take the bull— or, perhaps more precisely, the devil—by the horns. I said that I was sure that the devil had all kinds of lewd thoughts on his mind, that he made her think about sex, that she ought to undress and expose her body, etc. She said that was exactly what the devil tried to make her think of, but the devil also slowly discovered that the influence of God and the magic of God was not the magic of the devil. She really described the struggle within her mind, except that in the beginning of the hour it was in a rather delusional sort of way. Remaining within the delusional metaphor, I insisted that the only way to face the devil was to look at all the dirty things and thoughts he had on his mind, and still to prove to him that one can clean his dirty devil's mind and make him come nearer to God, perhaps. She wondered why the devil hated God, and I said that he didn't hate God but wanted desperately to be accepted again by God. Therefore, if he cleansed his mind, she could make him a promise that God might forgive him and he might return to God.

She then spoke about the devil appearing as all kinds of personages, such as different movie stars, etc. It seemed clear to me that she was now ready for the interpretation that I intended. I told her that sometimes the devil also appeared to her the way that I do, so that she believed that it was not Dr. E. whom she met but the devil. Indeed, she had said at one point during that session that the devil had now slipped into me. This came at the moment when I suggested that she must listen to the thoughts of the devil, and that I myself, when I listened to the devil, found that he sometimes put thoughts into me which had to do with sin and sex and naked girls, and whatnot, but that I laughed off these thoughts because they did not dominate me; I dominated them and the devil knew it.

At that moment she slowly became released and spoke of the possibility that the devil could be stronger than I realized, but she did not quite believe it. She spoke about the devil trying to take away from her the holy pictures that she had at home, and the Bible, and all the things she had of God and the angels. In their place, he tried to give her dirty images. I then said that he would like to do this with me, but he could not do it, and I pulled out of the drawer some holy objects that Teresa had given me in the past: a medallion of Jesus, and also one of St. Michael. She was quite taken with that, and I suggested that if she ever met the devil looking like me, she could easily find out it wasn't the devil. She herself supplied the answer, namely, that the devil would not dare touch holy pictures. I added that he was afraid of them as we would be of touching fire.

I was now well established, and she wondered whether it was not a great burden to me that I, who was not a Catholic, got all these gifts and Catholic pictures from her. I answered that I had learned about Catholicism through her and understood it through her and, therefore, it was really not a burden to me. We then ended the hour on the notion that there was no danger in the gifts I gave to and received from people, if we liked each other. Only gifts that one thought might come from the devil created difficulties. I constantly tried to bring home the point that we must face the thoughts of the devil, for only in that way could we take his power away from him, and reduce the danger that he could turn our thoughts into action. She asked me whether I believed in the devil, in his physical reality. I said that I believed in the devil very much in the sense that he sometimes possessed her mind. She then said that she doesn't believe either that the devil existed in reality but, rather—and she now gave up the idea of all of it being a mere dream created by God—that he existed in the mind only, and as a very powerful influence there. She had almost come to a conception of inner struggle without projection, but it was at the point when reconstituting took place that we had come to the end of our session.

As she brainwashed the devil, she actually cleansed herself of "dirty" thoughts. In this way, she identified with the therapist's interpretations and demands, and she slowly accepted her projections as inner awareness, as an inner struggle.

The material is not free of processes of magical influencing, such as facing me or the devil with holy pictures to paralyze possible hostile action against her, just as she feels influenced by God who paralyzes her actions.

We might say again that the "personality" of these introjects is characterized by the dominance of projection as far as the devil is concerned, and by the dominance of repression, if we are to understand the nature of the deity.

I wish to interrupt the discussion of clinical material to suggest an epigenetic scheme of defensive and adaptive apparatuses, as far as the psychotic psychic functioning is concerned. For this purpose, I have developed a graphic model of the psychic apparatus, using a three-dimensional cylindrical representation of certain inner relationships to clarify some puzzling aspects of the special difficulties of schizophrenics. As we know from Freud's early efforts, spatial models usually suffer from shortcomings and should never be taken too seriously. Mine is meant merely as a pictorial aid to restate graphically, as it were, what cannot be stated fully through clinical description.

This three-dimensional model is an attempt to combine features of Freud's topographic model of 1900 and his structural (or tripartite) model of 1923. The top of the cylinder represents the highest layer in the hierarchy of psychic apparatuses: the ego and all its apparatuses for secondary-process functioning—inner and outer perception, reality testing, judging, capacity for action, etc.; the conscious derivatives of superego and ego-ideal functions; and the conscious derivatives of id functions. The top circle is meant to be a graphic replica of Freud's model of the psychic apparatus as illustrated in The Ego and the Id. The lowest layer of the cylinder represents undeveloped self-organization, the undifferentiated phase at the early beginning of the psychic apparatus. Functions to be developed would "exist" there only as dispositions, as Anlagen. If one were to slice through that cylinder at any point, one would cut out and bare an earlier layer of the structure, which could be related to the history of the psychic organization as well as to the nature of current conflict material. The current material is frequently produced by means of regression or progression up and down the ladder between the undifferentiated phase and the highest organization. This material may be explained in terms of dominant psychic functions which could be "located" in this spatial model and would permit the creation of an epigenetic scheme of defenses and adaptive devices, similar, perhaps, to Erikson's use of a table for his eight stages of development. The mantle could be opened and this cylindrical model could then be compared to the picture of the psychic apparatus offered in the topographic model, when Freud refers to system consciousness, system preconscious and system unconscious.

Such a model might allow us to develop notions about the genesis

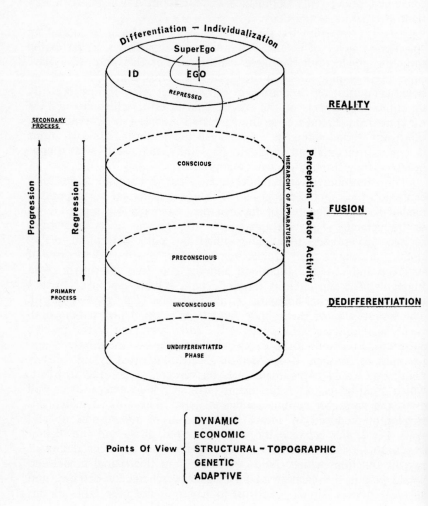

SYNTHESIS OF TOPOGRAPHIC & STRUCTURAL MODEL
OF THE PSYCHIC APPARATUS

of defenses and adaptive devices, and to classify clinical material in terms of phase dominance, defense dominance, adaptive-device dominance, reality-testing dominance and the like, in terms of the particular problems that we have with such patients.

We could look at clinical data in terms of ego fluctuations, instinctual fluctuations, superego fluctuations, object- relationship fluctuations, etc. At one stage of development, for example, we might speak of a therapeutic transference relationship that is under the sway of introjects. At another, we might refer to a transference relationship that is under the sway of permanent object representations and stable capacity for object relations.

If our assessment could predict the dominance of certain features of the psychic apparatus, we would be able to predict behavior both in and after therapy.

We might find that the clinical material which features Teresa's attempts to come to grips with her situation would require us to color certain parts of the model described, while others would remain white, indicating that they are unused and perhaps forever unusable. Freud suggested that nothing that ever entered the mind is destroyed, and that we can find the memory traces of every event in life. He compared the psychic apparatus with the eternal city of Rome, an analogy which has inspired this attempt at a three-dimensional model. He also mentioned the possibility that certain traumata could destroy mental functions which make the process of recovery of memory—the restoration or earlier conditions—impossible or very unlikely, in the same way that earthquakes, fires, wars and deliberate removal of parts of a city destroy many traces of its past.

The question that faces us is whether Teresa may ever be able to develop a transference relationship which is not inundated by regressed psychotic processes, by early precursors of object relationships. That question places the therapist in the position of a gambler who does not know that he plays with crooked dice and that the ordinary probabilities of the game are unavailable. Does the study of the material indicate that we are dealing with certain irreversible features, so that Teresa's "passive ego" can only build fluctuating, often psychotic, transferences, which will drive Eurydice back from Orpheus to Pluto in Hades lest she see the light of day? Will they drive her back from God to the devil and vice versa, and not truly permit her to exchange the assembly of unstable introjects, that meet and dissolve like an unreliable, agitated, shifting mob, for a stable assembly of duly elected representatives?

Let us return again to clinical material to indicate some of the questions that research has to answer. One may think of Teresa's picture of God and devil as object splitting, but we have suggested that the material indicates that she has pre-ambivalence, a state of affairs that exists before the negative and positive aspects of the objects are fused. One may use the term "splitting" after self- and object-representations have been established. Splitting is a regressive function. We deal frequently with states of mind in which there is presplitting, and in which there is still no synthesis of good and bad fragments of the parent figure. In one session, for example, she saw herself looking at Christ's feet, and suddenly had the fantasy that He had devil's feet. In this kind of image the positive features of the introject were stronger but somehow fused with certain negative features. The disassociated part—the sexual and evil part, in both Him and in herself—was now attached to the positive part of the transference, strong enough to defeat the negative. One might think of such experiences as precursors of synthesis, as painful attempts to set in motion a synthetic function, albeit a psychotic version of it, but nevertheless an active attempt to fuse positive and negative elements, and to gain insights. The glueing of part-objects precedes their genuine integration.

The 730th hour provides an illustration of Teresa's attempt to give up the idea that she is in a dream world, and to get distance from the dream. She tried to analyze the dream:

> She had been reading something which interested her, and she spoke about it in nightmarish terms. She saw in a magazine the surface of the moon, and while it was not exactly a nightmare, she objected to the color which was greenish and gave her an eerie feeling. That brought her to her wish to tell me about her nightmarish dream, which she said was not exactly a nightmare either. It seems that the dream took place somewhere in a house, perhaps the Home where she lives; some of the people seemed to remind her of the girls she knows at the Home. They were preparing a meal, a Mexican meal of beans with cheese; and she proceeded to give painstaking, obsessive descriptions of every detail of the meal so that I felt sure that these were her way of embroidering the dream with secondary elaborations. There was a guest, a lady, perhaps a young girl, who seemed strange and uncanny, because as they offered her the meal, Teresa thought the lady did not accept the food. She really wanted something else, but it also seemed that she was quite polite, and that she did accept some food but did not really fully participate in the meal. She did not remain with the others but went from room to room. Finally, all the people saw to their great amazement that the strange but kindly woman had disappeared but not in the usual way. It seemed that only her flesh disappeared, only her body, but they still saw the dress or whatever outfit she was wearing. Teresa modified the dream somewhat, but this was essentially the message: that they, the

girls, together cooked a meal, and that she, the woman, did not actually accept the meal, and even as she ate it, she indicated that she wanted something else. Finally, she withdrew and disappeared slowly in this strange way, perhaps rising to heaven.

Teresa tried to analyze the dream, to understand it; it was she who suggested that perhaps the woman was herself. I remembered, of course, that she had often thought of herself as a ghost, as someone who would go back to heaven, and I stressed the notion that she was dreaming that a person not satisfied with the food offered her had turned into a ghost and had disappeared. It was this interpretation of the old comparison with herself as a ghost that now made her work on the dream, and she stressed constantly that this was a *kind* lady. I spoke about this in terms of her having seen herself in the past as an evil ghost, but now she had become acceptable, a kind and good ghost. When things on earth did not go right, a part of her returned to heaven. Since she was a kind lady, God did not punish her but wanted her to go to heaven. As she pursued this topic, she also wanted to describe certain TV movies about vampires she had seen. She dwelt, of course, on the dreams she had had in the past, seeing herself as a strange and evil woman, the mouth smiling but ready to bite; as a vampire who would suck the blood out of people, kill them, and turn them into vampires. I used the current turn of events to show the struggle in her between the vampire ghost and the good ghost, and the fact that she now saw herself as a good ghost. We then spoke about the magic gesture that permitted God always to triumph over the devil and force him into retreat. Every vampire can be forced into retreat, and she could be turned into the good Teresa if she were exposed to the holy picture, the image of St. Michael, etc. I said that therefore this fear she had that either of us might be the vampire that sucked the blood out of and turned the other into a vampire could be overcome because we knew that God could out-do the devil and outtrick him. She sort of joined me in this en-deavor and said that in the past she had frequently refused to tell me these stories because she had been frightened by them. She felt now that she should not postpone them anymore but should use the next two or three sessions in order to solve the whole mystery of the vampire dream, and tell me the story of the haunted ghost in the castle, etc.

While God and repression won once more over the devil and pro-jection, we found that this inner election battle was a kind of cliff-hanger. The net result was not the re-establishment of autonomy, the victory of genuine insight, but demonstrated that the integrated and synthetic functions of the ego were comparatively feeble and were al-lowed only short-lived activity. They did not restore healthy adaptive devices, and she ended with the passive promise to use the next two or three sessions in order to solve the mystery, while postponing dealing with the tasks of life. Waelder stated that the humanistic goal of psychoanalysis is to bring about "enlarged consciousness" (11). In the case of Teresa and similar patients, we see that this achievement cannot be maintained; that the suggestion that they "follow the yellow brick road" which will lead to victory over the witches and help Dorothy wake up and return to her family does not seem to hold. Teresa's "yellow brick road" led her to a point where she could reproduce her dreams, did not accept them as reality, and even "analyzed" them. But as she continued to follow that yellow brick road, it turned into a Moebius strip (Ch. 25, this vol.), and outside became inside again. As she recognized the young woman of the dream as herself, and saw the flight mechanism, the ghostlike escape into the heaven of passivity, she was thrown as if by a sudden impulse, an outburst of negative activity, into the hostile role of the bloodsucking vampire. She tried to master this role by projecting it onto the eternal protagonist, the therapist, now turning into the devil. We can now better understand her image of the Christ with devil's feet, and the meaning of these primitive devices of pre-ambivalence.

Although the eternal struggle between the forces of hell and heaven continues and the further use of additional material might give us refined insight into the vicissitudes of the therapeutic struggle, we must sooner or later decide on a cutting-off point. We must do this even knowing it will allow us no more than tentative and unreliable assessments—clinical judgments and decisions which will be based on human error.

I have been using the pictorial representation of the psychic apparatus in order to think through the material in terms of the different metapsychological points of view. They can only give us partial answers, rationales which leave us puzzled and are soon discovered to be near rationalizations. The search for technical leverage is not unlike the struggle of the patient, who moves between heaven and hell, and who uses the earth not as the foundation for action and for living, but as a point of departure, upward towards salvation in passivity or downward towards the temptations of hell. We are drawn towards an attempt to explain the patient's imbalances through the different metapsychological assumptions. We may speak of deneutralization and defusion of drive energy; about ego defects and permanent inability to attain object-constancy or self-constancy; about lack of synthetic function and other adaptive apparatuses, and the like. I suppose it becomes clear that the old view of the ego as simply a mediator of conflict cannot give us the technical answers to such puzzling cases, and that we must think of the ego also as a problem-solving agency; not only as a restorer of inner equilibrium, but as an adaptational force.

Experiences with this patient have convinced me more and more that she never lives completely in the autistic world of her own fantasies. Even the most dreamlike adaptation in the consulting room shows the impact of the therapist's interpretations or other devices, helpful or unhelpful as they may be. Teresa is actually always responsive to the press of the environment, of reality. Even though she escapes into heaven or hell and never seems to have her feet planted firmly on the ground, the representatives of reality are not entirely ineffective.

The recent investigations by Fisher, Luborsky, Shevrin, Klein, and others as they repeated the old Poetzl experiment on subliminal perception are relevant here. A dream reported by the experimental subject helps him to remember in dreamlike fashion, via symbolic language and the primary process of the dream, the impact of the perception which he could not fully capture while he was awake. The experiment exposes "reality" for but a short moment so that the organs of perception, the adaptive and synthesizing apparatuses of advanced ego positions, seem to be side-tracked, while primitive ego apparatuses seem to register the material that was exposed to the eye of the subject. It is as if the memory traces were not strong enough to allow for more than subliminal perception.

The patient's response to the impact of the environment, the therapeutic environment of her current life situation, sometimes gives the impression that we did not expose her long enough or forcefully enough to what we had to say, that we have missed the point of "imprinting," and that we should do things more powerfully and harder. This seems to agree with the frequent impression of therapists that they must be intrusive and forceful with such patients, and that they must "feed them introjects," an interesting countertransference reaction which each of us has often enough experienced. But it has also occurred to me that it is frequently the *patient* who has not exposed us well enough to *her* "dreams." We are not sensitive or skillful enough to set into motion the more primitive ego apparatuses in ourselves which would permit us to register the cues from the patient long enough so that they could lead to technical action. Toying with the Poetzl experiment, I think of the patient as the one who exposes us, albeit too briefly, to her dreams. They register in our higher apparatuses but not potently enough also to register in those apparatuses of the therapeutic self which would permit, so to speak, perfection downward in the hierarchy of the psychic apparatus as well as perfection upward.

After all, if we speak of the "expansion of consciousness" as a goal for the patient, we must also speak of expansion of consciousness as a goal for the therapist. This expansion refers not only to Freud's dictum: "Where id was, there shall ego be," but to the necessity for developing an expanse of a wide range of consciousness, the restoration of the continuum horizontally and vertically.

As far as the therapist is concerned, we might as well reverse Freud's dictum and say that if we want to help such patients, we must some- times suggest that where ego was, there must be id as well. We must be capable of perceiving the patient's communications on all levels. There are moments when we have sufficient contact with these patients and experience the therapeutic work as less elusive, where we actually join the dream and help the patient wake up and join us, even if only for brief moments. I had such an experience with Teresa.

Again she was struggling with devil and God, and describing the terrible temptations of the devil, who pulled her down when she wanted to be an ideal good person. I described the struggle between her and the devil like a tug-of-war between two teams, each trying to pull the other to its side. I said that I wanted to be on her side, and help her pull the devil to her side as well, so that he would have to follow her rather than destroy her. She described the effectiveness of prayer vis-à-vis the devil, of positive dreams where the devil was defeated and where she was pulled to heaven. This brought to mind the death of her grandmother, a lovely, giving woman whom she lost when she was eight. In the coffin at the funeral, she saw the grandmother who had been "fixed up lovely," but as Teresa looked at her grandmother she could also sense a bad smell. She herself sometimes smelled like that— full of all the chemicals that were put into the grandmother, the smell of death. At that moment it was as if she had a nightmare—or was it a wish?—because that loving grandmother seemed to pull her so that she, Teresa, would be dead as well. And dead is what she wanted to be because she would be like the grandmother—perfect—but she would also be dead. But then God created a miracle, and he only made her dream this because she was really not dead; she was alive.

Suddenly she started to laugh, and finally confessed a fantasy about the therapist, which she thought was ugly and funny and crazy. She saw him as a merman, and it became clear that she was describing his lower fish body and the fact that the upper part was naked. Ever since I started working with her, she has often looked at me and, rather than making me into a catalytic agent, has sort of made me into her personal *Picture of Dorian Gray*; that is, her other self. I instantly said that I, too, had a fantasy about her, namely, that I saw her as a mer- maid. I remembered the Christ with the devil's feet, and realized, of course, that the sexual transference fantasy hidden behind her example had put into the image whatever the psychotic ego could in order to ward off the full sexual implications, by creating a tempting merman who was only a fish. She described herself as a mermaid who would eat fish and live in the "wide blue sea." She then continued the fantasy and suggested that she saw herself on water skis, being pulled by someone on a rope; then she described the lower part of her body as not quite a fish body: somehow there were legs attached to her. For a few short moments we enjoyed a game where I pulled her on water skis, but she started to laugh and described how the rope broke and she was rising on her water skis towards heaven—flying towards the clouds and then disappearing.

Here we clearly see the impact of the comment concerning the rope-tugging contest. Her response was one in which the contract and contest between us—facing the erotic implications of the transference fantasy—again broke as she flew heavenward.

I should add that during all these years there has been a little vase on my desk which pictures Copenhagen's Little Mermaid. Teresa had seen that mermaid many times, as she often desperately checked the desk clock to see whether the hour was ending and she could leave the painful therapeutic world to go "towards the heavens," but she had never commented on it. Now, she was amazed when I called to her attention that the little mermaid actually does have two legs, that only her feet have fins to help her swim. There is nothing in this room that did not somehow register in the world of her fantasies, but never in such a way as to have permanent impact on the solution of tasks. Whatever reality offered—the help of the therapist, the supporting figures in her environment, countless working and learning situations to which we tried to expose her—was always used either to get her back into the past or propel her forward into fantasy Utopias, that are, after all, a return to an idealized negative or positive childhood. One might say that she was so overwhelmed by the past and by hopes for the future that she could never allow herself to connect them by means of the present. The present is only a stepping stone to the inner world, but it makes itself felt like the picture in the Poetzl experiment; it makes its impact on the dreamer but hardly ever on the waking person.

Can we join our patients in their elusive pursuit of reality, that hunt for the present, for actuality? As we move with them toward their purgatories, their hells, their dreams of heaven; as we accept their flights backward and forward in time, we may discover the technical means, the theoretical insights to fortify the professional self-constancy which is required. In the meantime, we must be moved by the faith that it is not the patient's ego defect, but the gap in our knowledge which is the cause of the dilemma, and we must also believe that the questions we ask someday may and can be answered. Such optimism must sustain our humanitarian attitude and scientific interest, as we attempt to meet our therapeutic task.

REFERENCES

1. CARUTH, E. & EKSTEIN, R. "Interpretation within the Metaphor: Further Considerations." *J. Am. Acad. Child Psychiat.*, 1966, 1:35.
2. EKSTEIN, R. & WRIGHT, D. "The Space Child." *Bull. of Menninger Clin.*, 1952, 16:211.
3. ———. "The Space Child's Time Machine: On 'Reconstruction' in the Psychotherapeutic Treatment of a Schizophrenoid Child." *Amer. J. Orthopsychiat.*, 1954, 24:492.
4. —— & WALLERSTEIN, J. "Observations of the Psychotherapy of Borderline and Psychotic Children." *Psychoanalyt. Study of the Child*, 1956, 11:303.
5. —— & WALLERSTEIN, J. 'Choice of Interpretation in the Treatment of Borderline and Psychotic Children." *Bull. of Menninger Clin.*, 1957, 21:199.
6. —— & WRIGHT, D. "The Space Child—Ten Years Later." *Forest Hospital Pub.*, 1964, 2:36.
7. —— & CARUTH, E. "The Working Alliance with the Monster." *Bull. of Menninger Clin.*, 1965, 4:189.
8. FREUD, S. *The Ego and the Id* (1923). *Standard Edition*, 19. London: Hogarth Press, 1961.
9. ———. "Negation (1925)." *Standard Edition*, 19. London: Hogarth Press, 1961.
10. SCHLESINGER, H. "A Contribution to a Theory of Promising: the Making of Promises; Primary and Secondary Promises." Unpublished.
11. WAELDER, R. "Psychoanalysis and Moral Values." *Bull. of Phila. Assn. for Psychoanalysis*, 1968, 1:25.

CHAPTER SIXTEEN

One Step Beyond*

In presenting this magnificent essay on the phase of re-evaluation for termination of Teresa Esperanza's analytic treatment, Dr. Ekstein has again shared with us his unique and inimitable faculty to perceive scientific, intellectual and clinical issues with a sweeping panoramic vision. He now adds to his series of significant and valuable psychological scientific contributions in this presentation of a model for the integration of psychoanalytic psychotherapy with clinical research. These have been—in conjunction with training—the component arms of the Project on Childhood Psychosis from which this research material has sprung.

Those of us privileged to have shared this experience with him have watched the therapeutic progression of Teresa Esperanza, beginning with the initial diagnostic evaluation. Then, filled with an inner terror of unspeakable degree, she was shackled by complete helplessness in her search for the mother who was neither within nor outside her. Her initial therapeutic revelations about herself were of a lost creature, somewhere on an island, completely cut off from the mainland of normal living. She was an ice maiden, frozen with the terror of her internal rage, managing to survive—but not truly alive—merely maintaining the "refrigeration" and emotional distance necessary to manage her survival. In sharing Dr. Ekstein's profound commitment to research and scientific pursuit, we have followed the enormous saga of Teresa's long journey in search of mental health about which she initially had little or no comprehension. She perceived the treatment as a rescue mission by an Olympian god whom, in her psychotic despair, she really saw as

* Seymour W. Friedman is the author of this chapter.

219

doomed to fail in his undertaking. She herself had barely any hope of his success despite her overidealized, effusive outpouring of faith in his capacity to perform miracles.

Dr. Ekstein christened her the therapeutic pseudonym of Esperanza —the Spanish word for "hope," which he doubtlessly had hoped Teresa would have made her own. He did this as he realized that his first move must be to introduce her to the possibility of additional options for life other than frozen and moribund despair. Encased in it, she never could have emerged had it not been for his steadfast effort in and commitment to introducing and restoring her to life. In the course of this, he has given almost a decade of his own professional clinical life so that he might become the necessary infusion—the graft—which such psychotic patients seem to require of and from their therapist.

We have seen how Dr. Ekstein regarded Teresa as a completely unique individual. The diagnostic classification of psychosis served only as an opening wedge to the later understanding of the myriad of complex and perplexing manifestations of her psychotic personality for which the only predictable order is disorder. He had only his creative ingenuity, wide-ranged imaginativeness, clinical experience and psychoanalytic theory with which to create an instrument to establish contact and from which he could derive a technique for eventually effective therapeutic work. From the beginning, Dr. Ekstein recognized that he would have to convert the patient's deficits into resources. He approached Teresa with a therapeutic contract in which they would both form an alliance with her monster (1)—a deadly creature within her from whom she fled into her frozen state. This monster was the representation of the archaic precursors of a superego, and was derived from the ingredients of the very id forces against which it struggled and so desperately attempted to control. The monster had dominated her life as an alien and dangerous enemy, but Dr. Ekstein suggested that together they would help the monster to become an ally that would lead to re-integration and to a new, viable synthesis of the good and bad within her. And we have heard how the monster himself became an agent of her developing capacity for higher level ego function.

We have followed patient and doctor through the phase of the alliance with the monster—her creature; through her obsessive preoccupation with herself as dead; and through her descent into Hades in her search for Orpheus and love (Ch. 13, this vol.). Throughout the journey, we saw a gradual, although limited, kind of differentiation taking place within her, between the psychotic introjects that were becoming integrated into objects. We also saw a gradual formation of the self, which although still unreliable and unstable, had achieved some degree of self- and object-constancy and some equilibrium between good and evil, between fusion and diffusion. Teresa was thereby able to achieve a growing and changing perception of her objects from the earlier creatures and monsters to angels, good spirits and deities. She was able to experience something good, where heretofore her memory had convinced her there was only the bad, the destructive, the untrustworthy.

We have now come to a phase where termination and re-evaluation have become part of the overall process. She has progressed to the point where she considers the idea of termination, but has been unable to act on this wish. The therapist has also come to a point where he, too, would like to see her able to terminate. He wishes to help her take the proper action within the therapy, as well as within herself. Able to utilize social resources that could help her move into the world, she could fulfill her promise to herself to leave the psychotic dependence symbolized for her by the therapeutic situation. This had been her life for years, and now she seeks to find a new life in the reality and actuality of the outside world.

At this point, however, the therapist is faced with the dilemma created by the very nature of the therapeutic process. This process had enabled Teresa to leave her primary-process internal world, dominated by creatures and monsters, by helping to develop the beginning capacity to institute delay over impulse and impulse-action, and to substitute thought for impulsive action. However, this has resulted in a kind of paralysis, immobilizing her into a static existence which removes her from the world and makes realistic living still impossible for her. In the therapy sessions preceding the current re-evaluation, the patient began to toy with the notion of termination, although still without the capacity to do more than play with such thoughts. We have yet to see what else the therapeutic process has infused within her, completely dependent as she has heretofore been upon the therapeutic program for the total direction of her living. This may well have contributed to her dominant attitude of passivity and to the fear of action as being destructive.

Thus, the therapeutic process has actually brought about her allegiance to thought, although not necessarily to goal-oriented thoughtfulness. The latter alone leads to action rather than merely to an allegiance to the promise that can never be fulfilled, which had been her inner situation in the past. The promise itself reveals an incorporation of a facet of the therapist with which she has not yet been able to identify as a representation of secondary-process, goal-directed thought and action. Her promises still reflected her primary-process thinking in which she equated fulfillment with its declaration (5). We can see how the patient, in her literal and concrete thinking about the therapist, could well have interpreted and perceived him as the representative of inactivity and passivity, of non-action. This, after all, is implicit in a model of psychoanalytically oriented treatment and in the role of the therapist. We might almost say that both the therapist and the patient did their work too well. The therapist did not wish her to act like him; rather, he had hoped she would identify with the intent and purpose of reflection as being the agent that makes thoughtful action possible. But Teresa had indeed identified with the hopeful promise of the therapist, and had accepted him as a new object with whom she established a working alliance. However, he had not been able to incorporate his essential meaning. Moreover, she had been unable to achieve the necessary degree of intrapsychic development with differentiation of self and object which could have enabled her to exercise the judgment necessary for the intellectual action that puts an end to postponement and leads to the choice of motor action (3).

In other words, Teresa has not been able to achieve that level of intrapsychic function that would make it possible for her to judge, plan or act on a secondary-process level, and to move from goal-oriented thought to purposeful act. Her capacity to maintain separation and individuation remains so tenuous that acting on outer reality is immediately impaired by her fear of destroying it, or of being destroyed by it. In his paper, Dr. Ekstein presents us with the question as to the nature of this anticipated and feared destruction: what are the dynamic and economic processes involved; what are the mechanisms that make action appear—or be experienced—as a destructive rather than as an adaptive process?

We need examine carefully the implications of such techniques with this patient as that of an alliance with her monsters and of maintaining distance through interpretation within the metaphor. On the one hand, they have enabled her to reach the level of progress described in the paper. However, this paper also suggests the need to search and research for ingredients that might not have been provided which would have furthered the process sufficiently to enable her to be governed not only by the reality principle, but also by the actuality principle. That is, the ingredients which would encompass an adaptive use of her newly developed capacity for secondary-process thinking in living vis-à-vis external reality. The current adjustment is marked by an apparent commitment to passivity and inactivity, to paralysis as a way of defending against the impulse and chaos that are precipitated by external demands. Instead, she maintains her life as if it were a dream free of the pressures of external reality. She has now come to form an alliance with those good objects, the angels and good spirits. They, with God at the head of the hierarchy, have become representatives of repression and of inhibition of the impulse rather than of transforming it into action. Why is it that she has identified almost all activity with the command of the devil, thus seeing it as something which might destroy the very basis of any safety and security within herself and within the world?

The therapeutic process has both been governed by and has led to Dr. Ekstein's insights concerning a model of the personality which is derived from and combines both the topographic and structural models of Freud. In this new model, the beginning undifferentiated psychic organization is schematized as moving along the axis of a cylinder. In minute stages it progresses toward the optimum and maximum achievement of differentiation and individuation of the psychic agencies into the separate components of ego, id and superego. This enables a stable differentiation of self and object, as well as of inner and outer life, which guarantees against a return to the annihilating symbiotic fusion that destroys the individuation and identity necessary for optimal personality development. Dr. Ekstein's application of this model has shown how the patient's thoughts and language communicate to the therapist the inner functioning of the psychic apparatus, and invite him to join the patient in the necessary symbiotic relationship. It also shows how they provide the ingredients for the therapeutic process and for the growth of the intrapsychic organization.

However, in presenting his paper, Dr. Ekstein is also raising the issue of basic approach to the treatment of such a patient and even more regressed patients. He is asking if the approach to severely autistic and symbiotic children should be through thought and language alone. Perhaps the primary source of contact and therapeutic nutriment which would meet the particular needs of the most regressed aspect of their functioning must be derived from more primitive levels than thought and language. In order to approach these patients through their strength, we must not approach them through projecting islands which are advanced outposts of their development with little connection with the totality of their regressed mainland. Even though we consider the thought disorder as the hallmark of the psychotic process, we may have to reconsider that the thought organization may well represent a structure which has a relatively weak connection with the rest of the intrapsychic organization. This possibility leads us to wonder if our concepts of treatment of the psychosis are perhaps focused too exclusively on the more sophisticated higher intellectual processes which are involved in the observing functions of the therapeutic ego. We may need to postulate further regression of the therapist's experiencing ego that could be of sufficient depth to meet and to understand the inner workings of the most archaic organizations of the more regressed patients. Such regressions of the therapists might then enable us to enter into the patient's inner world at a point where we can contact their essential self—their mainland—rather than their isolated islands of ego functioning.

One of Freud's postulates significantly defining psychosis has to do with the loss of reality testing and the imposition of the psychotic person's inner reality upon his outer reality, thereby substituting and creating his own reality (4). This postulate of psychosis, meaningful as far as it goes, considers psychosis from the viewpoint of reality. It does not fully enter that inner world of the psychotic, even though profound understanding of the inner world of the extremely disturbed personality has been demonstrated in Freud's writings.

To carry these germinal insights one step further, we may need to look at psychosis from more than one viewpoint. Not only must object relations and thought organization—including the functions of memory and perception—be considered, but also the vicissitudes of the basic impulse, as it erupts into the behavior, apparently devoid of thought and reason and lacking any emotions except for primitive affect energy discharge. We may need to consider as a basic assumption that the psychotic process starts with the eruption of the impulse into external reality, and that the very process of treatment concerns itself with the taming of this impulse. This leads to the civilizing of the human being that is accomplished in the processes of maturation and development in the normal and neurotic personality organization, but which is besieged by so many difficulties in the psychotic organization.

Freud's conceptual model of psychoanalysis, so aptly presented by Rapaport, describes the partial discharge of the drive representation as occurring along three parameters: affect, ideation and conation. In the primary model, the impulse under the domination of the pleasure principle undergoes partial discharge in the form of ideation or affect discharge as a result of the inevitable imposition of delay in the path toward gratification. As the capacity for delay is internalized, secondary-process thinking, tamed affective responses, and goal-directed action become possible under a new principle of organization: the reality principle. Affect may well provide the energic motivation that enables the thought organization to become integrated with goal-directed action. The range of affective experience, similar to that of thought and action, also occurs along a hierarchical order from primary- to secondary-process form of expression. We must examine more carefully how, and in what way, the role of this hierarchy of affects can be brought into the theoretical conceptualization of the treatment process, and can become integrated into more effective treatment techniques. This is particularly true with the psychotic patients. Their personality disintegration is so grave that the psychotic adaptive, or in the long run maladaptive, effort fails to build an apparatus capable of controlling and regulating the impulse, the eruption of which might be said to represent the psychosis. The essential nature of psychosis is then reflected in the archaic and regressed state of the personality organization in which disparate components have neither achieved optimal differentiation and individuation, nor have been assimilated into an integrated and synthesized personality organization.

To make contact with these aspects of the deeply regressed psychotic patients, the therapist may have to make himself available to the most regressive aspects of the patient. As Dr. Ekstein has suggested, the therapist's expansion of consciousness may well need to reverse Freud's dictum so that where ego was, there shall id be in the service of the therapeutic ego. The process of such a therapeutic regression becomes necessary in order to achieve the form of primitivism that echoes and mirrors that of the psychotic patient. This may require that the therapist in order more effectively to contact the patient must meet his needs on the level of the most primitive emotions. This may involve even a kind of bodily action, as primtive and as repugnant as this might be to the therapist.

Dr. Ekstein has suggested elsewhere* that he believed the key to reaching a certain extremely regressed autistic child (with the kind of malignant illness about which we often expressed complete nihilism) might even require the therapist to lie next to the patient and cover himself with the very feces of the child. While resting mutely, devoid of thought, accepting completely this primeval archaic experience with him, the therapist would, nevertheless, at all times maintain his self and his therapeutic role—would not himself become psychotic. This most trenchant, powerful and insightful action-metaphor expresses and communicates that perfect symbiosis that protects the omnipotence of the autistic child and conveys the therapist's heroic commitment to lasting service to his patient. It is a most creative synthesis of the therapist's capacity for archaic regression and the highest order of sublimation in the service of the therapeutic ego. We are reminded here of the practice of the gorilla which protects its young by covering them with a coating of its own feces—certainly nature's most primitive way of providing warmth and closeness, albeit repugnant to civilized standards.

All this, of course, would create immense and perplexing difficulties in the treatment of these patients. But Dr. Ekstein has ended a decade of dedicated, skillful practice of psychoanalytic treatment of one patient. He now asks of us—as he does of himself—to evaluate what has

---

* Private communication.

and has not been achieved, in relation both to what had been hoped for and to what can still be strived for. We may have to consider the possibility that certain essential elements of the personality organization in the psychotic may literally get wiped out, and that there may be no replacement possible for them. Therefore, to some extent, we may be faced with an irreversible process that leaves a deficit which cannot be replaced or compensated for. However, unsure of this at our present stage of knowledge, we must, as Dr. Ekstein has suggested, be moved by the faith that it is not the patient's defect alone that confounds our therapeutic efforts. Our hopefulness must still remain our best guarantee of discovering the means to help these patients. And this hopefulness must combine with techniques that deal with all aspects of the psychological organization, affect and action, as well as thought organization and object relationships.

Our present knowledge only touches upon the importance of the role of the development of the self, following its individuation and differentiation from the object. This is considered the very first task of the personality organization. We need to study further the qualitative development of this self and its growing capacity for synthesis and integration of negative and positive images, of aggressive and libidinal elements. This is its second great task. We might even speculate that psychosis represents that stage of psychic organization in which the raw impulse, without drive representation, is totally dominant and continually erupts into behavior with which it confronts and confounds the world as it reveals its regressed and primitive aspects. The nature of the ongoing psychotic process may reflect the process of transformation of this deneutralized drive organization into the type of psychic organization that begins to delay the impulse and creates psychic structure. Those beginnings of the ego, even as they are capable of regulating the instinct and adapting it to reality according to the actuality principle, are also characterized by the fragmentation, disintegration and bizarreness which characterize the psychotic personality.

Returning again to Teresa who is entering hopefully and with hope into a closing phase of her treatment, we are reminded of what Dr. Ekstein has written elsewhere (2): an ending is also a beginning. At the termination of treatment we are greeted once again by elements of the illness which, like characters in a play, appeared first in order of their importance but return for their closing bow in reverse sequence. In his closing therapeutic work with Teresa, Dr. Ekstein has presented to us the seeds that can become the prologue to future research. Perhaps what we have best learned from Teresa is that our succeeding work must help us to touch those deeper layers of the self that possibly need to be contacted through more immediate affective and conative channels. We must explore further in what way the level of affective functioning can also be helped to progress from a primary-process level of primitive discharge to a secondary-process level of a modulated range of feelings. It may well be that the step from reality and paralysis to actuality and action cannot be made without also having developed one step beyond, so to speak, from the stage of deneutralized untamed affect discharge that makes both the thought and the act so dangerously destructive. For to the extent that Teresa needs the borrowed fantasy, she also tells us she fears her own thought, just as she fears her own self and must therefore borrow, but cannot identify with, that of the therapist.

Dr. Ekstein has often suggested that in the normal growth and development of the learning process, the child moves from the stage of learning for love to that of love of learning. Freud has defined mental health as the capacity to love and to work, and Dr. Ekstein has carried this definition further into a process whereby the healthy person moves from working for love to love of working. We might now suggest that there is the precursor to this in the psychotic child. It is the process of developing from living for love, where one must identify with the passive, anaclitic role, to the love of living, which is accepting the role of an autonomous, active, thoughtful and feeling human being: the goal for all our patients.

REFERENCES

1. EKSTEIN, R. & CARUTH, E. "The Working Alliance with the Monster." *Bull. of Menninger Clin.*, 1965, 4:189.
2. ———. "Termination of Analysis and Working Through." In *Psychoanalysis in the Americas*, Robert Litman, ed. N. Y.: Int. Univ. Press, 1966, 217.
3. FREUD, S. "Negation." *Standard Edition*, 19. London: Hogarth Press, 1961.
4. ———. "The Loss of Reality in Neurosis and Psychosis." *Standard Edition*, 19. London: Hogarth Press, 1961.
5. SCHLESINGER, H. "A Contribution to a Theory of Promising: The Making of Promises: Primary and Secondary Promises." Unpublished (1964).

CHAPTER SEVENTEEN

Notes on Treatment of Teresa: Assessment via Psychological Testing*

At the very beginning of treatment, Ekstein (2) notes that Teresa perceived her inner world as "finding herself isolated on an island in an engulfing world of fantasy. . . . She speaks about her symptoms and uses the phrase 'I am in the middle of an island. I don't know what to do. That is why I need your help. After all, you are the only one who can help me.'" Ekstein predicted that treatment would consist in "building bridges or connections from the island on which she found herself to the rest of the world so that she could venture out into . . . the world if she wanted to." If this analogy of islands, that is, islands of functioning, correctly pictures the inner state of Teresa's psychotic world, then one should not think merely of building bridges or causeways from the island of autistic isolation and confusion to the mainland of reality testing and adjustment. Islands do not float but are, in fact, connected with the mainland, albeit separated by the seas. One might, therefore, think of raising the land mass enough above the level of the sea so that, with true stability established, the tides and storms of the psychosis will not continually ravage and flood the islands. This notion seems to be expressed by Ekstein and Caruth when they suggest (3) that psychotic patients "suffer from certain basic ego deficits resulting in islands of psychic structure that are disconnected and fragmented," a simile borrowed from Knight (4).

---

* Joel M. Liebowitz is the author of this chapter.

In speaking about the treatment of such patients, Ekstein and Caruth go on: "In treatment we seek to integrate and synthesize the islands of psychic functioning through a kind of psychological grafting, metaphorically analogous to the use of fill to build a causeway between separated islands. If successful, if the degree of compacting is high enough, there will appear little difference in the completed structure from the natural formation. Nevertheless, we know all too well that underground movements will always be more dangerous here than where no fill has been necessary." The authors seem to suggest that, at best, one can help certain types of psychotics to cope more appropriately with the inner chaos by layering adaptive capacities "on top" even while the chaos remains on an internal, lower level.

This analogy of islands is being examined in order to see whether it can be considered a useful concept relative to the treatment of certain psychotics. This assessment will be attempted by reviewing successive psychological testings of Teresa during treatment. Specific reference to one TAT story will be made in this evaluation of treatment via the analogy of islands, but there will be no attempt to follow in depth the response content. TAT Card One, which concerns a child's relationship to a broken violin, permits the conceptualization of this broken violin as the borrowed and broken ego, that is, the flooded islands. The excerpts that follow are merely time samples and do not give a complete sense of a process. Nevertheless, for comparative purposes, they do give a clear understanding of the analogy of building islands and bridges to the mainland of reality testing and adaptation.

Teresa was first evaluated by Eiduson (1) in June of 1960 when she was fifteen years, two months old. At this time Eiduson described Teresa as "much more comfortable with fantasy material and involved deeply in it. In addition, the psychological test picture is of a girl who is fending off psychosis through becoming like a nine-year-old child—being simple-minded, withdrawing any libidinal investment from the outside world and remaining close to and wallowing in fantasies of the latency period in which she found herself protected and happy." Eiduson goes on: "A tremendous withdrawal from reality makes it so that she scarcely takes in data of the world around her. Further, she is at the mercy of aggressive impulses, feeling herself constantly devoured by the enormity of these, and preoccupied with them, despite her efforts to cut them off by restricting her life . . . like a little girl."

In assessing these statements one pictures a withdrawal to an island of safety and protection. This first evaluation makes clear that Teresa was panicked by the seas of the psychosis which surrounded her, and her attempt to defend herself was to withdraw to an inner world. On this safe inner island she hoped to find some protection perhaps by being and feeling like a nine-year-old, but she was now stranded there unable to bridge the seas which surrounded her. Consistent with the early therapeutic material, Teresa relied upon some magical powers to save her and could not conceive of building a bridge of her own capacities. In her story to TAT Card One, she speaks about a boy whose violin was broken and says, "One day he sat down at his desk and he stared at the violin and he was thinking, 'Oh, I wish the violin was fixed.'" The story ends with, "He is going to get the violin fixed and then play it as always." There is no evidence as to how the violin will be fixed but merely that some repair work will be done, perhaps by magic. In Ekstein's comments about his first meeting with Teresa he described her as feeling that he was an angel sent by God to help restore her back to health by a miracle (2).

In March of 1962 Teresa, now sixteen years, eleven months, was again evaluated. Eiduson indicates, "She seems to be given to panicky and hysterical reactions but these are considerably more encapsulated and circumscribed than they were previously . . . Confabulations and contaminations appear with little auto-criticalness despite the fact that she is at other times extremely cautious about 'thinking in a crazy way' and now is particularly sensitive to the tricks that the mind can play. . . . Major areas in which change appears is in the perception of people, in the interest of establishing object relationships and in the open giving-in and the acknowledgment of dependency needs. Altogether, Teresa is much more sensitive to people" (1). To the TAT card Teresa talks about a boy who has studied the violin a great deal and is given his own instrument for Christmas. The violin breaks and the father fixes it, but the boy plays the violin and the string breaks again. When the parents come home later the boy had fixed the violin by himself. But, Teresa is not certain how this took place, only that the boy somehow got the violin back together. As she says, "I don't know how. He was a smart little boy. He had a good mind. He worked the string someplace with a needle that was there and that was fine."

This is a striking difference from her response to Card One in 1960. The present story involves still a bit of unexplained reparation but also the beginning of a relationship. It is true that in this relationship the other person, the father, does not have the capacity to maintain himself as a continually good object. That is, the violin breaks after the father had repaired it. However, in the story Teresa entertains the notion that one can perhaps rely upon others. In the end, however, she returns to herself as the only one who can really take care of herself, but the idea is expressed that the little boy could fix the violin by himself. This seems to reflect a growing sense of her own inner capacity, her own growing sense of ego ability. This is further indicated in the test report

(1): "Teresa is becoming aware that she is on an island separated from a mainland of people and latent opportunities to establish object relationships."

In the 1964 re-evaluation when Teresa was eighteen years, nine months, Eiduson says, "One is struck by the greater core of reflectiveness in what she does, which pushes her to try to continually re-orient her thinking into reality appropriate channels. . . . It turned out that these channels are unmistakably correct and conventional . . . There is increased ego development in the direction of better judgment, more adaptability, more conventional thinking and more social sensitivity . . . Teresa's enhanced sense of judgment, criticality, and increased attention seems not to have modified the psychotic thought processes, but rather provides a kind of new outside layering which keeps the manifestations of the psychosis in check and has the additional purpose of providing gratification in and of themselves." Eiduson also notes that Teresa is more organized and that the ego abilities are now more apparent. Eiduson describes a layering of capacity, that is, a layering of ego adaptability on top of the existing psychosis. To use the analogy that we are following, the fill seems to have lasted and held and there is a capacity to stand on it and function intermittently above the waters of the psychosis. These emerging ego capacities may be pictured as islands that have been built up within the psychotic seas and, as Eiduson suggests, the fact that their existence seems to be gratifying and satisfying perhaps encourages further filling. Eiduson continues, "There is no question that important 'therapeutic messages' have gotten across to her. One message that she can spell out quite logically is the difference between thinking aggressive thoughts and acting them out. . . . All such sophisticated notions are apparently sufficiently integrated into her personality so that she can derive help from them in controlling her own behavior." It would seem that Teresa has adopted "messages to live by," as if she had borrowed a piece of Ekstein's "ego" and is attempting to make it her own in much the same way that a young child takes the admonishments of a parent to help him control his behavior. That is, imitation and injunction are there but not true internalization.

In Teresa's TAT story, the violin breaks and this time, instead of repairing the broken violin, the boy accepts another violin from his father. Thus, instead of working with the defective inner material Teresa seems to feel that to become whole again she must take what is good from someone else as a kind of ego transplantation or graft. But, Teresa goes on in this story, "This boy played all the concerts and everything, all the music on one violin. He had only one violin and he kept playing on it." The emphasis on the fact that there is only one violin suggests the tenuousness of the ego capacities. Yet, it does seem apparent that Teresa's solution for the moment is to take what is offered by others and make it her own rather than try to work with her own inner "bad" material, that is, her own inner broken ego. The change noted in the psychological testing is confirmed by Ekstein who notes "Teresa is sometimes capable of establishing a feeble bridge between her inner world, her delusional preoccupation, and her attempts to communicate with the psychotherapist. She does this by means of what I have called borrowed fantasies . . . metaphoric allegories borrowed from television shows or movies to which she is addicted. . . . The show becomes the brittle and unreliable bridge between her chaotic inner world and the vague desire to talk about that inner world . . . One can see then that underneath the unconscious, the reality-oriented attempt to master small tasks and to be committed to short-term goals, is a powerful psychic system which is characterized by the inner struggle, the alternating commitment to life and to death" (Ch. 7, this vol.).

In 1966, twenty-one-year-old Teresa was again re-evaluated. Eiduson indicates in the report, "She is, however, much more aware of being a very different, very odd and very isolated person, and her very studied attempts at adopting appropriate and relevant behaviors suggest how much awareness of this latter there is." Eiduson goes on to note two important differences between the current testing and previous evaluations: "The first is a pervasive sadness which seems to be derived from two things: one, this awareness of difference which seems to be accompanied by a feeling of hopelessness about outcome. . . . At the moment Teresa seems to feel the inevitability of being mentally ill." By 1966, that is, Teresa seemed not only able to recognize and perceive what was happening within her more clearly than before but also to despair of ever being well.

To the TAT card Teresa says "Um, well, he wasn't really miserable like I think, um, but there was one time I guess he felt, um, something, um, was missing and, um, he always wished for this most, most than anything else he could wish for or imagine or think about . . ." Teresa continues in this story, "So this beautiful interesting violin his father had given him, he was so happy with. Well, he was in his bedroom, this is really how it happened. I'll tell you a story. While he was in his bedroom he was trying it out and his father had taught him how to use it and his father was giving him special classes certain days, not every day, but it was around the afternoon 'til night, 'til not so late . . ." Teresa talks about the boy doing his homework with his violin and concludes the story by saying the violin breaks but is then fixed again. "It was a very delicate violin, too, if you want to know. I want to say that this is one reason why it broke up easily." Now, Teresa's solution appears to be to rely upon others who can teach appropriate lessons. She seems more willing to borrow the ego, the adaptive capacities of the object—the therapist—in order to help herself cope. This borrowing of ego can be analogous to the use of fill in the gaps between the fragmented islands of ego functioning and perhaps to re-inforce the base upon which she stands. Consistent with this, her TAT story reflects, more clearly than ever before, relationships with people that involve affect and meaning. Feeling unable to do it on her own, and even, perhaps, that she cannot do it at all, Teresa seems to be saying that she can learn lessons of adaptation well and can apply them with the fragile self that she feels she is.

Confirmation of this increased awareness and capacity is noted in the treatment hours themselves. Ekstein and Caruth note: "Her first attempts to move from a kind of autistic psychotic position into a world of secondary-process functioning, of reality and actuality, were communicated through a series of psychotic acting-out episodes, following which she developed some capacity to move from a primary-process level of functioning to a beginning capacity actually to perform tasks and promises on a minimal level. She has achieved now a kind of pseudo-normal facade of seeming adjustment. She is able to handle everyday details of budget, transportation, minimal encounters with peripheral kinds of social experiences, etc." (Chapter 26, this vol.).

I saw Teresa for her 1969 evaluation, when she was twenty-four. I saw her first while she was in the midst of a psychotic episode that resulted in a temporary stay in a neuro-psychiatric hospital. I then saw her two months later when she was far more organized and able to function more effectively. At this second meeting Teresa recognized me from the previous session and she was, throughout the session, charming and pleasant. Unlike her behavior in the first meeting, she was able to accept structure and limitations in the second. Even though she had certain primitive, adaptive mechanisms, such as using her fingers to count, she was not overly self-conscious about these. Instead, she seemed to turn the deficit into an advantage; for example, she told me in a rather charming way that she uses her fingers to count and then asked if anyone could really refuse her the fingers for this effort. My test report (5) noted that the content and the present evaluation are quite consistent with previous evaluations, even with the changes that are seen. Her responses are shorter as if there is more inner control although the control seems to be of the immediate situation rather than a lasting confidence in her ability to master and cope. That is, the feeling within her appears to be that one does not need to rely wholly upon angels (introjects) but can go to the parent (object) for resurrection when one feels divided and impotent to unite oneself. Teresa seems to recognize her impotence even as she recognizes that perhaps the strength of repair from which she may borrow may lie with the strength of others.

The TAT story that she tells is about a little boy who keeps pestering his father for a violin. Instead of the boy not knowing where the violin comes from or the father giving the boy a violin, the boy finally asks for the violin himself. The boy is given the violin, which is described as being shiny and gold, and the feeling between father and son is the shared anticipation of the moment when this child will become the great violinist to the pleasure and pride of both child and father. "So one day after the father hired a special professor, he was practicing but at the end he got tired and accidentally broke one string." Teresa described the boy as being very sad but the violin was fixed and "He said be careful next time. So the little boy was careful and kept practicing and grew up and became a great musician and the father was very proud. And he was always careful with the violins and wouldn't break them." The report states: "One also sees learned adjustments, imposed ways of dealing with demands. It is as if she has a bit of borrowed ego (the islands of functioning) that she tries to make her own and so, with a half-internalized and half-external ego, she attempts to cope and adapt. In this regard, she has developed 'models to live by," that is, "homilies' and 'phrases to reason by' that serve as external reminders of correct behavior. The ability to integrate, to synthesize is still for the most part beyond her and Teresa is generally passive and overwhelmed in the face of the inner chaos of the psychosis. But there are islands of strength within the psychotic seas and when the seas diminish, seemingly of their own accord, one can see islands more clearly than ever before."

The metaphor of islands and causeways relates to the two parallel processes that seem to occur. On one hand, there seems to be a process of filling, a layering of a crust of ego functioning over the psychotic seas. This, in turn, seems to have been possible because of the capacity of the mainland (therapist) and the island (Teresa) to link up. It would thus seem that the therapeutic relationship afforded Teresa the safety and opportunity to take a chance on layering a crust, on filling the seas. At the same time, one can conceptualize this link between therapist and patient—between the mainland and the island—as being the base of a firmer structure than the one that had existed earlier. For indeed, one can imagine that without this sense of firmness and security arising from the relationship, no ego layering, no filling, would ever have taken place. The analogy of islands in terms of the conceptualization of Teresa's inner psychotic world does seem justifiable. Generalizations from one case are risky, but one may suggest that perhaps the treatment of certain psychotics does follow the pattern suggested throughout this treatment. That is, one may have to imagine treatment establishing a link from the islands of autistic functioning to the main-

ınd of reality testing and adjustment so that once this link is estab-
shed a layering of a crust from the mainland to the island may indeed
ıke place. The firmness of this layer is demonstrated by recent events
ı Teresa's life. Although she had a breakdown several months ago,
zen two months afterwards, she had reconstituted herself and was
ır better organized than she had been before the breakdown. It may
ıe that very much like real islands that sometimes get flooded by the
iolence of seas and storms, the waters eventually recede and the land
ınass holds firm. One does not have to begin rebuilding the island all
ıver again but merely replace the fill that has been carried away by the
ısychotic disruption.

REFERENCES

. Eiduson, Bernice. "Psychological Test Reports, Teresa Esperanza, 1960, 1962,
   1964, 1966." Unpublished.
. Ekstein, Rudolf. "The Opening Gambit in Psychotherapeutic Work with a
   Severely Disturbed Adolescent Girl." Children of Time and Space, Action and
   Impulse. N. Y.: Appleton-Century-Crofts, 1966.
.. ——— & Caruth, Elaine. "The Working Alliance with the Monster." Children
   of Time and Space, Action and Impulse. N. Y.: Appleton-Century-Crofts, 1966.
.. Knight, R. P. "Borderline States." Bull. of Menninger Clin., 1953, 17:1.
. Liebowitz, Joel. "Psychological Test Report, Teresa Esperanza, 1969." Un-
   published.

Part Four
BUILDING OF AND WORK WITH THE SUPPORT SYSTEMS

In most institutions I know of the basic approach, even to the psychotic child, is to encourage him to see the world as it really is, which is exactly what the psychotic child cannot do. Instead, our task as we see it is to create for him a world that is totally different from the one he abandoned in despair, and moreover a world he can enter right now, as he is. This means, above all, that he must feel we are with him in his private world and not that he is once more repeating the experience that "everyone wants me to come out of my world and enter his." How, then, is this done?

BRUNO BETTELHEIM

Reflections on the Need for a Working Alliance with Environmental Support Systems*

We would like to examine some of the therapeutic implications and consequences arising out of the peculiar nature of the interaction between the schizophrenic child and his past and present environment. This is his universe, as one youngster labeled it, and it is a true merging of his inner world and introjects with his outer world where introjects are the substitute for objects. The schizophrenic child and his environment form a kind of undifferentiated unit, analogous to the matrix of the maternal symbiosis in which there is a placental-like interchange between the inner and outer worlds of the child. This interchange is immediately effective in equalizing that which is within and that which is without so that, in effect, differentiation is wiped out and fusion can be re-established. A relative lack of differentiation within the psychic organization is paralleled by a lack of differentiation of psychic structure from the environment. Consequently, instead of internal conflict, the predominant conflict is seemingly between the patient and the environment, which has become the externalized projection of his opposing impulses. This is why the inner life of these children fre-

---

* Seymour W. Friedman, Elaine Caruth, and Beatrice Cooper are the co-authors of this chapter.

quently seems to mirror and to echo—to reflect but not reflect upon—what they have experienced both in the past as well as in their presen environment. Their external world seems also to reflect and mirror—to resonate with their inner reality. We may say of these children tha they look into reality not to find what is there outside themselves, bu rather to find outside themselves what lies within. And all too ofter the real objects—the current reality figures in their lives—do act ou or, more correctly, counteract out, within the countertransference and out of the hate that is engendered in the countertransference (2), ir ways that confirm the child's most frightening and dreadful projections And as the child succeeds in finding or provoking the objects in hi outer world to echo the images of his inner world that are the archaic unstable introjects from his past, he thereby confirms the validity o and strengthens his allegiance to this inner world.

The psychotic child seems to experience reality without distinguish ing shadow from substance, inner from outer reality or self from non self. Our understanding of such a reality requires trying to comprehenc the experience of a world emptied of all but one's own thoughts—which, undifferentiated from their concrete imagery, merge with reality and, mirroring the mind, cannot be distinguished from the mind. Sucl an inner experience is similar to the man who does not know if he dreams he is a butterfly or if he is a butterfly who dreams he is a man

A case in point from the clinical reality of the consulting room is Rena (1), a severely regressed schizophrenic girl, whose violently de structive psychotic acting-out can be understood as an attempt to restore and at the same time break away from the negative maternal symbiosis This symbiosis is like an inner straitjacket in which she is entombed and restrained from her impulsivity, but which, at the same time enthrones her with a delusional omnipotence that is maintained by the mother-child symbiosis. In a psychiatric re-evaluation* after a number of years of treatment, Rena was described as an extremely sick schizo phrenic adolescent. Her illness was manifested by her marked thought disorder reflecting the ego dysfunctioning under severe disintegrative threat, with disorganization, blocking, incoherence, irrelevance, persev eration, condensation, neologisms, word salad, echolalia and autistic logic. At times she manifested hallucinations, false perceptions, and misidentifications. Thought content, expressed in diffuse, fragmented verbalizations, was concerned with many themes, including religious theosophy, color and primitive sexual acting-out behavior. Emotional expression was characterized by blandness and apathy, with shifting and apparent disharmony between affect, response and external stim-

---

* Conducted by Robert A. Solow, M.D.

ulus. She manifested numerous peculiar ritualistic mannerisms, stereo-
typy and catatonic posturing. In action she demonstrated unpredictable
behavior, ranging from the use of the toilet, to incontinence and fecal
smearing, and from withdrawn passivity to wild activity. When overwhelmed by any kind of disintegrative threat she resorted to violent
assaultive behavior, excitement, apathy and confusion.

Psychological evaluations of the child and her mother were also
undertaken at that time. The results illustrated the way in which Rena's
fragmented inner life mirrored in a bizarre and magnified fashion the
inner world of the mother, almost as if to recreate the original matrix
within which she had developed and from which she had never grown
away. Psychological testing indicated a very regressed schizophrenic
girl whose state of disintegration and fragmentation created an overall impression of an animated but not quite animate psychic collage,
as it were, with fragments of various aspects of psychic functioning
seemingly stuck together haphazardly. No underlying cohesiveness or
identity was formed even though one could occasionally get a cue of
the remnants of some personality organization. When she spoke—
with words, actions or bodily and facial gestures—one felt it was but
one of many voices, as if she had a reservoir of isolated, imitative and
stereotypic memories (of an echolalic and echopraxic-like nature).
Although the observer could often identify what Rena wanted to convey, it could not easily be related to whatever was going on externally
with her. In similar fashion, she perceived, which is to say, projected
onto, those around her as a multitude of fleeting, shifting extrojects
and part-objects. These momentarily became the source of gratification
of a primitive, instinctual, devouring organization that had never become
subordinated to more advanced ego control, and which was incapable
of postponement or anticipation, except for very fleeting moments of
isolated secondary-process functioning during which were revealed
extremely primitive impulse-delay mechanisms.

Psychological testing described Rena's mother as being in a state of
extreme distress, torn apart by an intense ambivalence which could not
be warded off through the brittle defensive structure available to her.
She was particularly helpless in relationship to the maternal figure. Still
entangled in her own negative symbiotic fusion, Rena's mother vacillated between seeing herself and/or the other object as omnipotent
or impotent, as possessing goddesslike endowments or animal-like
defects. She vacillated between her image of Rena as desecrated filth or
as consecrated goodness; she felt deeply identified with certain images
she had of her daughter, but felt totally alien to others. In short, her
perception of the girl was as fragmented, contradictory and unsynthe-
sized as the girl's own inner experience. She could accept in her daugh-

ter only the good, the beautiful and the precious—the godlike feature
that were a projection of her own omnipotent fantasies. She simulta
neously rejected the deeply disturbing, damaged, impotent, animal-lik
aspects, the denied, fragmented bits of self-representation which sh
projected onto the girl and which the girl had taken in, but in th
unpredictable fashion of an eternally revolving kaleidoscope.

Psychological testing highlighted how, separately, neither mothe
nor daughter was able to achieve any integrated, synthesized personalit
organization. Clinically, however, we observed that, together, thei
respective fragmented personalities seemed to achieve a kind of homeo
stasis which allowed for an apparent capacity to maintain a goal o
purpose until their unity was threatened, as, hopefully, would com
about after years of treatment. The mother had been able to support a
extremely difficult, expensive, demanding, draining treatment progran
of many years. She could manage this, apparently, as long as she per
ceived it as restoring the original symbiosis and eliminating those aspect
of the psychosis which, in fact, allowed the girl the only separate, albei
psychotic, identity she could achieve. When this separate identity be
came strengthened through the transference to the analyst and by the
utilization of auxiliary therapeutic agents (hospitalization, an occupa
tional therapist, etc.), which provided a nonpathological environmen
towards which she began to move, both mother and daughter startec
to act out disruptively. This interference with the treatment progran
made unavailable those supportive professional services that had begur
to substitute for the mother's external nurturing function, just as the
transference had begun to substitute for the internal mother represen
tation.

During her six years in treatment, Rena had required constant anc
intermittent placements, from home to hospital, to a kind of halfway
house where she lived with her own nurses; then back home in the
care of an aide, then to another hospital, and so forth. The pattern she
appeared to follow was one in which she would begin to move away
from the negative maternal symbiosis, then become terrified at its loss
Driven to recreate it, she would provoke the environment to counteract
out in the image of the bad mother, from whom she was forced tc
flee and towards whom she was equally impelled to return. The de
structive, psychotic acting-out thus maintained the delusional megalo
manic position by destroying the opportunity for individuation and
separation that the hospital environment potentially could have pro
vided. Her tremendous impulses towards symbiosis would constantly
make impotent any persons in her environment unable to withstand
the devouring demands that turned them into anaclitic or symbiotic
part-objects existing solely for immediate impulse satisfaction. Few

people could withstand the powerful psychotic struggle and acting-out that emerged in her battle both to maintain and to break away from the negative maternal symbiosis. Her struggles fluctuated towards and away from entering into a new growth-producing situation, a positive symbiosis with the environmental therapeutic agents which, in collaboration with the therapeutic symbiosis, might lead eventually towards individuation, separation and psychological development.

Her years of treatment were characterized by these powerful and contradictory impulses, which always managed to overwhelm whatever transitory nuclei of ego organization and control that might momentarily emerge out of the evolving positive therapeutic transference. The lack of any synthetic ego function—of any integrated personality organization—led inevitably to the lack of an overall direction in her treatment. All that could be seen was an unsynchronized internal autonomy of part self-representations or self-images, so that she seemed to have no purpose or direction that could be sustained. It was as if her inner processes were so fluid that there was no lasting differentiation between impulse and defense. She was without capacity for cathexis constancy, so to speak, so that any force propelling her in one direction seemed immediately to create its own counterforce of equal magnitude in a different direction. She indicated her desire to leave the hospital, for example, but then led the therapist to a locked gate, communicating thereby her feelings that she could only leave by breaking out violently in psychotic fashion, rather than in the doctor's fashion, which is through the treatment process. She sought to go for a ride with the doctor but led him to a strange car for which there was no key, metaphorically rejecting the "car" for which were available both key and chauffeur in the form of the treatment process and the therapist. Over and over she asked him for what he did not have or else caused the environment to destroy what he did have for her by provoking ejection from that environment. Her own lack of synthetic function seemed always to diminish the integrating power in those who treated her, thereby leading to a disintegrating impact upon the separate elements in her total treatment milieu. Her inability to make use of her environment ultimately turned it into a depriving one. Feeling helpless to take, she made those around her helpless to give, and thus she restored the oneness of nihilistic impotency between her and the environment. This, paradoxically, strengthened the delusional omnipotent inner power and control that guaranteed the psychotic existence and survival.

It is because of such experiences that we wish to explore and define conditions in a *controlled environment* which can provide the kind of autonomous structure that will sustain itself against the impact of such a patient's destructive impulses, without controlling the patient or the

illness, and respecting the need for autonomy, albeit a psychotic delusional one. In such an environment, the people continue to function as
whole autonomous objects, and can supply the necessary positive nutriment from reality—the external creative obstacle that can enable
growth, like the foreign speck in the oyster shell which becomes the
"organizer" for the pearl.

Let us describe an hour with the girl at a moment when she appears
to have momentarily passed the maternal symbiotic barrier and is ready
to enter into the new, positive symbiosis with the therapist. It is an
hour of rebirth which she subsequently maintains for several sessions.
It leads to a momentary level of integration at such a peak that she is
able to say: "I am so sick. How can I help you to help me?" But all
this is followed by a violent regression engendered by the panic at
leaving the maternal symbiosis. Even the relationship with the therapist
is dreaded as a potentially engulfing fusion threat. In the first hour
of this sequence, however, she is found in her hospital room by the
therapist in a severely regressed condition. Naked, disheveled, her
mattress torn up, she is in constant need of a male nurse during her
violent periods which alternate occasionally with moments of childish,
regressive submissiveness. This alternation forces the nurse, too, to
become like a part object that is either experienced as controlling her
or else as ministering to her most primitive instinctual needs.

Coming at his regular time, the psychotherapist assumes that her
behavior with him is not merely the expression of chaotic impulse but
rather is psychotic acting out in the service of communication, but on
a primitive appeal-and-signal level. She greets him with her body
crouched over at right angles, and is encased in her bedspread while
she tears her nightgown to shreds. He interprets her need to hide from
him within her secret, autistic world, but reassures her that it is safe
to leave it to be with him, or to let him enter it with her. He constantly
reaches out for affective contact despite her attacks and withdrawal.
Finally, during a momentary level of higher functioning, she bursts
out, "I don't want to hurt your feelings." He interprets her desire to
protect him, how she gives her whole life to do so, just as she feels
her mother gave up her life for her. As he speaks of how she must
punish herself out of her fear of hurting him, he interprets the conflict between the wish to have him, and the fear of this wish which
turns so quickly into a need to destroy him. He speaks of her undifferentiated love-hate that makes her want to push him out yet grab on
to him simultaneously. He restrains her violent assault but maintains
the physical contact, until finally the tide goes out and true contact is
established. For a brief moment she can give up her fear of losing or
destroying him and hence can truly keep in touch with him. This

has come about because she had been unable to provoke the assault from him that would have destroyed her but which she constantly invites—feeling powerless and destroyed when she herself is not the all-powerful, megalomanic destroyer.

Thus, with the psychotic tide momentarily at low ebb, cleansed temporarily of the bad object, she gently places her face in his hands as he leaves. Momentarily reborn, with the good object within her revived through the contact with the lifegiving therapist, she requests a bath. It is as if she is cleansing herself of the bad object, the psychic afterbirth, the filth, which is one of the many images assigned to her by the mother. This knowledge gives us some dynamic and generic explanation of the process which we interpret in terms of her fear of destroying or being abandoned and/or destroyed by the lifegiving object. This object, however, is experienced as a corpse which has been destroyed by giving life to her, so that she must give up her own life in return. Like Edgar Allan Poe, she it attached to a dead and deadly host that she feels she has killed; she can only feel the object as a corpse in whose womb she sleeps, and so eventually she must be destroyed herself. As she approaches the object—that is, the lifegiving contact—she assumes both the object and herself to be the negative, bad objects which must destroy each other. The therapist needs to approach her as if she were a dead body that he is to revive by supplying everything the previous dead womb could not. As he becomes an intrusive force, and unwinds the winding sheets, as it were, she becomes like a desiccated mummy and falls apart, a primary-process version of horror mysteries.

Nevertheless, we see evidence that there also exist some elements of an observing ego that reflects about the deadly struggle within her and says that she does not want to hurt him or speak of hating him. We can hope, therefore, even while knowing this level of secondary process cannot yet be maintained, that somehow each peak is an indication of ego function which will eventually develop.

By this time, however, the girl's chaotic behavior has already fragmented the help potential to her in the hospital situation. The administrators have begun to demand that she be withdrawn from the hospital, although they insist that if they could have handled her entire treatment they might have been able to maintain her. Thus, within the countertransference, we see how they have been turned into the image of the negative mother whose voice Rena constantly hallucinated as a threatening injunction that she must destroy the therapist rather than leave the mother. We can speculate, perhaps, that the girl has sufficient ego structure for her chaotic behavior to be a kind of psychotic acting-out in which she communicates her thought that she and her doctor are up against an impossible situation. The succeeding hour starts with her maintaining momentarily the regressive position of the newborn baby who can let the doctor take care of her and feed her, as she requests that he give her some water. This necessitates their going out in the ward, where she loses the momentary contact during which she had previously expressed compassion for him and a desire to protect him from herself. On the way to get the water, she becomes violently combative in the hallway, as if, in fear and terror, she must fight the hostile forces around her to get the very sustenance she needs for survival. It is almost as if she must prove to the therapist that the world is an enemy that will turn on them both, that he is helpless to protect her, and that she has only her rage to help her keep alive. Thus, during this hour we see contradictory impulses in which she says, at the same time: "Feed me, don't go away"; and "You can't feed me—powerful forces in me and the world will destroy us both."

We might say, therefore, that this girl preserves her delusional, psychotic identity through the psychotic acting-out which, at the same time, destroys her opportunity for true individuation and identity. In addition, her environment, also, is inevitably driven to counteract out with an equivalent force to maintain its delusional control over the girl, even as it is unable to maintain its self-control as an autonomous therapeutic source under the impact of her illness.

Our work with such severely disturbed adolescents and our recognition of the intra-relationship with the environment have helped us recognize the need for understanding the interaction of the multiple therapeutic agencies in the environment which often are involved simultaneously with such patients. We have come to realize the importance of the collateral work with the parents, as well as with the variety of professional therapeutic systems such as private nurses, day hospitals, full-time hospitals, occupational therapists, educational therapists, and so forth. For the very nature of the illness of the schizophrenic makes the contacts with these support systems more of an "intra-action," since if he moves away at all from the maternal symbiosis, it is often only to seek to re-establish it with new objects in the environment. We have seen how the impact upon the environment of the illness of these children is frequently one that totally destroys the integrated yet autonomous functioning of the various agents involved with the patient: the parents, substitute parents, the social worker, occupational therapist, hospital personnel, and so forth. The very lack of synthesized function within the patient is reverberated to and is mirrored by the objects in the environment towards whom the patient develops pathogenic transferences which led Freud to say such patients formed unsuitable transferences for the usual office practice.

Specifically, we are describing the need for a *controlled environment*. That is, for a therapeutic environment that has an autonomy which cannot be destroyed by the patient, and which permits the autonomous functioning of its members as whole objects within a structure unified by the mutual purpose of treating the patient. This concept of a controlled environment may be contrasted with that of a controlling environment. The latter, like an externalized superego in the form of authority figures, seeks to control or manipulate the patient rather than to help develop within the patient the self-control of an autonomous, active ego.

This concept of a controlled environment represents a kind of dialectic synthesis of opposing attitudes towards the treatment of the mentally ill, from the earliest harsh attempts to overpower and restrain the mentally ill by means of chains and snake pits; to humane efforts like Pinel's who struck off the chains; to those of Szasz who would close the hospitals and in thereby denying the existence of the illness, would essentially eliminate its treatment. But neither destructive hate nor helpless love is enough; only the insights that develop out of scientific understanding and not merely out of a moralistic or humanistic value system can permit the creation of an adequate treatment program.

Our knowledge of schizophrenia is now such as to make imperative the incorporation of our understanding of the function of environmental support systems into our model of treatment for this disease, which is characterized by a lack of organized, stable, synthesized structure. The fragmented, disorganized, unstable state, in which parts dominate the whole, also describes the impact of this illness upon the environment, which is driven inevitably to mirror the patients' inner fragmentation whenever they begin to externalize their feelings of panic and helplessness.

In order to maintain its delusional omnipotent control, which alone guarantees its psychotic existence, the schizophrenic personality must assume omnipotent control over the object, the therapist, the external environment and any part of the world that becomes its living space. It must impose its own design and organization upon everything from which it draws out the nurturance necessary for its very survival. It thus destroys the capacity of the environment to feed the starving potential for normal living. Instead, the environment is required to feed the pathology with part objects that are in the image of the illness itself, and in this way sustains the helpless, nihilistic, autistic core which creates the world in its own image. Not only the therapist, but the total therapeutic environment must withstand such onslaughts against its integrative capacity to provide a comprehensive, unified program. The child's therapist, the caseworker, the hospital personnel must remain united in their mutuality of goals even as they retain autonomy over their respective functions; that is, they must remain whole objects capable of sharing a purpose while simultaneously retaining individuality of function. Without such an understanding of the need for a total and unified treatment program, the respective healing agents are in the position of the blind men, in the fable of the elephant and the blind men, whose limited and limiting perceptual apparatus leads them to equate the fragmented parts that they perceive with its total identity as a unique creature who encompasses all these various aspects. Thus, even though each "may be partly in the right, in the end they all are in the wrong."

An optimal treatment plan for a schizophrenic child should be derived from a full evaluation of his total intrapsychic and interpersonal structure and functioning. The severity of the illness and its accompanying distortions and deficits of functioning have led to the recognition of the necessity for an integration of the intrapsychic model of treatment into a model involving the totality of the available support systems. It must be organized, however, around the dominant ethic that we deal with a human being whose basic integrity and identity are respected even as his illness is recognized and treated. Restoration of the capacity for inner choice and freedom to function remains our primary goal. Through the understanding of the therapist and the insight of the patient, we can hope—to paraphrase Freud—that where unsuitable transferences existed, treatable ones can be developed. For this we must have available all our total armamentarium of therapeutic facilities in order to offer a rational, unified, united and autonomous treatment program as a substitute for the irrational, disintegrated, symbiotic and ultimately helpless "anti-program" that the patient's illness has heretofore both created and responded to in those around him.

REFERENCES

1. FRIEDMAN, SEYMOUR W. "The Diagnostic Process during the Evaluation of an Adolescent Girl." *Children of Time and Space, of Action and Impulse* by Rudolf Ekstein. N. Y.: Appleton-Century-Crofts, 1966.
2. WINNICOTT, D. W. "Hate in the Countertransference." *Int. J. of Psychoanalysis*, 1959, 30:69.

CHAPTER NINETEEN

Casework with Psychotic Children and Their Parents*

Our clinical investigations concerning casework with parents of borderline and psychotic children have revealed a number of predictable patterns which define the task for the process to be worked through. A decisive question for the psychiatric social worker is whether it is possible to integrate the psychotherapeutic treatment of the child with her own understanding of and constructive influence on the reality factors in the total family situation. We try to study the connection between psychotherapy and casework, the bridge between the child's inner life and his environment. We are presently attempting the formulation of a model of the total treatment situation of the psychotic child which takes into consideration the internal therapeutic process, as well as the process involving the total support system (Ch. 8, this vol.) such as casework with parents and the use of external treatment facilities.

We deal with illnesses which seem constantly to divide and conquer existing treatment forces rather than permit them to function integratively. The very incapacity of the patient and his family to make use of a positive environment can turn it, in the end, into a depriving one. With this basic premise in mind, we believe the casework process with parents must take into account the nature of the intense mother-child relationship. The purpose of this communication is to clarify the meaning that separation has for these parents and their children as they attempt to move toward some form of individuation.

In work with parents of psychotic children, we have observed their

---

* Beatrice Cooper is co-author of this chapter.

terror when they see their children's therapy leading to possible physical or psychological separation. Fusion of parent and child frequently reaches a degree where neither has a clear concept of self, and each looks to the other to reconstitute or restore himself. In seeking clinical help, such fused parent-and-child people have reached the point where they ask for release from the terror and hopelessness of the symbiotic tie. Yet, in the process of separating, they expose the depth of their need to maintain this tie.

Benedek (1) and later Mahler (3) have noted that reciprocal interaction between mother and child determines the psychic process in the offspring which, repeated from mother to child, constitutes a psychodynamic link in the chain of generations. The mother functions within that symbiotic tie on two levels. She is the nurturing mother and, simultaneously, the child she nurtures is the extension of herself. The mother's attitude toward the child gradually changes in the normal course of events, and their mutual emotional feeding reaches beyond the relationship; each seeks objects to substitute for or to represent the original love relationship which does not remain static. But if she never becomes the "mother of separation," individuation cannot take place in the child.

What is the task of the social worker who deals with these parents as well as their children? Our view of the nature of the fusion existing between psychotic children and parents is that they are psychically so joined that separation seems to threaten total or partial destruction. Yet a separation process is necessary in order to create and strengthen independent psychic functions. Thus, the therapeutic process has the inherent in-between goal of separation, which is both desirable and necessary for recovery. We suggest the caseworker for such patients has a professional in loco parentis function; temporarily she becomes the parent of both—a kind of arbiter between siblings—and she remains that until individuation growth permits her to phase out.

The necessary separation applies to those merged psychological processes which make it impossible for mother or child to function either independently or harmoniously. They fear they will have no strength of their own. In the process of helping them to separate we help them to discover their own inner capacity for separation. Thus, concomitantly with the therapist's work with the child, the social worker's job is to provide structure by means of which the individuals can change this aspect of their social functioning; and she offers this help via an interpersonal reality- and task-oriented relationship.

The life histories of most of our schizophrenic children reveal that for them change has never grown out of a new awareness of choice, or from the development of greater capacity for enriching life experiences. Rather, it has often come about because of violent family crises which manifested the inner dilemma. Thus, as Searles has described (4), the schizophrenic child patient has an inner conviction that further change will bring additional loss, disruption and suffering. Also, everything within the personality of the adult, with whom the child has the closest relationship, has resisted change because the status quo is often experienced by the adult as the only means of maintaining the family's roles. When the parents are not overly involved with the child, all too often they are narcissistically absorbed in themselves. They vacillate from intense over-involvement to sudden withdrawal because they are afraid of the child's independent development. The child, too, fears his inner self; and his fear of what he might find within himself is heightened by the parents' ascribing omnipotent powers to him, the nature of which he does not comprehend. He experiences these powers as somehow flowing from himself but not an integral nor controllable part of himself. He develops the deep conviction that he somehow possesses a strange and involuntary malevolence which is totally to blame for the disruptive and destructive changes in daily life with his parents. He suffers, we might say, from *negative megalomania* (Ch. 7, this vol.). An 18-year-old schizophrenic patient thought his mental time machine determined the present, past or future of any interpersonal relationship. He felt he could render his mother helpless by thinking of her as a dependent infant; an oppressed, abused wife to her first husband; or an old, obsolete hag—characteristic thoughts which, by the way, often also crossed the mother's mind as she faced the daily struggle with her son. Projections and introjections fused within that *symbiotic sac* (Ch. 6, this vol.) encasing both.

An illustration of the process of separation is the case of 16-year-old Danny, an adopted child and a dedicated hippy by desperate conviction. His whole appearance resembled a Jesus with long flowing hair, an emaciated body, a pontifical and suffering facial expression. Usually barefoot, he could not bear tight clothing and his shirt hung unbuttoned over his body. He was impulse-ridden and suffered from a schizophrenic character disorder. He described himself with wistful pride as the youngest drop-out in the Los Angels school system: when he was eleven he left the sixth grade after successfully provoking the school authorities to insist on his departure. Since he had superior intelligence, his parents could not believe that Danny could not tolerate remaining in any school or cope with the tasks which school presented. The school finally said he would not be permitted to come to school unless he cut his hair. He then "chose" to keep his hair long as a rationale for not being allowed to go to school. He needed this rejection in order to believe that he was actually "all right" and could attend school if he wanted to; his being a drop-out seemed then to be an ego syntonic rebellion rather than a symptom.

In their respective individual therapies, his parents came to recognize that they were not able to support their son's treatment at home because they continually manifested their conflicts in ways which worked against his therapy. They tried desperately to get him out of the home and into a residential treatment setting, but their efforts failed. They accepted the need to work with the social worker in addition to continuing their individual treatment. When we began to work jointly with the whole family, a brief hospitalization was necessary in order to prevent Danny from acting out some destructive fantasies. After two days in the hospital he wrote a beautiful poem—the only one he had ever finished in his quest to be a writer—which described the state of the symbolic attachment to and autistic detachment from objects. (Premature "hatching" often leads to depersonalization instead of individuation (3).)

> I walked down an early morning road and saw the rain and heard the chattering of squirrels. The thickets of thorns and briars hid them and the early morning colors clung to my eyes as a filter which only could see the rain and the moss like mists.
>
> Step lively now and don't think of her white sheets and the ivy colored brick buildings of the city. To rest in her arms was worth all the wind and the autumned colors that shrouded the crescent landscape and that pull in my body now. I feel like an autumn leaf in this freedom of a wilderness and this hinterland is my life now; and my tired feet will vouch for that. So beautiful and detached from the mother tree, isn't that the story of an autumn leaf as it sails a crooked sea of rain.
>
> I saw no stars; and a wind-ridged sand on a diamond beach. And the gulls screamed at a crescent of light that sipped at the water's white-capped horizon. It was the wind that was bothering me now and I cried in the rain and laughed at the feeling of being the only one alone and the only one up to his knees in road mud.
>
> The ceaseless line of glass-boxed buildings all but lost in the fury of the torrents littered my garden with the chaos of industrial dragons; digging, charring, building, tearing down the old and lame, gasses, bricks, steel, electricity and the millions upon millions of cogs; people, yes only the people.
>
> The autumn leaves have crumpled and a soul has been beaten and a world misses nothing but the sound of its mechanical voice.
>
> Only a raindrop feels as I do; only the woods are deep and green enough and only a sun may break the nighttime's chill.
>
> The blurs of movement astound my senses and the animal sounds play symphonies with the breeze. I pause and listen. I may never take part.

In other times and places streams of cold melting snow have soaked my feet through heavy hiking boots. Now my boots are dry and only the sliding beauty of one twisting, flowing stream is my road. I sit on the bank watching my army canteen fill in the rushing rambling stream and listen to the squirrels complaining and laughing amongst themselves as if in jest. The water babies flash their silvery tails in the glint of sun light as they laugh and sing to the never-ending harmony of the flowing water.

I felt tired so I sat on a fallen tree and prepared myself for a good nap and a warm evening.

In this poem he described the danger of separation from the mother. He stressed his absolute dependence on her which was so frightening because it took away all self-initiative. When he faced freedom he had only chaotic impulses and no capacity for work or love except the pseudo-freedom of helpless, hopeless drifting. Even the hospital wasn't a safe place; he ran away, frantically telephoning the social worker to find him because he was lost in the wilderness.

Back at home, the more he pressured his mother to keep him occupied during the day, the more their relationship deteriorated. Rather than face the fact that the two of them were imprisoned by each other's symptoms, she desperately continued to seek private schools for him that would provide at least a physical separation for a few hours a day. He experienced the mother as someone who would provide at any cost, and the father as the authoritative, denying person. The father accused the mother constantly of giving in unconditionally. She accused him of never giving, always rejecting, always keeping the boy from having the relationship with his father that he so desperately wanted. After several years in the therapeutic process, they began to see how the boy was driven to create disagreements between them because he needed external situations which would undermine his plans for seeking the independence which in actuality he feared.

When they developed some insight into this pattern and no longer fell victim to his provocations, Danny began to make considerable progress. He accepted moving temporarily out of the home. He would see the social worker, who helped him with funds to make this move possible—one of the tangible services in casework to help change an individual's way of coping with reality. Danny's separate bank account required him to see the social worker weekly for her counter signature. Initially, she went everywhere with him: to the bank, to the Department of Motor Vehicles, to the grocery store, etc.; not as the ambivalent, controlling mother but as a protective helper who supported his otherwise fluctuating drive for independence.

Away from home, he felt the need to fill his time instead of sleeping away the days while his roommate went to classes, and began to collect marginal young people without family ties. Some of them experimented with pot and LSD, as did he. Gradually, as the apartment's purpose became distorted into a hangout for homeless dropouts, he became overwhelmed and asked the social worker to help him rid the apartment of what he had unleashed. This resulted in his breaking up with his roommate, necessitating a return home on the very day his mother learned of her own father's death—for her a death and resurrection simultaneously. Because of his appearance, he was not invited to the funeral; yet he felt he belonged there more than anyone because he saw his grandfather, whom he admired and loved, as an intellectual rebel, a replica of himself.

Gradually, the parents in establishing conditions for his living with the family disengaged themselves somewhat from setting up explosive interactions. Needing the safety of the home, he managed to keep just within the limits of these minimal parental conditions, channeling demands for what he considered freedom through the social worker. At all points of differences, the parents dealt with him through the worker, too.

From time to time, both the boy and the parents would shortcircuit this method. They wanted to act impulsively and avoid the social worker as a delaying force in order to restore the original chaotic bliss of the symbiotic arrangement. Each of them would then return to her to negotiate the crisis they had impulsively generated so that they could once again arrive at a workable arrangement. His mother began to understand the cyclical nature of her intense involvement and sudden withdrawals from her son. This behavior was connected to her earlier relationship to her own poet-father and her over-controlling mother. Danny's mother said, several days after her father's funeral: "Danny belonged there more than anyone; he was more his child than anyone else's."

In providing a casework program for Danny and his mother, an elastic structure was established, so that while Danny negotiated and fought against change he saw that nothing was destroyed in this process. He gradually became involved in the process of coming to the Clinic regularly, of organizing himself and his life so that he was able to make himself continually eligible for financial support which was offered through the caseworker. In so doing, he gradually identified with the structure—the very thing he had fought. When he demanded more funds, he would recreate with the social worker the same kind of struggle he had with his mother. The difference was that the caseworker was consistent either in granting or denying his request, depending on his reasons for it: how he expected it to accomplish his aims, and whether it would tend to help him achieve greater independence from his mother. In our "negotiations," we let him know that we were concerned that he attain greater capacity to make it on his own resources and not borrow his mother's. The latter were constantly changing and had always proven unreliable: e.g., when he became too demanding, she would disappear to a resort area to regain her strength in desperate isolation.

In the process we showed him that just as his mother had always held onto him by having him economically dependent on her, he bought relationships with other people in the same way. He paid more than half of the rent on the apartment that he had shared. He borrowed his parents' cars to provide friends with transportation because he was afraid that without these borrowed means he had nothing to offer and would lose their friendship. He wanted unconditional love and yet he offered conditions, alibis or reasons why he could never go through with an actual work or learning experience. He said, "It would frighten me to have to 'commit' myself to school and know that I would have to go there every day, because I might find out that I couldn't stand it, that maybe I'm not as smart as I think I am." Efforts to help restore his power to function threatened him because he feared the destruction of anaclitic object relationships, the loss of the provider, and the discovery that he could not maintain himself.

We created a flexible structure, and he was helped to see that his unreasonable requests—his demands that things be given to him unconditionally—created a replica of all he had known which had always increased his anxiety. Eventually, he himself would beg for limits so that he could use them in his relationships with other people and thus have some sense of self-boundaries. He could then go back to his former roommate and say that with more equality in their arrangements they could share an apartment. He stopped using his parents' funds merely to make himself eligible for the friendship of exploitive persons.

The casework process was, in essence, a continuous negotiation in which the patient used the social worker as a go-between to test out his capacity to function. Because he had not yet developed inner capacity for organization, he needed her to become temporarily his external organizer. At the same time, he fought her because he could not tolerate the idea. Thus, she became a kind of arbitrator between him and his parents, and between forces within himself.

After an absence of one-and-a-half years Danny returned to school. He always wore or carried some article of clothing belonging to his father, such as a scarf or jacket—a beginning identification perhaps with the formerly hated parent. He hoped returning to school would please his father, which was his way of restoring himself with his father so that he could get such privileges as the use of the family car. He also talked about his wish not to become sexually involved with girls until he could love on a deeper level because he "had enough trouble" understanding himself. In the past, he would pressure his mother to drive him to rendezvous with a teenage girl. They made love in the back seat of the automobile, while his mother "disassociated" herself by reading a book as she sat in the driver's seat. Now, he identified with the hero of the screenplay "The Pawnbroker," whose past, which he saw flashing before him, caused paralysis so that he was unable to act in his present. The pawnbroker came to his senses, as Danny put it, when he painfully put his hand through the sharp needle spindle that held receipts of pawned objects.

> It made me sick. I felt like vomiting. I could hardly move. It made me think of when I was five and I fell into a hole. It wasn't the pain that bothered me; it was that blood gushing out all over. You can hold back on pain, but you can't help seeing the blood. I thought by now I had overcome the fear of blood, but now I see I've got two problems—still my sick hair and my fear of blood. You can hold back feeling pain but you can't stop yourself from seeing blood. I know I couldn't fuck a girl who was a virgin because it would be hurting her and making her bleed. I would be hurting myself because I would be hurting the person I would want to love.

Evidence was manifesting itself that exploitive, anaclitic and symbiotic impulses might someday give way to a recognition of the other person, and to the establishment of a self-organization.

Two years after ending an active treatment program and depending only on occasional consultations, Danny has established a more normal, almost conventional life. The long hair had been "sacrificed" on his 18th birthday when he came home from his self-chosen hippy exile. He accepted a work situation which demanded skill and, passing an apprenticeship, has maintained it ever since. He married, gave up drugs, takes some university extension courses in the area of his work. Of course, one might hope he will allow himself someday to move beyond mere adjustment towards real inner freedom. But he has achieved a real separation from the parents and the old treatment situation, which was a partial replica of the basic parent-child bind.

The following material illustrates some of the problems in beginning a casework program with parents who have come to experience the symbiotic tie with their sick child as a hopeless form of tyranny. At the same time, they view the child's struggle towards separation in threatening and negative terms. In such situations, we need to develop a mutuality of purpose based on some individual autonomy of functioning. Such parents tend to pressure us to create a "perfect" environment—in which the original fusion is maintained. We strive towards a reality that can become an enabling, facilitating factor, and towards creating psychic zones in which a dialogue of common purpose with the parents is possible. A process must be initiated which will create a therapeutic environment whereby the parents can free the child for therapy, and the child, similarly, can free them for a separate relationship with the social worker. They can, thus, work through a beginning separation without feeling it will lead to psychological death (2).

Since such parents have an overwhelming need to make the social worker as omnipotent as they have made the child, the beginning casework can be crucial. We have found it effective to focus on how the social worker can help them in organizing their *external* lives. This provides some structure which helps them accept treatment requirements and they find themselves better able to cope with their *internal* disorganization. They may struggle against the structured program, but in that very process they develop some inner autonomy which enables them to function better.

In this case, Kay, the twelve-year-old middle sibling, an Alice-in-Wonderland type of girl, was living with her divorced mother. Each parent had applied separately for psychiatric help for Kay without the other's knowledge. The main problem seemed to be her long-standing phobia of attending school, although both parents were also concerned with her general unhappiness and great difficulty in relating to family and peers. The patient's deeper disturbance, masked by the phobic manifestations of fear of school and avoidance of relationships, could be characterized as a subjectively unwanted but needed symbiotic relationship with the mother. In a desperate and pathological effort to maintain self-sufficiency and to guarantee security and survival, Kay developed a strong fantasy life along with overt attitudes of contempt and disdain for others. These constituted a defense against interpersonal relationships, and were also a manifestation of inner feelings of omnipotence associated with the creation of a somewhat bizarre private religion, a kind of ego-syntonic delusion.

During the beginning phases of casework, the mother spelled out her anxieties in undertaking treatment and her guilt about having created the sickness in her child. She felt the onset of the illness was brought about when she had had a spontaneous abortion, when Kay was about five and her youngest a boy of two. She had to rely on the maternal grandmother to care for the children. She said that sharing her precocious Kay with her mother was her way of doling out pleasure to her. Her husband had questioned this move but hadn't had the strength to stop her. In retrospect, she realized he constantly questioned the harm that the maternal grandmother, with her puritanical ideas and concepts about cleanliness, might be doing to the child. But fearing emotional abandonment, which she had experienced in her own childhood, and feeling that her mother and Kay had a kind of rapport, her assumption in turning her child over to her mother was that she was both making up for her own deprivation and preventing deprivation for her child.

We came to understand that the parents had always regarded Kay as their "special" child. She seemed to have been an extension of the mother, of which both parents were aware in that, for them, she was never an individual in her own right. The mother maintained an internal symbiosis with the child as a reflection of her own unresolved deep dependency needs and pathological symbiotic relationship with her own mother. She inwardly regarded the child with awe, feeling as if she could never do enough for her, and needing constantly to win her approval—almost as if Kay were the parent figure and she the child. She had built up within herself and the child a kind of unreliable accountability to one another, so that each felt unable to function without the other. Thus, the child was given the hopeless task of completing the mother's life. The child actually had told her mother, "You do not have a right to have any kind of life without me because you did such a rotten job and you are such a failure as a mother. You have to make it up to me now!"

Outwardly the mother appeared to be articulate, confident, feminine and charming: traits which had been appealing to the father who needed a strong woman to sustain him. He had been taken with her apparent competence in their common profession in the advertising field, admired her capacity to manipulate others, and saw her as a bulwark upon which to lean. However, the appeal of these attractions declined during the marriage. In time, her compulsive defenses decompensated and she found the ordinary housekeeping routines of work to be mountainous burdens. She became outwardly enraged with the children and, in a sense, failed in her function as a wife and mother by temporarily deserting the father. This finally led to a divorce about a year and a-half before they came to the Clinic; she got custody of the children. The father had remarried.

Both of these parents were highly intellectual people who had gone beyond the college level of education. Outwardly, the father showed a facade of strength and confidence. He had experienced his own father as a brilliant and educated, but selfish and unfulfilled man who had deserted the family when he himself was ten. He had been left in the care of a dominating professional mother who constantly reminded her son of his father's evil, and stimulated in him a sense of masculine weakness and feminine identification. He retained his deep attachment to his mother. To him, Kay was special because she seemed to be the only one who loved him, which gratified and fulfilled his need for love from a feminine figure. His behavior demonstrated fusion of identities in the family, with no individual member retaining his own identity but each being obscured and overshadowed by others. This was significant for Kay. She never emerged as a separate individual but always appeared particularly lost in and sacrificed to the parental needs, purposes and goals.

In spite of the father's overt apparent dedication to the treatment process, his subsequent moves clearly revealed his original determination. This was to stay clear and free of a binding and meaningful commitment in any form—whether of money, time or personal investment in the patient's need for help. His efforts to engage the family in a treatment situation proved to be in behalf of his own disengagement.

The beginning casework process involved both the mother and father in separate interviews, in which the social worker entered a triangular relationship—the pathological trinity—substituting, so to speak, for the patient. Within a very short period the parents were funneling the emotional impact through the social worker rather than the child, who had previously served in this way. The social worker could experience how both parents expected her to be the omnipotent one to replace Kay, who had carried this burden for so long. They did this in a subtle, seemingly positive way, with a degree of sophisticated acceptance of the value of treatment. They even expressed the wish that once they were freed of their current chaotic situation, the father would be able to work more efficiently thereby increasing his earnings and providing the financial security needed for a maximum treatment program.

Both parents essentially presented the difficulty in terms of their feelings of helplessness in the face of the child's insatiable, tyrannical demands upon them. They couldn't bear the extent to which Kay involved them; yet the very nature of her illness indicated that they would need to be involved in a long, intensive treatment program. At this point they preferred to see themselves as really turning Kay over to the Clinic, with themselves in the roles of siblings getting advice on handling the tyrannical peer. The abrogation of the parental role is frequently a sequela to the bewilderment and puzzlement of parents of such children.

At this time the mother and children were living a considerable distance from the Clinic, as well as from the father and stepmother, which required much freeway driving which the mother dreaded. The child's first therapy appointment precipitated a frantic state of emergency on the part of both parents who advised the social worker that after the interview with the therapist the child had run away. The mother tried to involve the father in her efforts to locate the child, and in the crisis the social worker was also immediately called upon to rescue them and the child. In reality, the child hadn't run away at all but had wandered out of view while the mother was making a telephone call in the hotel lobby. Somewhat disoriented, Kay was seated in the corner of the lobby, crying, and was approached by so-licitous adults who attempted to comfort her. It was the mother who had become panic-stricken, had felt that there was no one to turn to in the entire city, and had decided to call the police and/or the father. When mother and daughter were reunited, they comforted each other in expressing their depressed feelings about the beginning treatment process. The mother played the role of the stronger parent figure and verbalized her anger towards the father for not being the one respon-sible for bringing Kay to treatment. Secretly, both parents had made false promises. The mother told the child she would need to come but once; the father said Kay could move in with him; both parents had assured the Clinic that they were ready to begin.

The mother actually undermined the beginning of treatment by telling the child that Kay needed someone besides the mother: that it was "quite possible"that the mother could get killed in an automobile accident. In this eventuality it was important for the child to establish a meaningful relationship with the therapist. She thus allowed for the implication that if the child fully identified with treatment, she would be causing the mother's death. This clearly illustrates the ominous way in which the mother viewed the separation that treatment would bring: a death sentence to the mother-child relationship. The child remained silent on the way home, dressed the next day for her therapy appointment, but disappeared again before they were to leave. She had locked herself in the bathroom but meekly came out when the mother shouted, "You must come, we both need help!"

This complementary acting out of their shared inner conflict indi-cates that both mother and child experienced the beginning of the therapeutic process with the fear that it meant the loss of one another. The beginning issues were clear: could psychotherapy take place in the face of such an environment; and could the social worker influence the environment in such a way that manipulation would be replaced by insight?

What slowly emerged in the subsequent casework interviews was the mother's need to know the Clinic was available to her and her daughter because of her overwhelmingly chaotic state and feelings of helplessness. Outwardly, the mother had functioned well from time to time as a professional person, and had taken several graduate courses. She had been intermittently running in and out of the house long enough to have sporadic contact with the children but not long enough to give them adequate or consistent maternal care and support. The children never knew when the meals would be served, whether there would be any food in the house, whether their clothing would be laundered, or whether the mother would be home at all. At the time that treatment was starting, they were suffering from illnesses which required medical attention; the apartment was in a shambles and infested with bugs. The children lived with a depressing sense of shame about their mother's malfunctioning. She had gotten into over thirty car accidents within a one-year period, incurring thousands of dollars of indebtedness. All of this had come about despite the fact that the father did send adequate support money. The mother's functioning had deteriorated severely along with her daughter's. Consequently, she regarded the beginning therapeutic program for Kay as a source of relief for herself and as a strong, supportive outside force to help her organize herself.

In treatment, both mother and child revealed more fully the extensiveness of their pathology. The child gave the picture of an almost full-blown paranoid schizophrenia; the mother appeared to the social worker as an hysterical, pathological liar, searching for someone to believe the state of her helplessness. The technical issue for the social worker was a twofold one. She had to avoid reacting to the pathological environment and avoid attempting to become an even better manipulator than the mother, and she had to try to understand the mother's sense of ineffectualness which had led to an intolerable "double bind" for mother and child. The child was pleading, "I need a better functioning mother." The mother's plea was, "The child's tyrannical hold on me makes me less and less effective and is destroying me. I can no longer function, not even outside the home as a professional person. I am literally making the walls of my home come tumbling down." Our task together, then, was to help this woman begin to discover whether there were any alternatives for her, and to introduce the possibility of change as something not to be feared.

We began with recognizing her dysfunctioning, and that we were here to strengthen and support her. We would not be used by her to blackmail the ex-husband into giving her funds to meet her emergencies but would help her begin to meet these emergencies with her available assets. She wrote letters to her creditors and we discussed budgets. From interview to interview it became more fully clear that she had very little concept of using money in a planned way. Everything was done out of impulse or in response to the greatest pressure at the moment. This included using the children to arouse guilt in their father for not being more generous. We tried to show her the consequences. By doing this she had fostered a lack of reality-understanding for them; it made their father appear to be responsible for their plight when, in fact, he gave the family an adequate amount each month. The same unrealistic attitude on the children's part coerced her repeatedly into meeting their exorbitant demands for expensive purchases, which had added to her financial crisis. She began to alter her approach, attempting to communicate directly with the father instead of indirectly through the children.

As she began to trust the social worker enough to discuss her car accidents, her need to deny so much in her life became clearer. She essentially regarded herself as a dangerous person who, if allowed freedom, could be destructive to the social worker as well as to the other significant people in her life. Also, if she really allowed the caseworker to be entirely helpful to her, she would become vulnerable to her fears of rejection by the social worker. In helping her to budget and work with money realistically, we also began to help her see symbolically that there perhaps was a way of budgeting her aggressive and libidinal needs. The social worker very deliberately allowed herself to be used as a functioning mother who could help her learn how to budget her life, but would not meet all of her needs. The social worker structured the times when the mother was expected to see her, and the times when she would be additionally available. By refusing to be completely available, she compelled the mother to restrain her overwhelming impulses until such time as they could be discussed with the caseworker.

We soon discovered that the mother had little capacity to carry over insight or make any connection from one interview to another. She would experience the relationship in such a way that she would try to act like the social worker. Her strength would fail and she would revert to her usual impulsive, chaotic and ineffectual ways. She would then become extremely angry with herself and the children, running away and leaving them for several days. Ostensibly she used the rationale that she had to visit her aged mother who lived some hundred miles away. The children would be left without food at home and only a few dollars with which to purchase meals. Upon her return, no one was able to express openly any feelings about what had happened, but then there would be a blow-up around some unrelated factor and Kay would behave explosively towards a sibling, clawing at her brother's face or destroying her sister's dress. The mother would then describe to the social worker how proud she was that the child was able to express her feelings!

The social worker could suggest finally that she begin to examine how she really felt when Kay acted abusively towards the other siblings. One day, after returning from a visit with her mother where she had experienced her mother's characteristic, repetitious tyranny, she suddenly found herself experiencing Kay in the same way. She was then able to ask the caseworker what she was doing to cause both her mother and her daughter to fuse in her mind. What did she do that they could both treat her with contempt? Why was it that she could feel stifled and guilt-ridden like an imprisoned person who had no right to have any kind of a self because all of her self belonged to them? We also became aware that the reward she got for returning to her own mother was the tasty, nutritious balanced meals which her mother invariably prepared for her. This, of course, was related to one of the major ongoing reality problems she had in providing similarly for her own children.

She then began to express her angry affects toward all of her children. She felt that they, like her mother, were forcing her to turn her whole life over to them, and that she had no rights as an individual. It was because she felt so inwardly involved with them that she behaved at times so very inadequately as a mother. When this happened, the children were put in the position of having to call upon their father and stepmother for help. The mother would experience this as proof that the children were being cruel and mean and hurtful. She also saw Kay as having a problem in needing to deny herself any pleasure and, thus, destroying the mother's pleasure. However, she rarely could express openly any feelings toward the child. Instead, she acted them out by literally leaving her without available food for several days, knowing full well on some level that this was an anxiety-ridden, terrified child who would suffer intensely.

The caseworker helped her to understand and deal more effectively with Kay's negativism (refusal to eat her meals with the family, to leave her room, to come to treatment). The mother could begin to see it as Kay's attempts to survive and maintain whatever identity and autonomy she had in the face of imagined and actual threats of being overruled, effaced or neglected. Thus, the mother began to stop reacting to it as a form of conscious stubbornness on Kay's part or, as she described it, "playing games." This reduced the mother's feeling of inadequacy, and she no longer strove with futile, intellectualized arguments to deal with Kay's rationalization that "the rottenness of society" was the reason Kay preferred to remain in her room.

The psychiatric caseworker's strategy in working with Kay's mother was not to be critical of her as the other people in her life had been. The caseworker accepted her and tried to strengthen the forces within her that yearned for adequacy and organized expression. It soon became clear that she enjoyed working outside the home but had felt that Kay's illness imprisoned her at home, even though, in fact, she didn't stay there. She knew only extreme forms of maintaining relationships: over- or under-involvement. The social worker gradually was able to deal with her feeling that there were only two choices available to her. She had accepted either fulfilling her own needs as an individual and, in so doing, abandoning the children; or else giving up her own needs totally and sacrificing herself for the children although the resultant resentment and anger this generated made her perform inadequately anyway.

As her right to be a working individual began to be reinforced, Kay's mother found a job, not in her professional capacity but in a related field. She began earning funds and making some moves toward paying off her debts instead of maintaining total dependency on her ex-husband. It was at this point that the child was able to turn to her father from whom she had separated herself for a six-month period. Although she had been unable to attend school for several years, she now told him that she needed desperately to enroll in school. She put it that she felt freed of worrying about her mother; since her mother didn't need her any longer, she could now go to school. Once mother and child were outwardly functioning—the mother at work, the girl at school—the mother began to reflect on how her life was totally intertwined with that of her daughters—the three of them living out a triad of adolescent fantasies, the girls, for example, plotting ways in which the mother could meet and become the paramour of men of great wealth so that all three women could live lives in keeping with their extravagant illusions. She was then able to see how she and the children were using their improved functioning primarily to feed their fantasies, and she began an earnest effort to differentiate between mirages and realizable goals, between what her daughters insisted she wanted and what she truly wanted for herself.

In summary, although each member of Danny's family was involved in individual therapy, the casework process helped them to experience the way in which they manifested their intrapsychic conflicts in their daily interaction. The several processes proceeded independently; the focus, being different, permitted the parallel treatment. One without the other would not have been sufficient to deal with constant impulsive discharge of interpsychic and intrapsychic conflicts. The casework process enabled the parents to reflect before they acted or acted out; the boy could delay or negotiate, and begin to allow for reflections which he could bring to his therapist. Each could begin to grasp how specific behavior caused his difficulties to follow certain patterns. In becoming aware of the connection between overt behavior and inner problems, each was better able to understand the frustrating, self-defeating ways in which he had attempted to resolve inner conflicts.

In the second case, it soon became evident that the mother had no basis for structuring any kind of planned effort. Her life was dominated by her inability to see any options but extreme choices and the mutually pathological bonds that existed between her and her most disturbed child. The social worker's task was to help the mother accept the reality of her divorce and prepare herself for some sort of stable life so that Kay's treatment could take place. The casework process began with the tangible services of the psychotherapeutic program at the Clinic. It worked until child and mother could begin to separate and individuate so that the mother would not remain a sibling but could become a parent who no longer experienced her child's helplessness as her own. The social worker provided the link that made it possible to maintain a stable limbo situation long enough to permit the growth of some form of independent functioning, directed toward a life ruled by adaptation rather than by chaotic impulse.

REFERENCES

1. BENEDEK, THERESA. "The Psychoanalytic Implications of the Primary Unit: Mother-Child." Am. J. Orthopsychiat., 1956, 4:389.
2. FRIEDMAN, S. W. "The Diagnostic Process During the Evaluation of an Adolescent Girl." In Children of Time and Space, of Action and Impulse by R. Ekstein. N. Y.: Appleton-Century-Crofts, 1966.
3. MAHLER, MARGARET S. On Human Symbiosis and the Vicissitudes of Individuation. N. Y.: Int. Univer. Press, 1968.
4. SEARLES, HAROLD F. Collected Papers on Schizophrenia and Related Subjects. N. Y.: Int. Univer. Press, 1965.

CHAPTER TWENTY

Parallel Process as It Emerges in Casework*

When children are accepted for treatment as part of the Project on Childhood Psychosis, it is required that the parents agree to be seen in a casework relationship. This is a usual requirement in work with children; where the treatment of severely disturbed children is carried out on an out-patient basis, however, the character of the casework relationship has some unique characteristics. The intensity of the disturbance and the unstable quality of the family relationship expose the treatment process to constant crises and threat of disruption. This problem requires that the therapist and caseworker maintain an unusually close collaborative effort to help the parents sustain the treatment and to avoid disruption. Such close collaboration has been part of the work done in the Project and has permitted the observation of the emergence of what Ekstein has called "the parallel process" (3). He, however, confines his discussion to the training setting, whereas, within the Project, it has been possible to observe the emergence of this parallel process with patient and parent or guardian. Thus, therapist and caseworker are dealing with the same type of conflict in individuals of different ages and with different modes of inter-personal interaction. Awareness of this parallel and the collaborative effort permits the therapist and caseworker greater insight, which can be extremely useful in maintaining the treatment. It is essential that therapist and caseworker remain clear as to the contributions of the techniques which they are using, because it is this complementary effect which is of value in the

* Beatrice Cooper is the author of this chapter.

out-patient treatment of the highly disturbed children within the Project. The caseworker must have full awareness of the conflict as experienced by the child as well as the parent but always be able to maintain a relationship with the parent on a casework basis. Under these conditions, the many essential supplementary tasks which cannot be done within the therapeutic framework can be accomplished through the casework process. With families where there are frequent crises characteristic of relationships based on schizophrenic pathology, the maintenance of the two roles provides a basis for understanding the crisis as part of an ongoing consistent process rather than as episodic, irrational and disconnected periods of upheaval. In this communication, two illustrations demonstrate the special casework problems centering around the parallel nature of the emergencies generated in parent and child in the struggle for the child's separation and individuation. No implication is intended that the emergence of parallel process is limited to work with disturbed children but rather that the awareness of this process can be of special help in such cases.

The first illustration* involves professional parents who became concerned about the degree of their seven-year-old son's unhappiness and jealousy toward the younger sibling. The psychiatric examination revealed him to be a deeply anxious child with low self-esteem and serious doubts and confusion about his sexual identity. This boy has obsessive-compulsive concerns about perfect performance; tremendous need for complete approval by the male father-image; obsessive-compulsive preoccupations and interest in numbers, words and the fear of secret thoughts that would lead to the loss of love and severe punishment by the parents. He shows an age-appropriate intellectual performance and a certain degree of maturity. Despite these, he gives an overall impression of a child who has not yet found security in a close relationship with his parents and inwardly feels himself to be lost and unacceptable with no real place in his family. The diagnosis of personality pattern disturbance with borderline features, manifested by impaired reality testing and impulse control, was made.

These highly goal-oriented parents expected their child to be as responsible and work-oriented as they. They had never permitted themselves overt acceptance of their original dependency relationships. The mother had been supporting the family while the husband continued training. She had functioned as a totally independent, self-sufficient and adequate woman who could not only handle her home, marriage and children, but also had sufficient sensitivity to become aware that this

---

* The author is indebted for this illustration to the therapist, Bella Schimmel, M.D.

latency child needed treatment. The mother came to treatment with a facade of strength, acceptance and understanding. In the initial phase of treatment, however, she instituted, by her own choice, a plan which would allow her to stay at home and be a full-time mother. It was at this point that she began to deteriorate emotionally. She found herself screaming at her youngster and wishing he were dead.

This crisis was a reflection of what was going on within the child who, in seeing his own therapist, was experiencing for the first time the question of his symbiotic dependency. He began having extended temper tantrums and pleaded with his mother to advise the therapist about them. He said, "I can't stop." The mother, in bringing to the caseworker in dramatic fashion her crisis and the boy's plea for control, indicated both the depth of their feelings of helplessness and the threat they experienced as the boy's therapy and her casework began to make overt the dependency the two of them had hidden so long.

In the process of our working together, we were able to help her see that her reaction was one of anticipated loss. This reaction was reflected in her developing acute symptoms which would make her feeling of dependency clear in terms of her trying to make herself the primary patient. This was her way of letting us know that she was ready to be involved in this treatment program. She knew only extreme polarities of reacting to her child, either as a distant mother or as an all-involved mother. She felt the child's illness and need for treatment had come about because she had had to be the provider in the family. This had forced the child into becoming prematurely self-sufficient and quasi-independent. She felt now that he should have the right to regress, have his mother available on a full-time basis and should experience what he never truly experienced before—being the baby who could depend on mother.

This self-imposed goal of attempting to make up now for earlier non-mothering produced her symptomatology since she couldn't tolerate this alternative either. At home, the child had regressed, couldn't control his temper tantrums, pleaded for a strong loving mother. He found, instead, that his mother, who appeared strong and adequate to the outside world, fell apart just as he did and couldn't control herself, let alone him. When he got upset over the loss of a school assignment, he would cry, kick at the door, and feel that all was lost. The mother would frantically search for the lost material in vain and then herself cry and feel as helpless as he.

This mother needed to use outside support, such as her professional position, her husband, or the social worker in order to help her maintain some emotional distance from the child. We tried to help her understand that the parent does not need to see her role as the child's organizer of his inner disordered life. From the outside it would seem that this child was indeed very separate from his mother. Inside, they were very much tied together in that both were looking to the outside world to be their organizers—the child to his mother and the mother to her husband or the caseworker.

This boy represented some part of the self of both parents which was unacceptable. The mother denied her own desire to mother or be mothered. What she had never received in her childhood she had denied to her first born. Her inability to give to this child grew out of her fear of the child's dependency, further complicated by her husband's need for her as his mothering figure. She was able to accept her husband's dependency, but denied anger toward him. She had to live with both her own and her son's lack of mothering and, like the son, grew up unprotected. From her point of view she had given the son more than she had ever received, and his need for additional mothering, for a strong mother to protect him from his infantilism, recreated the helplessness she had experienced as a child.

This woman was a mother who felt her husband needed her, and she wanted to help him so that he could become a strong man who could be the father for her. At the same time, her expressed need in regard to the child came out in terms of her wanting to protect him against the strict father. For such a woman, the basic personal and parental needs are denied under the threat of the loss of control to mold the child to meet her particular personality needs as they occur. The child becomes the living symbol to both these parents of their unmet dependency needs. When he literally cries out for control, through severe temper tantrums and jealousy toward the younger sibling, they are unable to give it, as it represents a breakthrough of their own cry.

It has been observed that so-called emergencies, which, in general, are but a reflection of the emergence of new unconscious material, are very frequent in the treatment of such families at the time when individuation and separation are paramount in the child's treatment. For the duration of these cases has many periods of crises experienced differently by the therapist, caseworker, parent and child. The first overt signs of change in behavior seem almost equally difficult for the therapeutic team and the parent to live with. This is the point at which the parents come rushing in, fearful and outraged, saying in essence, "You've made things worse," or "This isn't what I asked you for." In the beginning the parent can only comprehend that the child's illness requires treatment, the nature of which is unknown. Social workers and therapists are symbols for the child's illness and can represent for the parent people who become critical of their role. At times, the parent will make the social worker the perpetrator of all this.

We all know the period of wide difference between the therapist's objective therapeutic understanding of the beginning signs of emerging potential health and the parents' subjective concern about the form that this is taking. Realistically, this is a more difficult period in many ways for the parents. Their reactions conform to their goal of therapy which, in essence, requires that we eliminate from the child's behavior that which infringes on the parents' vulnerability, but maintain all the elements which have brought some comfort and gratification. This beginning emergence of an identity which is alien to the parents, as it were, both threatens and, in many instances, can precipitate greater disorganization of the parents. But this period can be used positively to retrieve aspects of their own projected egos, enabling them thus to tolerate the new phase of the separation process.

Another illustration* of the parallel process is in the casework with a parent substitute, an aunt, of a seventeen-year-old girl who had been brought for treatment because she was so difficult to maintain at home. The diagnosis of schizophrenic reaction, childhood type, with hysterical personality features had been made when she was fifteen years, four months old.

The aunt had spent considerable time and exhausted her funds in helping the child with her learning difficulties. When it emerged that an explanation for the learning difficulty could be the girl's underlying emotional disturbance, the aunt sounght psychiatric help. The child's father had disappeared early in her life and her mother had been psychotic almost since she gave birth to the baby, leaving the care of the patient to the unmarried aunt (1). The child was stuffing herself with food, hallucinating, masturbating and talking about alleged sexual encounters with the aunt's friends. Treatment was the aunt's attempt to control these symptoms and enable the girl to return to school. The impasse seemed to be the child's resistance to the aunt when the latter would deny her anything. The aunt felt the way to handle the child was to force her to realize that no one else would ever care for or want her and the way to improve was to accept that the aunt was her savior. From the first interview, the social worker tried to help the aunt prepare for the resistances to her niece being in treatment *and* improving. The aunt thought her whole life was motivated by her need to serve others. As she struggled with the meaning of a commitment to treatment and its many ramifications, it became clear that she wanted just enough help so that she could better manage and control the girl.

As the emergence of unconscious material came into consciousness,

---

* The author is indebted for this illustration to the therapist, Rudolf Ekstein, Ph.D.

by way of violent psychotic acting-out, the conflicts frequently developed around the issue of the adolescent's attempt to break from the over-dependent relationship with the parent-surrogate. Any movement away from the symbiosis carried with it the threat of forbidden sexuality. In the course of the child's treatment she was beginning to go to school by herself and would get close to the male bus driver. At the same point, the aunt experienced contradictory feelings in her object relationships and was, thus, fearful of her capacity to love. A part of her wanted sexuality, a part of her felt it was forbidden. She could not permit herself the unambivalent gratification of marriage but only the guilt-laden rewards of adulterous relationships.

While she wanted to compete with the child for her therapist, she simultaneously experienced the therapist as a fantastic sexual threat and forbade herself, by way of the child, to visit him. Our work with these people indicated that both the aunt and the child used their relationship to get back other relationships. If the aunt could use the casework process to maintain the child's treatment, she would make a positive constructive movement of ego-strengthening nature. She tried to get closer to the therapist by way of wanting to have intimacies with the social worker. Thus, around the time the child entered a private school and began to become aware of her attraction to young men, the aunt came in scantily dressed and talked about her quasi-sexual encounters with other professional people. She clearly demonstrated her anxiety about the transference feelings towards the social worker and diluted the relationship by having quasi-closeness with the nurse of the doctor from whom she sought medical care. Then she acted out her anger by blaming her impoverishment on the child's illness.

This came at a time when the source of the aunt's reaching out was that the child was being provided with other contacts: private schooling, teachers, schoolmates, etc., which were beyond her previously limited contact with merely the aunt. Paralleling this, the aunt, on her own, had entered adult education classes in a nearby high school to improve herself. This can be viewed on one level as an act of sibling rivalry to grow up or it can be seen as a healthy effffort of the parent-surrogate to prepare herself for the future independence of this child. The aunt's return to school and her decision to have more contact with people grew out of her new-found strength released through the casework process, which had focused continually on the social issue of how to maintain a child with treatment without the aunt herself becoming ill.

Such a process should not be called psychotherapy. This term should be limited to the process in which the goal involves a dissolution of unconscious conflicts and defenses and a re-integration into the conscious personality of new solutions and choices growing out of the resolution of transference resistance. The casework process is regarded as an auxiliary to the psychotherapeutic process. In this illustration, casework made the aunt aware that her hypothesis had been that of a tyrannical super-ego, such as that of an older sister who had to care for an unmanageable sibling. In the casework relationship she was enabled to see that there are alternatives between this role and that of being the permissive mother figure. These were the only two she could perceive and this resulted in her being constantly torn between these polarities.

It was noted earlier that one problem in such cases is to maintain the child in such a way that treatment does not disintegrate due to the social pressures involved in the proposed gradual separation from the parent. Whenever it would seem, through casework, that the aunt could free herself of the symbiotic position, a crisis would be precipitated through the illness of the child. This would give the aunt an alibi for not carrying through on an external change in their living condition. Whenever the aunt and child began to think of inter-dependence instead of intradependence, the child, in turn, tried to embroil the aunt into the treatment. Over and over again, the child acted in such a way as to bring the aunt into the therapy, thereby constantly recreating a destructive triangle. On one level, the aunt wanted to save the psychotic child and get help for her somewhat in the manner she had done for other relatives, which interfered with her own acting-out proclivities. On another level, she used the child as a way of introducing her own problems and her own pleas for help.

After several years of treatment, this impulse-ridden adolescent moved to a psychiatric day treatment center and was carefully supervised at home in the evening by her aunt who felt it was impossible to permit social encounters. The child had been describing to the therapist her abortive efforts to grow up, which took the form of a kind of flirting with work arrangements and efforts to attach herself to many different people. During this period she developed a relationship with a schizophrenic adolescent boy and tried to assert her independence through adolescent defiance by acting-out sexually (2).

In connection with some disciplinary issue the child was temporarily expelled from the day treatment center. In the process of informing the aunt of the basis for the expulsion, she learned about the child's sexual escapades and reached a crescendo of rage which caused the child to disappear during the next night for a lost weekend. In desperation the child tried to reach other people: her therapist, the volunteer of the clinic and the social worker. Unable to reach them, she experienced a panic and regressed to a level in which only her now revived negative introjects controlled her. She contacted the boy with whom the sexual play had taken place, behaved like an animal in heat, returning from time to time to the angry aunt, defying her physically, restraining and taunting her with magnified reports of her sexual activities and then running away again. The crisis culminated in the aunt's decision literally to throw her out. The child appeared at the clinic door with the aunt's instructions that the child was now the social worker's responsibility. The aunt defied the clinic now, a parallel to the child's defiance of the aunt. We had to try to help the aunt not to react pathologically to the child's need to provoke the world into becoming a replica of earlier hostile introjects.

This sexual acting-out was the girl's way of showing the aunt and therapist she was ready to grow up. But the nature of the acting-out impinged upon a basic conflictual area of the aunt's psychic organization. Thus she needed to eject the child totally and attempt to do so psychologically. She would no longer support treatment or have anything to do with the girl. The technical issue in such instances, where an overdependent relationship must be disrupted, is that treatment alone will frequently not suffice to maintain the total situation in which violence and chaos are almost inevitably engendered.

The problem of attachment/detachment is always violent. It is a reflection of the inner struggle between the unrealistic infantile desires and the negative hostile introjects which such patients create as their own monsters when the environment does not provide them. With such behavior, this child could turn a fairly calm and supportive aunt into a raging, screaming, rejecting mother. The patient creates a crisis in the treatment by provoking the relative to abandon her. The violent acting-out serves to split the symbiotic fusion between the child and the aunt and could be pictured as the energy involved in splitting the atom.

In the parallel casework process with the parent figure it became clear that the child's attempt to separate from the aunt and thus move closer to the therapist was threatening the adult. The aunt felt the only way of handling the psychosis was to control it completely, to suppress it. She had developed a close relationship with the social worker and felt that, in order to please the social worker, she—the one responsible for the child's care—had already altered her standards for looking after this child. She felt the social worker had influenced her over the years to tolerate the child's psychotic behavior as it emerged instead of suppressing it and had prevented or dissuaded her from retaliating. Session after session, she described how she would have liked to have behaved impulsively by grabbing the child and beating her rather than attempt to understand the illness. The child's coming for treatment was always seen by the aunt as a promise that the child would improve just enough to be manageable but never would be independent. The niece would be, as it were, a child-adult with no sexual impulses so that the aunt could live quietly. Instead, we stressed separation by introducing special schooling for the girl and having the aunt consider work as a way of freeing herself from the isolation of maintaining a sick youngster.

The acute need for the parallel process emerged, as the child struggled with the use of greater freedom, and the aunt became very frightened by its implications for her. The situation reached a point where the aunt felt that she could not control herself any more. She wanted to return to her old way of coping by having the child be afraid of her through threatening her with withdrawal from treatment, placement in the state hospital, or physical assault. It also became clear that the aunt felt powerless with the niece. For she could now see clearly how she used the youngster's illness as an alibi, a reason why she could not live a fuller life, why she herself indeed could not seek and find more satisfying relationships. Harried and conflicted, she would try to intimidate the social worker. Unable to dominate the worker, she began to feel threatened and dominated by her. She would reproach the social worker with the assertions that she felt that she was destroying her life.

However, as the aunt was able to develop insight into her need to maintain a controlling relationship, she could begin to understand how she struggled against the social worker in the same way the child had struggled against her actual domination. It was at this point that there was some tenderness in the relationship and the aunt was able to say quietly and calmly, "You don't know how it hurts me to be so cruel to you but I have to show you how desperate I am. I am drowning, and instead of holding out a rope to me you dangle it just beyond my reach." The realization that casework could lead to the aunt's separation from the pathological relationship with the sick youngster held both hope and intense danger. It was at this point, when she felt powerless to protect the child, that the child's threat to her was experienced. The aunt used the casework relationship to see what other alternatives she had for improving her life situation. She developed some understanding as to how relaxing control over the child could be mutually helpful, whereas previously she had felt that this would result in the girl's becoming more psychotic. At times she would continue to try to terrorize the social worker with angry outbursts just as previously she had tried to control the child with similar behavior. The social worker stressed that it was within the aunt's power to let the worker help her or not help her; that she had a choice not only in this relationship, and her relationship with the niece, but in setting her own goals and trying to reach them.

In such joint work it is especially important that the therapist focus his work with the patient on the intra-psychic conflict whereas the social worker must consistently focus on the inter-personal relationship between the parent and child. Casework can help parents develop awareness of detrimental interaction and to discover other alternatives in behavior that are available to resolve crises. While both therapist and social worker use a common basis for understanding the psychodynamics of the conflict, the different focus, when sharply maintained, dictates a difference in the selection and use of the material. Thus, the mother experiences the entrance of her seven-year-old son into treatment as a loss of the boy. The social worker deals with the material in relation to the way the mother felt about bringing her child to treatment within the reality framework. The social worker does not deal with her view of herself as helpless and lost which would have shifted primary emphasis upon her own individual needs, as would have been done if she were in individual treatment.

The social worker understands that the mother's current reaction is an unconscious conflict from the past but she deals with it in terms of its connection with what is going on now. The caseworker uses her insight and understanding of the parent's dynamics to translate them into their overt meaning for the parent in relation to the child's current difficulties. When the mother of the seven-year-old son works through her acceptance of his illness and his need for treatment, which imply separation, she must bury the illusion that her child is healthy. Both patient and client struggle with the acceptance of clinical truth and its social consequences, but the child does it in terms of himself, and the mother in terms of the child rather than herself.

In the second illustration, when the adolescent girl was struggling to become an independent individual, the aunt reacted violently to the worker and child as they indirectly were forcing her to face independence. The aunt's fury was fed by finding that the social worker did not make herself available to replace the disappearing dependency gratification. Instead of interpreting to the aunt the problems around her deep dependency needs, the worker helped the aunt find gratification by engaging her in the process of finding a school for the child so that the dependency could be channeled into a more constructive mode. At the same time it was pointed out to the aunt that the violent negative feelings were a drain on herself. With these directions the aunt shifted from her feelings that the social worker was someone taking her child away from her to feeling that the social worker was a savior who was finding an adequate safe school for the child. Although it was evident to the social worker that the shift was a reflection of the intense underlying ambivalence about the symbiotic position with the child, this conflict was not interpreted. Instead, the aunt was encouraged to think of ways to use the extra time which would be available to her. To establish independent goals for herself now, instead of relying on the myth that after the girl's recovery such goals would magically appear.

The casework process can thus be used to assist the parents to adjust to the changing relationship in a manner which anticipates and thus prevents their internal crisis which results in disruption of the child's treatment. The parents remain with the old conflict but find new ways to adjust to these and to the child who has been a focus of the conflict.

REFERENCES

1. EKSTEIN, RUDOLF. "The Parent Turning into the Sibling." *American Journal of Orthopsychiatry*, 1963, 33, 3:519-520.
2. —— & CARUTH, ELAINE. "Psychotic Acting Out—Royal Road or Primrose Path?" In *Children of Time and Space, of Action and Impulse*. New York: Appleton-Century-Crofts, 1966.
3. —— & WALLERSTEIN, ROBERT S., M.D. *The Teaching and Learning of Psychotherapy*. New York: Basic Books, 1958.
4. YAHALOM, ITAMAR. "Complementary Therapy of Severely Disturbed Children and Their Parents in a Day Care Center." *Journal of Jewish Communal Service*, 1964, 40, 3:289-297.

The Trap: The Child's Emotional Illness as the External Organizer of the Family's Life*

The psychotic child's illness often becomes the organizing but pathogenic principle for the family's way of life. Since the interaction between the sick child and the parents creates a psychological fusion state, our task in offering help is to initiate a process of nonpathogenic separation and individuation for the parents and the child. How can they come together when they fear fusion, fear that getting too close will result in the loss of differentiation of self and object? Mutual tasks unite people and serve to perpetuate the pathogenic aspects of the relationship. With an exceptional child, the object relationship for the parents and that child decides what patterns of strength will be called upon that will organize their lives and introduce both heroic and pathogenic features. The heroism of maintaining a psychotic child at home is carried out under such a tremendous task setting that strengths and capacity to maintain a treatment program emerge. This specific pathogenic organizing principle brings out in the parents the best as well as the worst. This communication will try to show *what causes the parents to react to illness*, what illness brings out in the parents. For regardless of the causes of the illness, it becomes both a new organizing factor and also a disorganizing factor.

---

* Beatrice Cooper is the co-author of this chapter.

The impact of the illness as it polarizes, as it develops a system of organization within the family, varies. With some parents the illness becomes a bond of united love to safeguard the child. Sometimes it drives parents apart in a bondage of hate, and the child makes the cleavage between the parents even bigger. In one family it pulled the parents together to the extent that the father, recognizing his wife's struggle in maintaining such a psychotic child, allowed her to bring a young man into the home. This was to help care for the child but also to provide her with a young lover: every concession was made allegedly in the service of rescuing the child. We recognize that in all of our cases there was considerable pathology shaping the specific pattern of functioning, but through the illness of the child it became even more powerful. The mental illness of the child will enlarge the existing pattern of parenting and make out of it a more violent aspect of pathogenic interaction, thereby initiating a vicious circle without end.

Treatment of psychotic children was always aided through the concomitant treatment of parents who came for help in coping with their sick child. Social workers used this as a place to begin and as a way of sustaining parents to be able to maintain long-term treatment of such children. As families came to understand the repetition of their old conflicts and its relationship to the current problem, living with a psychotic child, they were able to modify these patterns on an intra psychic level. They could see that there could be some degree of choice and that they need not continue the pathological relationship that imprisoned each family member.

Illness of a child brings out in parents massive reaction which may have consequences that will not aid treatment. The ordinary parental holding-onto the child may lead to patterns where holding-on and letting-go become pathogenic reactions. Holding-on may become a symbiosis so that parents and child cannot separate. The child may bring out in the parents an enraged wish to get rid of him—throw him out—but when one is ready to work on an actual separation the parents will hold on desperately to the child. In this way there is a magnified version of "individuation-separation versus holding on" (2) experiences all parents have, and the social worker's problem is to help the parents let go or hold on in nonpathogenic ways.

In demonstrating what causes parents to react, we begin with the study of families for whom the maintenance of the sick child at home has been based on a kind of denial of the severe pathology. Pathogenic fusion is experienced as ego-syntonic until it is threatened by the child who either seeks other kinds of arrangements or becomes so disturbed that it becomes observable to the outside world. Then the alibi for maintaining this arrangement can no longer hold up. During the diag nostic evaluation, we observe the family's attempt to explain why things are the way they appear. But as we accumulate data in the treatment process, our power to modify the dynamics or change the distress is hindered by a life-and-death struggle unknowingly to maintain the pathology intact. It is as if the family must maintain at any cost the symbiotically fused existence; as if to begin to separate, to differentiate, is equated with the threat of death.

At times the child-patient maintains an autistic position of isolation, so that the parents do not see the extent of the child's pathology. Since our schizophrenic patients cannot trust their perceptions, and are primarily oriented towards themselves, they are ridden with doubt and anxiety. They have little sense of wholeness or togetherness and are unable to rely on established, dependable objects. They have fantasies of destructive omnipotence or fear of excessive dependency resulting in the imminence of their annihilation. One lives at the expense of the other as the mother projects a fantasy of catastrophic danger hanging over the head of the child. Its source emanates from her, but the denial frees her to appear as his protector. She is the overprotective mother, the life-saver, the guardian; yet behind the conscious need is the latent need to keep the child from growing away from her. Thus, neither one is permitted an independent existence. Generally, the father has failed to provide strength to ward off the mother's assault on the child. The child senses the power struggle between the mother and father and worries, sometimes developing a fantasy of one parent killing the other. It then becomes safer, for example, to react like a deanimated machine and thereby to avoid any kind of identification with parental destructiveness, actual or imagined (3).

E. James Anthony (1) has written about changes in family functioning which resulted from a member falling ill. His study reviewed ways in which different families dealt with the impact of illness as well as the changes in the organization and function which ensued. His work indicated that the impact of the illness largely depends on the nature of the marital relationship which, in turn, reflects the characteristics of the early parent-child relationship. When it is symbiotic (the spouse substituting for the mother), separation or threat of separation may precipitate a life crisis which undoes the previous precarious accommodation based on dependency. When the marital union has an autistic pattern (with the partners living together but in separate worlds), the crisis is often provoked by some anniversary of a childhood situation involving identification with the parent figure. The accommodative response becomes one of increasing diversion until the progressive detachment is recognizable as a psychotic illness. Although the symbiotic and autistic categories represent a simplistic view of the field of psychoses, there is some heuristic advantage to dichotomizing the two types of crises which stem from two patterns of marital relationship and produce two forms of accommodation to illness. This accommodation, of course, may have both a positive and negative side to it. On the positive side, it allows the crisis to be contained within the family and resolved without recourse to outside help. On the negative side, treatment often gets postponed until the psychosis is far advanced, the capacity to use help reduced, and the burden on the remaining family members, especially the children, is beyond their emotional capacity to bear.

In our cases, psychotic children are very special to their parents, who suffer with them and adapt their way of viewing the world through, in part, the distorted way the child views it. Some of the parents have separated and divorced; some remain together in the same house as parents, not as marital sexual partners; some remain together bitterly resenting the need to maintain the marriage and the home as the only possibility for providing the psychotic child with structure. In one of our families the long-married couple is creative and humorous. But they experience the psychotic child's struggle to free herself from the symbiosis as possibly leading to the death of the father, who is constantly called upon to rescue the child as she encounters social dangers in her eerie wanderings through the hippie community.

We have earlier discussed the role of the parent in the treatment program for psychotic children, the meaning that separation has for these parents and children (Ch. 19, this vol.). We have stated that our therapeutic process has an inherent midway goal of separation, which is desirable as well as necessary for recovery. This goal aims at the separation of those merged psychological processes which not only make it impossible for either parent or child to function harmoniously, but arouse the fear that they have no separate strength of their own. We have said that casework with the parents helps to provide a structure by means of which individuals may change this aspect of social functioning. We would like to use several cases to illustrate the process by which we try to help families gain individual autonomy and alter their interpersonal relationships so that they don't draw on the pathology.

These families found various means of functioning. In some, the parents and child functioned as a single sick unit, disintegrating to the point where neither parent could function outside the home until separation through placement in a hospital had been achieved. In others, parents' intellectually superior functioning outside the family was unimpaired. They chose to further their careers and did not experience this as incompatible or inconsistent with treatment goals for the psychotic son. We recognize that the need to maintain the illness is different in these cases, yet we are aware of degrees of pathology inherent in the pecific arrangement with the psychotic child. Some parents literally xperience the psychotic child's suffering as if it were their own. The hild is tuned in on this intrapsychic level to the parents and, at that noment, acts out the parents' unconscious fantasies. For example, it requently happens that the parents reach the point where they deserately ask for placement—they can't endure the child any more. It ; then that the child literally runs away or gets lost, complying with he parents' wish for a kind of destructive liberation.

In one such situation, we were asked to evaluate a 12-year-old aughter of divorced parents living with the mother. Initially, the problem seemed to be the child's fear of attending school. But as we came ɔ understand the dynamics, we saw that the child's deeper disturbance ad been masked by a school phobia and poor peer relationships. In ctuality it was the outcome of an unwanted symbiotic relationship vith the mother in which the child expressed fear of separation from er. Subsequently, the child developed a fantasy life and external attitudes of contempt and disdain for others. These were both a defense gainst interpersonal relationships and a manifestation of inner feelings f omnipotence—bizarre religious notions of self-sufficiency to guarantee er survival.

This child was special to both parents, whose marriage literally was acrificed so that that the mother could maintain the oneness with the pecial child. While the mother felt that the child was unique and xceptional, she tended to reverse the relationship with her child so horoughly that the child would say, "I am not my mother." The arents, highly educated intellectuals, outwardly competent individuals, egan to deteriorate as the mother's compulsive defenses decompensated. 'he mother was a basically hysterical woman with a sweetness-and-light ttitude which tended to mask her disorganized home life. She was a ad manager with an occasional burst of efficiency. One minute there vas no food in the house; then there was an over-abundance of everyhing. She was totally inconsistent, giving everything or nothing. Beoming enraged at the child and her own failure, she emotionally eserted the father, which led to his pressing for a divorce when our atient was ten and a half.

In this family, parents and child were intimately fused. Confused arcissistic needs and self-esteem were derived from each other without upporting and enforcing each other's individual identity. The child's ttitude seemed to be a massive defense against the overt expression of sychosis, thus having the quality of defense as well as adaptation.

To the mother, the daughter was gratifying as an especially bright, erceptive, and creative child who would say charming and clever things. n reality, the child seems to have been an extension of the mother, which both parents recognized in their awareness that for them the child was bits and pieces of themselves. For the mother, it was essential to maintain a symbiosis with the child, reflecting as it did on her own unresolved, deep dependence, and perhaps somewhat pathological symbiotic relationship with her own mother. On the surface, the mother appeared feminine, charming, confident. Beneath this facade was the inner insecurity, the weakness, which in the past had appealed to the father, who had really needed a strong woman to maintain his strength. The father had also been left in the care of a dominating, phallic mother who constantly reminded him of his father's evil and developed in him a sense of masculine weakness and feminizing identification. Thus, the father remained with a deep dependent attachment to his own mother which he had to repeat with his wife. To him the patient was also special because this child seemed to be the only one who loved him which gratified and filled his need for love from a feminine figure. He used her as the one with whom he shared secrets.

The process of working together led to significant improvement but as in a Greek tragedy, fate caught up with the family in a most terrifying manner. We had begun to understand that some of the causes for the fear of separation began when our patient's brother was born when she was two. At that time, her elder sister had been severely burned and required months of intensive care by her mother. Consequently our patient had had to be largely cared for by the maternal grandmother. This left the mother with the feeling that she had lost the patient to the grandmother and could no longer do enough for her, let alone be as good a mother as the grandmother. The beginning sessions were a painful prediction of what the child's coming to therapy meant to the mother. She felt she was giving the child to the therapist because she feared her own death was imminent. This fear was associated with her fear of driving the long distances necessary to reach the clinic. For her, then, accepting treatment meant leading to her own death.

At the beginning of treatment, the twelve-year-old patient was living with her mother and two siblings. She had reversed roles with the mother by taking over the caretaking and housekeeping duties, and also by dominating, controlling, and ordering about the mother, who was given to excesses and often left the children without food or money. The mother feared and pacified the tyrannizing patient. The child, after a few months of treatment, had become withdrawn and seclusive in her room. She had severe temper tantrums and refused to let the mother remove food from the room, which had accumulated filth and dirt. The mother explained the patient's need for treatment to the child and the social worker as a precautionary security of a professional friend should the mother die. She thus introduced into the treatment situation from

he very beginning her awareness of the patient's primitive affect dis-
rder and the first vis-à-vis the mother of the patient's murderous, homi-
idal fantasies.

We helped the mother borrow our strength so that she and the child
vere able to separate from each other. She began to support herself in
er profession, and the child started to attend school again. In the
vork with the parents, we saw that they were mechanically competent
n the skill of living outside of the home, but could in no way deal
vith human realities. They had a magnificent social facade. As the
hild became involved in treatment, the parents attempted to make the
linic responsible for her emerging illness. They actually believed, as the
ather put it, that if a person caused someone to reveal his pathology,
hat person was responsible for the pathology. Much work had to be
pent in helping the parents recognize the extent of pathology in the
hild, so that each parent could interpret to the child why it really was
hat she was being brought for treatment.

In absorbing the process of being involved in a therapeutic process,
he parents revealed their own pathology. For the mother, this included
he extensiveness of her careless driving, resulting in many traffic viola-
ions, her phobias about freeways, and the necessity she felt to move
lose to the clinic as a way of holding on to it. The mother had begun
o date, to consider marriage, and to press for greater autonomy. She
irged us for psychiatric help for the other, elder daughter, who had
ccelerated her high-school program and was about to graduate early
n order to pursue a theatrical career. Whenever the children pressured
he mother and she felt she didn't have strength to hold, she sought
utside strength and authority, such as psychiatric help. She was under
articular stress because just as her professional functioning was sta-
ilized and her future seemed more hopeful, she was confronted with
er children's demands which limited and theratened her. The father
ccasionally would respond to her plea that he strengthen her position
vith the girls, but proved over and over again to be unreliable. She
ad finally yielded to the older daughter's request for psychiatric help
nd was actually driving her to an appointment with a therapist, when
he two of them, driving in a small car, were knocked off the road by
gasoline tank truck. Their car burst into flames as it rolled down the
ill, and they were engulfed. Somehow both crawled out of the wrecked
ar towards safety, only to be met by a wall of flames pouring down the
ill from the burning gasoline truck. They were hospitalized and under-
vent intensive care, but both mother and daughter succumbed. In spite
f her injuries, up to the end, the mother was coherent and displayed
uch remarkable psychological strength and orientation that even the
ospital personnel were overwhelmed as they saw this woman lose her

fight to survive. She had lived up to or, rather, died from her ow
prophecy.

Another family with a six-year-old psychotic child, a beautiful gi
had an adolescent son in high school who did quite well. The psychot
child's conception was unplanned and unwanted by the mother. H
inner security was threatened by the pregnancy because she felt
would keep her away from her own mother who had suffered a seve
heart attack and needed her desperately at that time. She feared, als
that at her age she would produce a defective child. Finally, the pre
nancy occurred when she felt threatened by signs of instability in h
marriage. Her sheltered and precarious balance might disintegrate wit
the addition of an intrusive object, an undesired infant. Thus, despi
her husband's opposition, she sought an abortion; she tried three tim
but without success. Both parents then used the child as a way of con
municating murderous impulses, while outwardly appearing lovin
and pleasant. Holding back inner rage and the wish to murder, th
mother felt guilt over the attempt to abort; the father over wanting t
punish his wife for creating a defective child in the attempts to abor
In addition, the mother feared losing her husband to his own mothe
who had just been widowed, and exacerbated her dependent, guil
provoking relationship to him. The elder child's need for surgical trea
ment for a knee injury was another factor in setting the feverish climat
in which the child was born.

This highly narcissistic, emotionally fragile mother throughout h
life had felt herself deprived and cheated, denied of her birthrigh
controlled by an older sister, and dominated by her mother. She ha
preserved her own inner stability and self-esteem by material gratific
tion and had warded off demands upon her for more mature and mate
nal parental responsibility. She and her husband came from a povert
stricken background, but the husband had an optimistic, hopeful att
tude and pursued his artistic work diligently. He maintained the fami
stability but felt himself to be the source of protection for the moth
and the guardian of her stabilitiy, which was his main concern an
which he felt was constantly threatened by the child's illness an
demands for emotional and financial support.

To counteract their hidden inner feelings about their child, th
parents saw her as beautiful in her infancy. While the mother succes
fully breastfed the baby, she experienced the child as satisfying. Lai
guage development in the child had proceeded so that she had indivi
ual words. Between the ages of two and three, however, following th
surgical removal of an eye cyst when the child was hospitalized an
separated abruptly from the mother, the child's speech regressed. Sh
became unable to communicate her needs and wants, developed intens

ear of separation from the mother, especially in medical buildings. With he development of her symptoms—hyperactivity, clinging, resentful defiance intermingled with caution, rocking to music, grimacing, and many other forms of bizarre isolation and seclusiveness—the parents began their odyssey of seeking psychiatric and psychological help. By the time they came to us, although the child was barely six, they had already gone through six diagnostic evaluations, a course of group and family therapy, and eventual placement of the child in a day school. Throughout the search for help, the mother had been desperate and hopeless. She felt the child's illness was an immensely burdensome one that deprived her of a more comfortable and materially gratifying way of life. Sometimes by sacrificing getting help that the child needed, the father maintained an optimistic and hopeful attitude with which to support the mother. He remained convinced that both child and mother needed help in their own right, and that he would successfully manage to get it for them.

At the time we began to work with the mother, she had made two suicide attempts and had had two periods of hospitalization. The subsequent psychotherapy had been interrupted because of the child's special needs for attendance in the day school. These two parents together committed themselves to a total treatment program that would help them individually as well as their child. The family mobilized itself in a positive way, accepting a very arduous program which required driving some fifty miles a day in order for the three of them to have this treatment. The father, in his ceaseless search for help for his wife and child, always perceived his need for help as coming from the outside, always saw external problems and pressures as disturbing his wife.

It was necessary to help these parents establish a common purpose so they could organize their strengths both to help their psychotic child and to bring cohesion and unity to their total life. The father's ambivalent plea for help and his attacks on the helping person or forces was a plaintive appeal as resentful and reproachful as the mother's. She constantly and ambivalently tested whether she could trust the helping resource as she projected her own fragmentation upon us. The significance in this particular situation was that at no time did these parents outwardly experience the child as disruptive, or destructive of their way of life, even though they experienced this internally. Their home was well maintained. They handled their finances carefully. They were able to provide the child with a kind of external structure which enabled her to take hold, so that, in her way, she knew they were constantly available to her. It was as if through the child they could become the reliable parents that they never thought they were or could be. Thus, through the sick child, they could be helped to establish themselves as positive parents.

While the mother was infantile and demanding much of the time she also was the good, compliant child who did what was expected of her therapeutically. Once committed to treatment, she kept the commitment—hers and the child's. She no longer had to make suicidal threats or gestures as a way of experiencing being cared for. At our Center the child was allowed to regress and be the psychotic-like Ophelia that she was. At home the parents—both artistic people—supplied her with art media so that she was able to identify with them and create illustration-type drawings, caricatures of their own artistic production, thus never behaving in such a way that her parents couldn't cope with her. The parents were frequently asked why they maintained such a sick child at home, but it is obvious and apparent that they needed the child, that they saw her as an extension of the best part of themselves not just the worst. It is through her that they may become whole, healthier people and, hopefully, she may benefit from it. For these parents, having a sick child is experienced more as providing something for them, rather than robbing, cheating, or threatening them. They use this child as the one who enabled them to acquire necessary parenting for themselves by way of seeking help with and for the child.

Perhaps the case history of a third family illustrates most powerfully the desperate and heroic struggle to maintain a family together. The 13-year-old daughter was brought to us when she was having difficulty in attending school; had rage reactions against the mother; at times blacked out and behaved bizarrely and then had no recollection of the behavior. She was driven into social interaction with hippie peers involving drug use. The elderly parents had been married some fifteen years before they had their first child, who was born neurologically damaged. Five years later, their second daughter, our parent, was born. She was a precocious, creative child, but upon menses developed the bizarre behavior which was later diagnosed as a schizophrenic reaction pattern; she was receiving signals from outer space, and fusing identity with a friend's.

At one point during treatment, the girl exhibited wild, chaotic behavior, such as going off to the hills where her illness was masked and expressed by a hippie-like way of life. Despite this, the parents went along with her getting up every morning at 5 and carefully dressing for her pretense of going to school, which, of course, she never reached. They reached a point of desperation, however, after the father suffered a heart attack. He would get phone calls in the middle of the night either harassing the girl if she were home, or from the girl herself, saying that he must help her, that she was in dire straits and needed him

) rescue her. He would have to wake completely, even though he
worked hard and long as a laborer, and go out to wherever she was to
escue her. She would express appreciation, tell him she would be a
good girl, and would then go into a quiescent period for a week or so.
Afterwards, she would break out into wild, chaotic, impulse-ridden
behavior once more, leaving her clothes all over town. She was con-
antly taking things without permission, or destroying objects such as
urniture that her mother had repaired, or grabbing makeup that be-
onged to the mother. In the absence of the mother, who was working,
he would mess up the entire house that had been left neat and orderly.

The mother wept for herself as the uncared-for and unloved child
he was, and wept for her child whom she felt she had harmed. She
xperienced her child as reviving the memories of her own mother, a
ymphomaniac. In the course of treatment, the parents said that they
eeded to get custodial care for her since they had lost all control over
er, even thought they recognized that illness caused the misbehavior.
They saw her behavior as breaking up their marriage. The mother was
ctually saying to the father: choose between your daughter or me.
Ie thought a man should not be asked to make such a choice, but if he
vere, his first responsibility was to his wife. The girl was behaving so
sychotically that they couldn't reach her on any level. They saw their
hoices as desperate ones: they would have to commit her through
uvenile Court to a foster home or to residential treatment. Before they
ad even come to us, when things had been even more desperate, they
ad been turned away by the State Hospital facility because the girl
vas not seen as sufficiently ill for such assistance.

The parents could see that the girl was asking for control, but they
ouldn't reach her so that she could respond to their united strength.
Thus, they would shift tactics. They would placate her for fear that
otherwise she would run away. They saw themselves as powerless.
Deeply attached to her, they recognized that in her illness she was
lienating herself from all her friends, her friends' parents who, in the
oast, had given her refuge and tried to understand her chaotic mood
hifts.

What is the impact of such an illness on a family? Here was a family
lesperately wanting to try to maintain the outpatient treatment, recog-
izing that the patient needed the home situation, needed the tie to
he parents. At the same time, they felt the tie was destroying them,
s she literally was destroying the furniture, writing obscene remarks
on the walls, living from time to time an animal-like existence with
orimitive behavior. In horror, the parents had to shriek out and rebel
hat they couldn't tolerate it any longer. Working people, they had
nigrated away from the ghetto and had strengthened themselves by

reaching outward for cultural and educational experience for source
of enrichment. The father had once functioned as a professional perso
in the mental-health field and had been a writer. His creativity ha
ceased at a time of threatened homosexuality and personal traum:
when he was faced with the fact that he was a father as well as a hu
band, a role he really was not able to assume at that time.

It was perhaps out of a need for compensation that this wild, undi
ciplined man then became the idealized father, the motherly-fathe
figure, who overly cared for his children. This applied both to his neur
logically damaged first child as well as to our patient. It was the latt
whom he saw as more like himself; with whom he felt such rapport th
he felt that a special extrasensory perception experience existed betwee
them. In this deep, close, intense relationship, the girl both bloome
and revelled as she approached puberty. In a subtle way, the wife r
sented the close relationship between the highly creative, intelliger
daughter and the husband, who could communicate on a level that sh
and the husband never could reach. Thus, there was an added factor t
the usual mother-daughter difficulties that occur at puberty, with th
girl literally wanting to assume the mother's role, and to depreciate he
And the mother was all too ready, because of her own dynamics, t
fall into this triangle situation.

We were able to strengthen the parents' concern for self-developmer
so they resumed their functioning in the community. As they exper
enced this fulfillment, the child slowly quieted down and used the soci:
worker to find herself a temporary home with a friend. She was ab)
to allow herself to "borrow" the friend's parents to structure her dai)
routine so she could return to school. She stressed how she must no
experience the adult world as pressuring or forcing her but enablin
her to avail herself to what the world had to offer, such as educatior
Mother and father were able to accept the daughter's indirect parentin
by the friend's parents, and thus a beginning separation in the service c
individuation took place. Actually, when the social worker was exper
enced as the more desirable, more effective parent by both parents an
the child, we found that nonpathogenic separation took place by mean
of the enabling process of casework.

The girl returned home. Although she could have gone about with
her friends, she chose instead to remain home, either quiescent, draw
ing, or voraciously reading books which she instructed her father t
get from the library. Gradually she began to paint over the bizarre draw
ings with which she had literally covered every bit of space on th
four walls and the ceiling of her bedroom. There were occasional explc
sions in which she appealed to her father to kill her, to beat her, t
destroy her. His response was one of calm compassion, in which h

verbalized he would not harm her. She would then become like a contrite, complacent child, offering to do chores about the house when the parents were away at work, in order to please them.

While she continued to meet on infrequent occasions with her friends, she did not, since these outbursts, go wild through the hippie community. The parents' insight enabled them to understand that they panicked when the child's erratic behavior reminded the father of his younger sister, who had been hospitalized some fifteen years. This sister, whom he had helped raise and felt paternal toward, was in her psychotic periods sexually provocative with him. Likewise, the mother felt helpless when the girl, abandoning her friends, went into a withdrawn, quiet period, because this isolation reminded the mother of her own earlier days. She had felt unable to go outside in the ghetto neighborhood of her youth for fear of hearing from her peers that her mother was a prostitute.

It is apparent that the child's illness was not seen separately from the parents' dynamics. They rescued the child because of the deep, basic relationship intrinsic in the illness of each. The bond between them was not something separate or external; rather it was characteristic of what we see as illness which can even burden the treatment as the parents' additional pathology requires their own treatment program.

We are working with families for whom separation and individuation are terrifying concepts. Symbiotic parenting or autistic parenting is frequently a consequence of the illness, a pathogenic protective device which the parents cannot give up when separation and individuation do become possible. The child's illness has reinforced this device, leaving the therapist the task of helping them give up a crutch which has become an obstacle to health rather than a support to the ill child. Separation actually restores genuine parenting—the love of a separated object. It frees the child-parent relationship in the way that giving up of the cocoon frees the butterfly.

REFERENCES

. ANTHONY, E. JAMES "The Mutative Impact on Family Life of Serious Mental and Physical Illness in a Parent." *Canad. Psychiat. Ass. J.,* 1969, 14:433.
.. MAHLER, MARGARET S. *On Human Symbiosis and the Vicissitudes of Individuation.* N. Y.: Int. Univ. Press, 1968.
. SEARLES, HAROLD F. *Collected Papers on Schizophrenia and Related Subjects.* N. Y.: Int. Univ. Press, 1965.

Part Five
RESEARCH ISSUES

This in turn raises a host of other questions to which we can at present find no answer. We must be patient and await fresh methods and occasions of research. We must be ready, too, to abandon a path that we have followed for a time, if it seems to be leading to no good end. Only believers, who demand that science shall be a substitute for the catechism they have given up, will blame an investigator for developing or even transforming his views.

Sigmund Freud

CHAPTER TWENTY-TWO

On Some Current Models in the Psychoanalytic Treatment of Childhood Psychosis*

To all those who are not irrevocably committed to one of the current oversimplifications.

ROBERT WAELDER

Fifteen years ago in a review of the literature on childhood psychosis, the authors concluded their summary of this important and still largely puzzling problem area of psychiatric illness on the following note:

> One may predict, then, or certainly hope, on the basis of accumula-
> tive evidence, that the period from 1956 to 1966 will bring further
> improved treatment techniques which may shift the emphasis from
> an uncertain prognosis for childhood schizophrenia to one in which
> there will be increased probability of recovery (3).

The optimism then expressed for the creation and development of improved treatment techniques in the area of childhood psychosis continued to sustain the impetus toward research and discovery and has motivated the authors and their collaborators to continue their research efforts in a group research endeavor. The exposition of the theoretical

---

* Seymour Friedman is the co-author of this chapter.

and clinical views set forth in this paper represents a digest of some major issues relevant to the psychological treatment of childhood psychosis within the framework of psychoanalytic theory, its principles of personality organization and its theories of treatment technique.

Epoch-making events in the history of scientific investigation provided a key of infinite potential leverage for the resolution of the dilemma inherent in childhood psychosis, that within itself are contained those irrational forces that stand in the way of its rational mastery. Although described by Freud as the three major narcissistic blows delivered by science to mankind, they nevertheless opened the road to increasingly new horizons leading to even greater restoration of man's self-esteem. These events were: the Copernican explanation of a helio-centric universe that replaced the Ptolemaic ego-centric view of the universe remindful of the infant's omnipotent fantasies; Darwin's genetic view of evolution as the antithesis of existing religious beliefs about the creation of man as a rational Homo sapiens undifferentiated from the unreasoning animal, which discounted the Linnaeus anthropological and theological concept of man as uniquely different from animals; and Freud, with the discovery of the unconscious, which challenged man's faith in his rational uniqueness and forced him to consider himself as not only biologically akin to animals, but also psychologically related as an organism driven by non-rational forces.

These three great advances in the history of science were essentially changes in a point of view which stimulated the observation of new data and the relationships between data that allowed for a more unified view of the world. Out of this new way of looking at the world and with the introduction of the concepts of the unconscious and the primary process came a more unified view of psychopathology in which the differences between neuroses and psychoses were severed and no longer regarded as essentially different and separate. The implication, implicit in Freud's view of the narcissism of mankind, that there is no basic difference between the psychotic and the neurotic individual, is still denied in many parts of the psychiatric world, although it represents a major trend in the development of psychiatry from Kraepelin through Freud.

Kraepelin's major contributions were in the area of diagnosis and classification of symptomatology. However, he also studied the progress of diseases and taught that there was a process to all diseases including schizophrenia, although he felt the prognosis was to end in dementia. Bleuler was particularly concerned with thought and affect disorders in schizophrenia, although he remained within the 19th century conceptualization of psychosis as equivalent to insanity and dementia. It is with the 20th century extensions of ego psychology that we have developed an understanding that the thought disorder implies merely that such patients operate under an order which we do not as yet comprehend. Freud's major contribution to the study of psychosis (after the introduction of the Tri-partite model in the "Ego and the Id") can be traced to his paper of 1924, "The Loss of Reality in Neurosis and Psychosis," in which he emphasized the structural aspects of psychosis, specifically the loss of reality testing and the loss of the capacity for normal object relations (4).

Looking more closely at the different emphases of these theoretical approaches, we can see how what appears manifestly as different ideological views concerning the cause of illness is rather a reflection of the latent views concerning the cause of the cure. Of particular importance here is the involvement of a hidden commitment to a specific treatment philosophy and technique. Freud's emphasis on reality testing and object relations is the expression of his commitment to an analytic technique based upon relationships, contact making, transference, etc. Kraepelin emphasized the process inevitably leading to dementia which thus reflected his underlying pessimism regarding treatment methods, particularly of psychotherapy. Bleuler, although stressing a thought disorder rather than the unknown order behind disorder, also expressed a nihilistic pessimism about the treatment of the schizophrenic. Psychosis is still frequently regarded as untreatable and attempts are still made to either deny its evidence or to get rid of the evidence through commitment to a pessimistic treatment philosophy. This situation is even more exacerbated in the case of childhood psychosis, which is not yet fully accepted as a valid part of the training of a psychotherapist. Treatment of childhood psychosis is still, metaphorically speaking, but a small island isolated from the main continent of child psychotherapy. To bridge the distance between the two and to provide for intercommunication and eventual integration of the two arts of treatment, we recognize the hopefulness and the promise in the attitude that psychosis in childhood is a treatable disease process. This view is scientifically supported by Freud's formulation of the psychic structure, as elaborated in the Tri-partite model, which permitted the unification of a psychopathology which would embrace both psychosis and neurosis.

Turning to the process of treatment itself we recognize that in the case of childhood psychosis particularly, as with all psychological illness, the treatment begins with the first appearance of the patient before the doctor and in the initial procedure of entering into a diagnostic evaluation. However, it is not the diagnostic evaluation as such, but rather the diagnostic process within this procedure which we see as related to the treatment process and as being a first and integral step in establishing the treatment relationship. In the diagnostic process we see an encounter or interaction between the doctor, the patient and the patient's family for the purpose of deciding what kind of commitments regarding treatment can be made by all concerned in the treatment relationship. Therefore we relegate to lesser importance those issues of classification and diagnostic labelling per se, but rather place emphasis on the encounter, the necessary diagnostic steps that are part of a process which leads to decisions about treatment. We would like to refer to this as a process leading to a social and psychotherapeutic diagnosis. Perhaps the phrase "Psychotherapeutic Diagnosis" is more applicable since it implies an assessment of how these very forces that led to the illness can be utilized as agents for the cure. The very work of establishing such a psychotherapeutic diagnosis should itself be therapeutic. The diagnostic encounter must not merely be the destructive one of discovering or being confronted with illness, but should also include a constructive contribution leading toward decisions and actions that cope with a situation and thus itself renders a form of curative experience.

The primary purpose of the diagnostic procedure is not to attach the correct label or name to the illness, but rather to find a way in which the child patient and parents can enter into a treatment program that can resolve the disturbing conflicts at the basis of his illness. Depending upon the age of the child and the intensity of his disturbance, the assessment must often evaluate the potential for acting-out, the depth of the illness, the suicidal and homicidal potential and the issues of possible hospitalization. Since, initially, the family and patient are likely to try to embroil the therapist in their battle over the patient's symptoms, it is necessary for the therapist to find a way to maintain an accurate distance which will allow him to evaluate the situation and, at the same time, to become sufficiently involved to establish a workable relationship with them.

In order to diagnose and treat these children the therapist must be personally committed and totally dedicated in his attempt to create a treatment environment which will fully accept them in their state of illness in order to provide a maximumly secure environment in which the illness can emerge and can experience maximal opportunity for change. However, our lack of knowledge at this point makes us unable to fully create an adequate receptive environment since the optimum conditions for acceptance of treatment for and by such children are not yet fully understood. During the evaluation procedure the psychiatrist is most often placed in the position of seeming to appeal to the child, reaching out to him in an active effort to create a trust situation under virtually impossible conditions, since the child's illness precludes any experience of trust. At the same time the psychiatrist is not yet ready to completely commit himself to the treatment process, and in a sense is operating within a social vacuum. The minimal commitment that does exist makes possible the evaluation of the patient and an appraisal of the possibilities for help by treatment resources existing in the community, whether by the psychiatrist himself, referral to another psychiatrist, an agency or hospital. This minimal commitment to treatment in this stage of evaluation parallels the patient's minimal commitment to treatment which may exist only to the extent that his symptoms represent a cry for help and a symbolic communication of his need for treatment. These children and their parents want treatment but fear the treatment. They fear the outbreak and the emergence of impulses, fantasies, fears and feelings which are an integral part of their illness. Their concept of treatment is to receive help to avoid relationships with people, to contain the impulses and instincts that are breaking through and to strengthen their defenses against the emergence of the illness in order for it to remain contained and controlled internally. As an example, one psychotic adolescent girl resolved never to have any more bad thoughts and sadistic fantasies about her mother and other people. Another 14-year-old psychotic girl expressed the desire that she be helped to avoid her sinful thoughts that were an integral part of the delusional system which she could not recognize as illness, but rather could experience only within the context of a religious fervor. Such goals set by these children may appear to be a resistance to treatment. On closer examination they can be seen to represent the wish for a magical and immediate return to health without having to work through a psychopathology. Such yearnings and desires to get rid of and to push away the illness should not merely be considered a resistance but often are valid communications about the patient's fears and needs which can be used as indications as to how to establish the initial contact with him and how to work toward a positive transference. In the patient's urgent request to condemn his silly thoughts, to suppress and restrain, even to forbid the expression of his feared impulses, he is seeking a superego re-enforcement from the examiner in order to achieve immdiate help for the underlying illness and thought disorder. What the patient initially seeks has actually been advocated by certain schools of psychotherapy as the essence of treatment. They advocate suppressing rather than treating the psychosis. In the philosophy of psychoanalytic psychotherapy set forth here, the basic aim is not one of suppressing the psychosis, although it is necessary to seemingly accept the initial condition of the patient for treatment. But, of course, the ultimate goal would be to help the patient relinquish such conditions rather than accepting them as necessary and final. Resistances all too often lie in the therapist rather than in the patient in adapting the techniques of classical analysis to the special needs of these extremely variant disorders.

Kraepelin (6) wrote in 1917 that it would be wrong to assume that the negligent, cruel and senseless measures that characterized the treatment of the mentally ill in the preceding century precluded the existence of more sympathetic and systematic measures that were more sanctioned in modern times. He pointed to the doctors whose rich experience or genius afforded the better understanding of mental disease and who developed sound methods of treatment because they viewed patients sympathetically and without prejudice. These were exceptional men, however, who alone could neither modify existing practices nor improve the lot of the masses. They were the seeds from which, under more propitious conditions, would spring the modern science of psychiatry. The seeds that germinated into the greatest fruition were those that blossomed into a philosophy and system that rendered its genius, talent and humanity teachable and thereby available to the many as a working instrument, rather than remaining the envied, exclusive possession of the fortunate few.

In order to understand a treatment philosophy it is necessary to have a basic model for treatment. Clinical reports from most current workers in the field of childhood psychosis lead to the inference that the treatment of the neurotic and psychotic child is basically different. We seek to present here a treatment philosophy and a model for treatment in which the psychotic and the neurotic child can be similarly dealt with, based on Freud's synthesis of the differences between these two major areas of mental illness within a single conceptual framework of psychopathology.

A scientific model is designed to provide us with a frame of reference by means of which a tremendous amount of clinical material or observational data can be utilized in such a way as to enable one to make predictions. The model permits us to think about a variety of data in such a way as to master these data, to predict, and to bring about a reconciliation of these data. The essential features contained in the body of a tremendous amount of data are made visible through the model.

The model of treatment to be presented is one which allows for consensual points by means of which we can communicate with each other even though we do not know what the other experiences. A model is created on that which is known. We immediately are confronted with the difficulty that this model has the purpose of looking at something which is not yet known. This problem is dealt with by creating a tentative model that is constantly being tested for its adequacy as it is being used. Research and treatment use of the model continue simultaneously, hand in hand. If it is found that the concepts delineated by the model do not work, one realizes that the logic is incomplete and it is necessary to add something new to the language. If the data do not fit the new model or require many unparsimonious changes, adaptations and modifications, it may be necessary to develop a new model that will better encompass the changes necessary to describe the treatment process in childhood schizophrenia.

Fifteen years ago, the senior author described a model of the treatment process based on the then current view that interpretive intervention emanated from outside of the treatment process and therefore did not include the impact of the process on the analyst (3). Today we recognize that treatment necessarily involves an interaction between patient and therapist even though the essential process is intra-psychic and the interaction very unique. Psychotherapy is not here being considered as an interpersonal process, nor as an interactional process, nor as a communication process alone. But we must recognize, in order to understand the intra-psychic process in psychotherapeutic change, that it is also necessary to understand the impact upon it of extra-psychic processes during the period of change.

In that model, the precursor of our present one, the basic observational data consisted of the interpretive process as the primary activity on the part of the analyst, and the free associative process as the primary activity on the part of the patient. The process of communication between the patient and therapist was set up under conditions which, unlike a social relationship, dictated a different set of rules, a different focus and a different function for each, even though they both shared the same long-range purpose: intra-psychic change in the patient and restoration of psychic functioning on an age-appropriate level. In psychoanalytic treatment the therapeutic contract defines the activities of the analyst as well as of the patient. Basic rules govern both. For the patient the task is to attempt to talk freely. For the therapist the task is to attempt to listen freely. Thus, the free associations of the patient are met by the freely suspended attention of the therapist which is focused on understanding such elements as transference, adaptive and defensive mechanisms, regressive behavior, unconscious communication, etc., which he will interpret. The therapist thus has a dual function in which there are elements paralleling the regressive and progressive elements of the therapeutic process in the patient. In this model we see that the transference development of the patient is matched by a countertransference potential of the therapist. The countertransference potential must be kept within the service of the treatment and be an identification to help the patient rather than over-identification to act out with him, which is ofen the fine line between controlled empathy and the loss of analytic equi-distance.

For the model of treatment, the basic observational data are the productions of both the patient and the doctor. The free associations of the patient are met by the interpretive interventions of the doctor. In many ways it would appear that the rules for the patient and the doctor are like mirror images. They are very similar in that neither can act as in ordinary social situations and the rules define all behavior within the analytic framework. The patient must reveal his needs but not act them out. The therapist must check his needs but not repress them and utilize them in the service of understanding instead of permitting them to deteriorate into countertransference reactions.

However, in dealing with children, especially psychotic children, it is almost impossible to maintain a classical analytic framework, at least with regard to the external conditions. The child does not free associate. The child does not understand the rules of the game. It is necessary to see how the basic classical model of treatment requires modifications in order to understand the impact of treatment on children, both neurotic and psychotic, and how it will be necessary to re-define the model for these special cases, and develop a structure which can be maintained or restored after innundating forces have been absorbed through interpretations or parameters.

The model of the psychotherapeutic process that has been discussed is based on Freud's topographic model of the personality presented in the *Interpretation of Dreams* (1900), and is derived from the hypothetical assumption of a mythical, ideal analytic patient who is stable and whose psychic organization provides the structure for the therapeutic process. This model, derived from the classic conception of analysis, will have to be adapted to the unique problems of treating childhood schizophrenia by supplementation of a model of the structure of personality. Rather than creating a dichotomy between the topographic model and the structural model of the personality developed later in *The Ego and the Id* (1923), we visualize the most effective model as one arising out of a synthesis of these two models into a unified one.

When treatment implications were based largely on the concept of psychosis as representing a breakthrough of unconscious forces which were conceived of as a wild jungle in which no structure, no logic, no time sequence, no evidence of reality testing could be found, treatment of psychosis, dictated by social pressures and needs, could consist only of sealing over the seething caldron and driving back the dangerous destructive forces. Clinical maneuvers designed to "put the lid on" these forces are, in our current psychoanalytic framework, not considered as treatment but rather as a kind of manipulation which leads to so-called restitution which, in fact, is an untreated, covered up disease process.

The structural model of personality portrays the psychic organization in terms of id, ego and superego structures which are best described in terms of their functions and processes, or as Beres (1) has recently suggested, as a functional model of the personality with emphasis on purpose, function, development and processes. The dynamic relationship between the psychic organizations makes obsolete the Pandora's Box metaphor, but rather stresses the conflict between impulse and defense, the wish and the reality testing capacity, impulsivity and delay functions. Such a model permits the recognition of the quasi-adaptive resolution of a conflict represented in symptom formation. It also recognizes that conflict can take place on any level of the organization. There are functional relationships between the different aspects of these personality structures, all of which can take place at different levels of the personality organization which is perceived as a hierarchy of structures. We suggest here that we combine these two models and conceive of the structural model as operating in depth. The various levels of consciousness may perhaps best be construed as different layers of psychic organization forming a hierarchy developing out of an undifferentiated archaic phase in which can be found latent dispositions which later develop into the organizers of more complex structure within the personality. Such an integrated model allows for a more refined and subtle description of the specific ego deviation suffered by psychotic children. It also permits the concept of fluctuating ego stages at various levels of regression and progression characteristic of the functioning of the psychotic psychic organization which is correlated with the particular form of integration of id, ego, and superego functions operating at a particular moment and at a particular level of the psychic hierarchy.

These concepts can be graphically illustrated with clinical data of a schizophrenic adolescent girl who, at the time of her diagnostic evaluation, fended off an open psychosis by regressing to the fantasies of the latency period in which she found herself protected from panic and terrifying fantasies by her inadequate psychic maneuvers. In analytic treatment this patient would repeatedly demonstrate how she could function on a marginal level within the limits of the secondary process only until the pressure of primary process material would overwhelm the capacity of the ego to control the flood of archaic material which lead to regression, to archaic and primitive levels of psychic functioning and reliance upon her psychic invention of the Creature, a delusional introject and precursor of the archaic superego, as an aid in organizing strengthening and sustaining her psychic functioning. This Creature became her delusional, terrifying, yet protective object that helped her to maintain some level of integration as she continued to deal with the archaic material that flooded her. Each such treatment hour then becomes comprehensible and an instrument for the treatment that follows when set against the model of treatment which we here present.

The vicissitudes of regressive and progressive forces and the manifestations of the Creature can be followed along the vertical and horizontal axes of such a model. We can follow the appearance of the Creature at those times when the patient needs to strengthen her determination to talk "nice" and thus avoid the influx of primary process material. In the struggle between her desire not to communicate, the "not nice" material interferes with the process of communication, and we see the parallel operation of the model in which the struggle between the progressive and regressive forces leads to paralysis. A progressive breakdown in her ego organization is accompanied by a breakdown in the level of superego structure. For as the flood of disruptive material becomes more primitive and archaic, it is necessary to counter this with more primitive and archaic defenses. Low-grade defenses are used to ward off low-grade primitive impulse derivatives. The Creature, in order to avoid danger, creates a virtual paralysis of advanced ego organization and in the end results in regression to the very archaic level from which the danger originally emanated. The rapidly fluctuating vicissitudes of these internal psychic forces, incomprehensible by secondary process logic and without comparable manifestations in normal and neurotic psychic functioning, find a basis for understanding in the synthesized structural model of personality which we here suggest.

The observation of the structure of the schizophrenic mind may be best conducted from the observations made during the diagnostic and treatment processes. Conversely, a process can only be studied if we recognize that there is a structure which moves through the process and is changed thereby. Any model of the psychotherapeutic process is therefore based on the assumption that we understand, or at least in part know about the structure of the personality which is undergoing the process.

In the analytic treatment of this psychotic adolescent girl, the breakdown of the initial higher form of integration leads to the introduction of the Creature, an auxiliary superego, actually a precursor of the superego, a projection of primitive delay mechanisms perceived as an external threat by the patient to bolster the weak inner control. Since the schizophrenic patient does not have available normal thinking as a form of trial action, delay mechanisms via the introduction of the Creature serve to ward off impulsivity and acting out, but without sufficient reality testing. Lacking reality testing and realistic discrimination, this form of primitive control device wards off impulsivity and self-destructive action but also indiscriminately wards off all action at any level and leads to a paralysis of higher ego functions.

Despite the regressive aspects of the Creature that is generally experienced by both patient and therapist as an enemy, a paranoid delusion and an external persecutor, this primitive precursor of the superego has the primary adaptive function of serving to avoid a complete breakthrough of the primary process, of instinct and archaic functioning. It also functions to ward off outside dangers. Derived from the primary process, this Creature also derives its energy from the sources of the id, even though its function is to wall off the id lest it overwhelm the ego. Paradoxically, the Creature is derived from the same material that it serves to counter-act, having similar origin but having been differentiated into a different purpose.

As the therapeutic hour of this psychotic girl continues, it becomes evident that archaic primary process material has over-run the primitive police power of the Creature and has inundated the ego's secondary process functioning. It is at this point that the therapist feels helpless to understand or to apply his therapeutic power if he insists that the treatment process be the same for a psychotic as for the normal or neurotic child. The unmodified model is not constructed around a schizophrenic child but rather takes a view analogous to the Ptolemaic view of placing the normal human being in the center of the psychotherapeutic world. The logic of the situation forces us to look to those necessary changes in the model in order to make it fit the special needs of the schizophrenic child. The failure to modify the model of treatment under these circumstances places the therapist in the situation of meeting the patient with his own psychosis, as it were, and the fiction of the post-ambivalent character which the schizophrenic patient can neither accommodate to nor simulate. The resultant failure in therapeutic effectiveness further arouses anxiety and terror in both the therapist and the patient and leads to a breakdown in the treatment process.

An understanding of the function of the Creature as well as its relationship to the function of the therapist must become an integral part of the therapeutic model. Observation and analysis of the patient leads to the insight that the Creature appears when the doctor is absent. When analyzing the various vicissitudes and functions of the Creature we can observe that it serves as a projected paranoid delusional defense against the archaic process and thus is a measure of the intrapsychic process; and that it describes a particular functional relationship to the doctor, a tension system between patient and doctor, and therefore is a measure of the interpersonal process. The Creature functions as a helper, as an agent to delay and to ward off the psychotic process, and as a tempter who brings about that very same aspect of the psychotic process which it also helps to defend against. Analogous to the functioning of a mechanical pace-maker which regulates the heart beat, the

Creature artificially regulates the heart-beat of the primary process in archaic functioning when the normal psychic pace-maker of interpretation by the therapist is ineffectual.

The Creature, therefore, is a primitive psychological device that works both for the delay function of the ego and for impulse discharge of the id. Its adaptive power and value make it a necessary adjunct to the therapeutic process and leads to the importance of the therapeutic philosophy of establishing an alliance with the monster, the therapeutic work of committing the Creature, like the therapist, to work in the service of the patient's recovery. In her desperate attempt to stem the flood of the archaic material which emerges as the hour proceeds, and her attempt to comply with the injunction of the Creature not to talk, express or let loose harmful primary process thoughts and impulses, the patient is led to communicate in what appears to be a harmless device of talking about a borrowed fantasy. These fantasies, even though they are introduced by external stimuli, are related to her inner world, thus providing the patient with a means of communication by which she can both escape from her own inner world and, at the same time, relate the content of her inner world to the therapist. She can thus disavow her connection with her own inner world, complying with the injunction of the Creature and escaping its threatened punishment. At the same time she acquiesces to the imagined therapist's requirement that she talk about the inner world. While maintaining an equi-distance between inner and outer world, between id, demands of superego and the remote and still unaccepted ego-therapist, the patient resolves for the moment the conflict that would otherwise inevitably paralyze her functioning. She maintains her position via the invention of the Creature in much the same way that the neurotic conflict is often temporarily resolved through symptom formation.

Continued stress on this achievement of integration, however, is disrupted by the increasing flood of the archaic material as the process continues, an inner threat and a threat to the therapeutic function. This is met by a defense of psychotic obsessionalism, manifested in the expression of a myriad of irrelevant details in a desperate attempt to avoid the seduction of the doctor, whose attitude expresses the wish that she tell him her thoughts, and a desperate frantic effort to hold back the breakthrough of primary process material. We see that the facade of an obsessive-compulsive defense is a desperate effort to maintain the therapeutic structure which is now being urgently attacked by the psychotic process. The breakdown of this facade permits more primitive aspects of her ego organization to appear. These fluctuations in ego states are characteristic of such patients who undergo shifts from higher level defenses to underlying free associative processes. Primitive autistic experiences of death and the struggle to remain alive, the desperate need for the helper to appear, at the same time the certain belief that such a helper cannot be trusted and cannot save her, emerge into open relief.

The eruption of the archaic primary process creates in the patient the feeling of having lost her mind, of being dead but half-alive. The impending thought disorder is manifested by the concretistic language and primitive archaic symbolism by which she begins to communicate the psychotic fantasies of total isolation in an objectless world where no one will accept her or believe her language. She is reduced to the terror of the underlying psychotic fantasy that, alone and isolated, she is but a living corpse.

Reich's (7) metaphor of an onion to be peeled as a rough description of the necessary working through of systematic layers of impulse and defense in order to get to the underlying conflict, although applicable for normal and neurotic psychic organization, is not applicable in the case of borderline and schizophrenic children in whom there is no stable personality organization but rather one that is fluctuating, unpredictable and unreliable. The onion metaphor is developed out of an understanding of the personality, and of the psychotherapeutic process consistent with the topographic model of the personality elaborated from the standpoint of ego psychology. Such a view of the therapeutic process was consistent with the view of Wilhelm Reich and Anna Freud in her early writings during the period when the beginnings of ego psychology assumed the ubiquitousness of an obsessive-compulsive personality structure in which impulses and instincts were assigned to a Pandora's Box-like unconscious against which were directed conscious defense mechanisms in order to keep the lid closed. The goal of psychotherapy was to make the unconscious conscious.

In the elaboration of the structural model and subsequent developments of ego psychology, the emphasis shifted to an understanding of the interchange of dynamic, economic and functional arrangements between the various aspects of the personality. Theoretically, we must deal with the issue of how the psychotic personality structure influences the various aspects of the model of the therapeutic process. The first prediction that may be made about such patients is the unpredictability about their ego organization. Methods of establishing contact and of making effective interpretations with expected predictable success in normal and neurotic patients do not achieve similar results with psychotic children. When the therapist is permitted into the inner world of the patient and is successful in restoring contact, he is paradoxically faced with the double bind that if the symbiosis is totally restored this, too, will terrify the patient and cause him to retreat. Optimal contact can be restored under those conditions in which the therapist conveys his understanding of the patient's language and at the same time avoids the terrifying aspect of that double bind by skillfully remaining in a position in which he does not enter the symbiosis too completely. To further differentiate between neurotic and psychotic ego organization significant for the psychotherapeutic process and method, we refer to Knight's (5) metaphor of the island separated from the mainland by the intervening sea of primary process. With a neurotic patient, the symptomatology is like the outer island separated from the main continent of adaptive functioning. With a psychotic patient, the small amount of adaptive functioning and higher level functioning is the outer island isolated from the main continent of psychotic structure. The uncanny aspect about the treatment of the psychotic patient is the way that the causeway between the island and the continent can be so easily inundated; what is predictable is that the fluctuations and shifting within the personality structure can rapidly occur in unpredictable fashion and under unpredictable circumstances. Such patients are able to maintain the object only as long as the object is present. This is similar to the situation of the capacity to retain the memory of the spoken voice only as long as the sound waves are present. As the sound waves die out, the voice recedes into an unstable, unreliable memory. The power of interpretation with the patient is limited by a similar unreliability. The voice of interpretation may appear powerful at first but does not persist and dies out. Its initial impact cannot be sustained and therefore no permanent reliable effect can result from its initial powerful impact. As neurotic defenses are restored, however, the patient can be treated, based on the model of the psychotherapeutic process applicable for the neurotic patient. Treatment with such patients requires not only constant island hopping, as it were, but a constant change in the kind of transportation utilized. To supplement Knight's model of the islands of fragmented ego functioning which have to be hooked together in the treatment of borderline and psychotic patients, we add the Moebius strip model (Ch. 25, this vol.) to describe the psychic organization of the psychotic patient, in which there is no clear-cut differentiation between outside and inside, between conscious and unconscious and between self and object.

   From the original notion of psychosis as a deficit of personality organization we have moved to the position of introducing into the psychotherapeutic work with psychotic children a notion of psychotherapy which is not based on compensating for deficits, but rather restoring the continuity in psychic organization which was destroyed by deadlocked struggles between the forces of impulse and the forces of delay and adaptation. We called attention in this paper to a variety of models or analogies and to notions such as, that the basic questions of ideology are hidden commitments to treatment philosophies; and that diagnosis must move from a labelling process to becoming part of the treatment process, i.e., must become psychotherapeutic diagnosis; that modern treatment techniques do not aim at suppression of the psychosis but at restoration of the continuity between primitive and advanced psychic organizations; that a treatment model for analytical work might be more useful if it represents a synthesis of Freud's early topographic model of personality and his structural views of later days. We must understand the problems of defensive adaptation not only in terms of metaphors and analogies which draw on orderly layers of personality organization, but also on metaphors which make use of instant reversals and opposites such as is represented in the Moebius strip or dialectic thinking.

Following Freud's uncanny gift of turning obstacles to treatment and insight into instruments of advance, we have advocated the alliance with monsters and dragons rather than following the demands of the patient and society which is to banish the devil. We have accepted delusional systems as artificial pace-makers and thus see them as positive factors in the life and death struggle of our sick children. We have called attention to interpretative innovations which permit the restoration of links between "islands" of advanced ego functioning and have adapted interpretative language to available psychic structure in the patient, rather than take for granted that they can adapt to conventional psychotherapeutic response. The catastrophic discontinuities in this category of illness force upon us experimentation with new models, the establishment of both therapeutic and research commitments in which the persistent life and death struggle of the patient is matched by the persistent commitment to the exploration of new treatment techniques based not on the over-commitment to a school of thought, but rather to a school of thoughtfulness.

REFERENCES

1. BERES, DAVID. "Structure and Function in Psychoanalysis." Unpublished.
2. EKSTEIN, RUDOLF, KEITH, BRYANT & FRIEDMAN, SEYMOUR. "Childhood Schizophrenia and Allied Conditions." Schizophrenia. L. Bellak, editor. New York: Logos Press, 1958.
3. EKSTEIN, RUDOLF. "Psychoanalytic Techniques." Progress in Clinical Psychology. D. Brower and L. E. Abt, editors. II:79-98. New York: Grune & Stratton, Inc., 1956.
4. FREUD, SIGMUND. "The Loss of Reality in Neurosis and Psychosis." Collected Papers, 2:277-282, 1924.
5. KNIGHT, ROBERT P. "Borderline States." Bulletin of the Menninger Clinic, 17:1, 1953.
6. KRAEPELIN, EMIL (1917). One Hundred Years of Psychiatry. New York: The Citadel Press, 1962.
7. REICH, WILHELM. Character-Analysis. New York: Noonday Press, 1961.

CHAPTER TWENTY-THREE

Levels of Verbal Communication in the Schizophrenic Child's Struggle*

He who has mastered any law in his private thoughts is master to that extent of all men whose language he speaks, and of all into whose language his own can be translated.

RALPH WALDO EMERSON, 1837

As has often been pointed out, although speech is central to the analytic process, few psychoanalytic studies have been devoted to language and its evolvement. What analytic work on language development exists reflects the history of psychoanalytic theory. We can distinguish six phases in the psychoanalytic conceptualizations of language evolvement (6). The early Freudian model of 1895, developed in the context of neurophysiological considerations, attributed the emergence of speech—the means of Verständigung—to the early helplessness of the infant, and has indeed been a useful first framework, allowing subsequent generations of workers in this field to fill in the details. This initial helplessness—that "primal source of all moral motives"**

---

* Elaine Caruth is the co-author of this chapter.

** As Freud described the baby's cry in the face of hunger, thirst or pain, and when outside help is required in order to relieve or satisfy his needs, and thus to restore a state without tension, he stated: "At early stages the human organism is

(10)—will again be of central concern in our present task of describing a developmental language profile, as it were, for the psychotic child.

In the second phase the conceptualization of language development was strongly influenced by prevailing theories of psychosexual development, and the origin of language was speculatively related to various sexual factors. Work in the third phase, utilizing reconstructions from the analysis of adults and children, stressed the preoedipal mother-child relationship and the importance of the "primitive love talk" (4) in terms of needs to be met by the "mother tongue." The fourth phase was under the growing dominance of ego psychology, the adaptive point of view, and notions of differentiation of psychic functions. Molecular considerations of speech mechanics and often too-literal assumptions about the origin of speech elements gave way to more sophisticated models relating the origin of speech to the development of ego functions. The genetic reconstructions of early preverbal experiences were utilized as blueprints for further investigation. The fifth contribution, developing out of the analyst's growing readiness to collaborate with and to learn from other behavioral scientists, came from direct observation of infants under both empirical and experimental conditions. A sixth source has been the study of language in schizophrenia and related disorders, particularly as they occur in childhood; this research has led to improved models of thought and speech development which permit us to see Freud's early and dramatic germinal insight of 1895 as one which has borne rich fruit and which invites new work in the same direction.

The following presentation centers around some new work in that direction. The data derive from the intensive study of long-term psychoanalytic treatment processes with schizophrenic and autistic children. We shall describe our attempts to redefine and delineate the variety and degrees of disturbances in communication that we find in different kinds of schizophrenic and autistic children. This venture into the area of psycholinguistic problems germane to psychotic children requires some ideas of the philosophy of linguistics and science, some concepts of psychoanalytic ego psychology, and some knowledge of the technical interventions one experiments with in trying to bring about a Verständigung—a system of communication—between oneself

---

incapable of achieving this specific action [the supply of nourishment]. It is brought about by extraneous help, when the attention of an experienced person has been drawn to the child's condition by a discharge taking place along the path of internal change [e.g., by the child's screaming]. This path of discharge thus acquires an extremely important secondary function—viz., of bringing about an understanding with other people; and the original helplessness of human beings is thus the primal source of all moral motives" (p. 379).

and the schizophrenic child. These notions may help us understand the meaning of the schizophrenic child's language and discover the latent order behind the manifest thought disorder, the communication illness of the patient who struggles with, for, and against language, just as he struggles for and against object and self in the prolonged autism-symbiosis conflict that characterizes the central difficulty of the schizophrenic child—the one which is re-created in and through the transference during the course of analytic treatment.

We are referring to the fact that autism and symbiosis may be understood as normal phases in the development of object relations (13). If these are successfully mastered, the infant gains the capacity to differentiate self from nonself and eventually to perceive the people around him as separate objects. The relationships he develops with them change in nature as his psychological development proceeds. This progression in object relations optimally moves from the initial objectless autistic state to the early symbiotic position of communion with the maternal figure, and then to one in which the child gradually begins to separate —"to hatch" in Mahler's words—from the object through processes of differentiation and individuation which lead ultimately to the capacity to achieve object and self representation, stable identifications, and to a psychic organization that is capable of functioning on the level of the secondary process and according to the reality principle. In the schizophrenic child, however, we see instead a prolonged and pathological version of the normal symbiotic-individuation struggle of the infant. The pathogenic symbiosis, while maintaining the delusional omnipotence derived from the fusion of mother and self, is also experienced as an engulfment and annihilation of the beginning self representation within the normally protective symbiotic sac.* In an earlier publication (Ch. 6, this vol.), we said: "We can thus visualize the psychotic state as one in which self and object representations are enclosed within the symbiotic sac, separated by a porous osmotic membrane. It is undergoing, without yet having achieved, separation, nor stable cathexis and differentiation of self and object. In this stage only primitive ego functioning exists. It is dominated by primary process and unstable impulse control, in which the thought disorder is characterized by the equations: thought = action; inner reality = outer reality; self = object" (p. 109).

However, the moves toward separation lead regressively toward the autistic position and thus inevitably to the loss of self in an empty, objectless world which may become seemingly static and immovable or may be a fleeting and fluctuating phase. The schizophrenic adaptation consists of the attempt to restore the symbiosis through fusion

---

* Comparable to what Mahler has referred to as the symbiotic membrane.

experience, as well as the attempt to achieve some kind of separation through an autisticlike avoidance of the object.

The following clinical material will demonstrate the specific ways these core conflicts of the schizophrenic child find different forms of expression at different stages of psychic maturation and development. We might even think in terms of a normal developmental line (9) of language from silence and communion to speech and symbolic communication. This would include such stages as babbling, echoing or echolalia, delayed echolalia, self-echoing, expressing, appealing, and finally symbolic communication. Specific developmental disturbances for each stage can be described, several of which are depicted below. The clinical data will also highlight the relationship between the development of early object relations and the beginning development of language.

Case 1

We start with a "classically" autistic, nonspeaking three-year-old, Nanny, the kind of child that Kanner, Bender, Mahler, and others would describe as autistic. Clinically, these children are extremely withdrawn; their relationships have a mechanical quality in that they use the other person like a deanimated tool. Language, when available, is not used in the service of communication but rather in a beginning attempt to contact the external world, still barely perceived as separate from themselves. We refer here to the imitative and mechanical, stereotypic, repetitive speech known as echolalia. These children do not seek symbolic communication through their language, but rather attempt to establish a symbiotic fusion relationship with the maternal figure. The imitative behavior of echolalia and echopraxia can be understood as an attempt to introject the object, but it occurs at such a primitive level of imitation that the child experiences no psychic differentiation from the object; he cannot swallow you because there is no stable, separate "you"; yet he experiences the process as himself becoming "you." Thus the inevitably unsuccessful attempt at incorporation leads instead to fusion or loss of self. Nevertheless it must be understood as the forerunner of identificatory processes in an as yet primitive, undifferentiated psychic structure.

We have previously described the difficulties of treating such children who must constantly destroy the very contact they seek, and whose efforts at establishing this contact lead to this loss of self in the fusion experience (7). They seem to have available only the "choice" between becoming the senseless, selfless, albeit delusionally omnipotent echo of the therapist, or else of rejecting the therapist who has become a terrifying engulfing threat. We then see a retreat to the precarious precursor of identity which the autistic position seemingly offers to such a child, whose pathogenic experiences within the maternal symbiosis have not allowed for the development of sufficient ego structure to move toward true separation.

In Nanny's treatment we could observe changes in her symptom of echolalia from an initial form of imitating without understanding to more advanced forms of delayed echoing that became precursors of descriptive language functions in that she would also verbalize her own activities in the third person. Her first echoing was comparable to the imitation games and imitative sounds of very small, preverbal children. At the beginning of treatment, the little girl seemed to be dominated by the peremptoriness and choicelessness of impulse as she wandered everywhere throughout the clinic, guided not by any intention or understandable and meaningful search, but driven but utter chaos, or so it would appear to the casual observer. As she wandered about, the therapist* would follow her, observing that chaos and seeking to discern the hidden order or meaning behind it. At the same time the therapist described Nanny's actions in very simple phrases. The therapist's "verbal echopraxia," so to speak, of the child's motor activity— a choiceful regression in therapeutic technique from more advanced technical interventions to a repetitive description of the child's actions —was responded to by the child with echolalia, her beginning way of taking the psychotherapist in, comparable to the peekaboo game between mother and child. The therapist would say, "Here Nanny goes, here Nanny stops." After a while it was observed that Nanny had developed rudiments of speech in the nature of echolalia, a mechanical and repetitive speech which seemed to echo some of the therapist's words.

Nanny, after acquiring echolalic speech, remained for a long time on this imitative level, without truly understanding the meaning of the words. After many months of effort, the child's mother reported that the echolalic speech had developed into *delayed echolalia*. She would comment, for example, "Here Nanny go," which could be understood as the delayed echo of the therapist, who, as we have seen, had chosen to establish contact with the child by describing her actions to her, much as a mother interprets the expressions of the infant in such a way as to echo the inner need they express. The therapist's remarks could also be understood as an immediate echo of the child's

---

* Mrs. Leda Rosow, M.A., has contributed this case illustration.

own action which was in the nature of a trial thought, albeit a very primitive one, expressing a beginning awareness and recognition of the self experienced through the action.

Shortly thereafter, while the mother was driving with the child, she heard Nanny say: "No, no, you mustn't do it" and "That's the way," imitating the therapist's words. The mother knew that neither she nor anybody else in the family had used these phrases, and that even the intonation was a parrotlike imitation of the therapist. From this report we surmised that the therapist had made contact with the child, who could now maintain an image of her even when the therapist was out of sight. We suggest that the therapist's phrases—one phrase of delaying and one phrase of approving—could be considered external organizers by means of which the child had developed a steering device, a kind of primitive red and green signal for restriction and for permission. A germinal delaying apparatus had been created which could serve as a beginning kind of internal control of impulse expression. In some mechanical fashion the therapist had been taken in, even though for a long time this attempt to introject the therapist would continue to deteriorate into a primitive fusing with the therapist's voice and speech instead of leading to more appropriate identificatory processes. We understood this as an attempt to restore the lost introject (in the absence of the object) by means of maintaining it as a quasi-auditory hallucination expressed verbally in the delayed echolalia. The child had turned echolalia into delayed echolalia, which can be understood as the expression of a memory in a mental organization which still lacked the capacity for symbolic and cognitive representation.

Later in the treatment, as the child and therapist were walking out of the building one day, they discovered that it was raining. The therapist said: "Nanny, it is raining." The child's response was, "It is wet." We understood that she had acquired the beginning of symbolic representative speech through a temporary identification with the therapist's symbolic functioning. In this one short sequence she paralleled the development of Helen Keller when at eight years she understood the meaning of the verbal symbol "water" through the persistent efforts of Anne Sullivan Macy and had thus acquired symbolic speech, that "unique hallmark of man." Both children had thus indicated their capacity to establish the continuity between the concrete experience and the abstract generalization.

In discussing the child's moves during a long span of intensive therapeutic work, we saw the following three steps: echolalia, delayed echolalia, and finally simple descriptive symbolic speech, accompanying her struggle for, against, and with objects, out of which evolved the capacity to master primitive speech functions. Once the therapist had become a sufficiently stable part of the child's inner world, there emerged a beginning "voice of the conscience," and the beginning of higher mental processes which could lead toward identification and superego development. The therapist, by her choice of initially echoing the child in an attempt to empathize with the child's autistic, deanimated world, had gradually gained entrance into that world as a kind of living tape recorder of the child's unspoken, unverbalized, and, as a matter of fact, preverbal needs and experiences. The therapist could then become a creative echo and ultimately translate these needs into a higher form of communication, after she and the child had first restored a communionlike relationship in which the child's need for reunion with the maternal image was restored via the transference.

We would now like to discuss that struggle toward understanding and genuine Verständigung against the background of Karl Bühler's Organon model of language. He distinguishes three functions of language: expression, appeal, and representation. This model is utilized in order to give a graphic illustration of the genesis of speech and learning of language. In the beginning, Nanny's imitation, her echolalic gesture, cannot be understood in terms of object relationship. Nanny does not consider the therapist a person. The child at this point is frozen in an autistic mode. Nanny imitates but cannot animate the therapist and she does not attach meaning to the imitative speech. She talks to herself via the speech element she had received from the nurturing person whom she has now joined within the symbiotic sac. If she could interpret her behavior, she might be saying: "As I become conscious for the first time of the fact that I am walking up and down, I become conscious of it through a kind of auxiliary ego, the eyes of the undifferentiated mother object. I-we have learned to imitate, and I-we start to observe myself. I start to become aware of motor activity as a part of me. I can do no more than echo language without really understanding it, but in doing so I get approval from the person who loves me and therefore I can acquire the beginning of language function."

In the establishment of communion between therapist and child, an attempt to use sound as a bridge between the nurturing person and the child is the first step in bringing about primitive understanding which leads to imitative speech. This kind of Verständigung is really reunion, a restoration of that early unity of feelings, and thus has appeal function. One could say that the child's first imitative speech is meant to restore unity with the mother, a unity maintained and limited by and within the symbiotic sac.

When echolalia develops into delayed echolalia, a kind of hallucinatory equivalent expressed in sound, it becomes evident that delayed echolalia serves as a beginning attempt to negotiate between impulse and delay. Nanny used delayed echolalia as a steering device to approve and disapprove of impulse expression. To that degree, she had internalized the therapist and was building up an introjected steering device, a crude ego function to make her independent of the therapist. Nanny restored the therapist by talking to herself when the therapist was absent, through describing her own behavior in similar approving and disapproving terms, but without really being able to regulate the behavior. Impulse was not yet modified by this primitive control device of description. Where impulse rules, there is no need for communication with the object via verbal language. Once she had started to experience the person, primitive precursors of object relations developed and she could begin to acquire the first elements of language. But such language was still only a signal. It was as if Nanny were saying to us: "I notice what I am doing and I remember whenever you approve or disapprove of it. It is almost as if you were there. But your disapproval or approval is as yet an ineffective signal. The language that I use does not truly guide me. It is a quasi-steering device after rather than before the fact. I still cannot remember our past experiences together to guide me before the act, but through the act and through the accompanying delayed echolalia I can restore them and begin to reconstitute or, more aptly, constitute the beginnings of a separate psychic organization. For me, language does not serve thought as trial action but only as *post facto* description."

Case 2

We now turn to an episode from the beginning phase in the treatment of five-year-old Danny, a somewhat more advanced schizophrenic child with both autistic and symbiotic features. Whereas Nanny had initially been almost totally withdrawn into an objectless, contactless world so that the therapist had had to spend many months seeking to find some means by which to intrude herself even into the child's awareness, Danny demonstrated more responsiveness to the therapist as an object, albeit primarily as a deanimated thing that he used as a tool both to satisfy his needs and to serve as a toy around which to weave his fantasies. Danny had shown signs of deep disturbance as early as age two, convincing his mother that he was mentally retarded. By the age of three the difficulties in feeding and sleeping and other signs of disturbance such as head banging, rocking, resistance to being held, and slowness in the development of language resulting in an inability to communicate emotionally with others, had led the parents to seek help. Supportive treatment on a weekly basis had led to some improvement in his language development and communication ability, reflecting a growing appreciation of his own identity previously experienced more as a thing than as a human being. Two years later, he appeared to be a seriously disturbed child, who, at the time of evaluation, demonstrated continuous activity of a primarily repetitive and apparently purposeless nature. He gave the impression of having difficulty in differentiating between himself and the external world; he appeared to have shut out most of the human object world, using it primarily as an inanimate tool in relationship to his own needs. His spoken language, usually of an echolalic quality, was scarcely intelligible, but he reacted appropriately to those commands which were satisfying to him. The initial diagnosis was infantile autism, although elements of minimal interhuman relationships were noted; e.g., he could indicate verbally certain basic needs such as "I want candy," his wish to remain in the office, or his desire for his mother to come.

Danny thus was psychologically more advanced than Nanny, who initially had been incapable of symbolic communication of her wishes and concerns. After some months of treatment Danny began to engage the therapist in a kind of continuous mutual echoing, as he indicated clearly his wish for the therapist to echo his "Hello dolly," just as he clearly was himself echoing, like a prerecorded tape of a tape, an earlier experience. When after many weeks he replaced "Hello dolly" with "Hello grandma," it became clear that he was re-creating with the therapist the memory of an earlier experience with a primary figure. He now revived this in the treatment* by assigning to the therapist the role of the delayed echo of the earlier object; and just as the earlier experience had not truly been a dialogue between himself and the object but had been experienced in a mechanical, deanimated fashion, so did he mechanically repeat the memory through the mutual delayed echolalia shared with the therapist. The therapist was allowed to enter into the fantasy not as a separate object but as a re-edition of the earlier maternal figure with whom there apparently had existed only a meaningless, contactless kind of interaction.

Normally, the infant's speech development proceeds via "echoing," that is, imitating the mother, within the context of an emotionally meaningful mother-child relationship in which the child echoes the mother, who in turn, through her loving "baby talk," echoes the baby in the early, satisfying preverbal communion relationship which slowly allows for the development of meaning.

In therapy, Danny was reliving such early experiences, but in his case they lacked the positive affective contact necessary for the develop-

---

* Morton Bramson, M.D., contributed this case illustration.

ment of true communication. He ascribed to the therapist the role of his echo, in the attempt to restore the memory of the earlier experience in which there apparently had begun to evolve some awareness of the object as somewhat differentiated from him although still partially fused within the symbiotic sac, i.e., "separated by a porous osmotic membrane ... undergoing, without yet having achieved, separation, nor stable cathexis and differentiation of self and object" (Ch. 6, this vol.). In Danny's assigning to the therapist the task of echoing him, as he himself echoed a seemingly meaningless phrase from a record, we see a re-enactment of the past: in response to Danny's delayed echo the therapist must become echolalic, just as originally the child himself echoed a mother who herself could not furnish any spontaneous communication with him but could only repeat—i.e., echo—words to him that did not truly convey any inner emotional meaning. Thus this play was an echo of what should have been a dialogue but which was in fact a monologue that the child had internalized and now was projecting. It was as if there were two introjects, or extrojects, talking together; although to the extent that Dany was not satisfied with the inner monologue and sought the external object around which to weave the fantasy role of one of the introjects, we realize that he was approaching the stage where he might become capable of a true dialogue.

In the nonpathogenic therapeutic relationship, a different resolution becomes possible so that instead of merely going through the motions of a relationship, similar to actions on a stage, there can eventually develop true contact and communication. In the early stages of treatment, however, the child's precarious precursors of ego functioning still needed omnipotently to control and maintain sameness with his surroundings, and the only safe "dialogue" was the prewritten monologue whose story is woven around the therapist, who must act it out with the child as if it were their shared memory.

Danny initially made contact on the level of the desired communion, the preverbal language of the symbiotic phase in which there is still "connection"—to use the language of an eight-year-old borderline schizophrenic child, Johnny—rather than symbolic communication. We might think of the child's development with respect to the capacity for object relations as a process moving from autism to complete fusion, to increasingly greater degrees of differentiation and individuation within the symbiotic sac, until finally, emerging from the symbiosis, there remains only the "connection"—the post-neonatal but still unsevered umbilical cord, so to speak, prior to the final severing and separating. As a consequence we understand that thought and language development proceeds in a parallel fashion.

Case 3

The above-mentioned borderline schizophrenic child, Johnny, had an extremely labile, fluctuating psychic organization. Occasionally he was capable of higher levels of object-related communication. At other times he was dominated by regressive conflicts over differentiation and separation which, in the transference, were reflected in fluctuating fusion experiences and deep regressive shifts to primary process thinking and language. At such moments Johnny ordered the therapist to "copy" —i.e., echo—him. Johnny's more advanced psychic organization enabled him to observe these massive but still partial regressions and to experience the threat of object loss, which he attempted to forestall by "regressing" the therapist with him as she echoed his psychotic thoughts and language. In this way he apparently could experience fusion with her. For example, he would start to bandage his own finger and end by bandaging hers, without concern for or awareness of where he ended and she began (Ch. 25, this vol.). His request that she echo him reflected an attempt to exert some modicum of ego autonomy over the passively experienced regression "in his private thoughts" and language, a regression which he actively tried to impose upon the therapist (chapter 26). This child was able to communicate his feelings of being "disconnected" as he graphically portrayed on the "connection board" (his word for blackboard) or in his repetitive attempts to connect up various train-track layouts, which he rarely completed in time to run the train, just as it was initially difficult for him to maintain and complete a connected secondary process train of thoughts. On the "connection board" he projected his changing self and object representations or, more aptly, images, as they fluctuated from connected to disconnected, from teeny mouth to devouring monster, from Jonah to the whale. When these archaic fantasies took over, he sought to fuse with the therapist, who, by copying or echoing him, became a projected reverberation—an echo of this threatening inner world into which she had intruded. Moreover, since she now was one with him, she was less likely to fly away and disappear —one of Johnny's prevailing fearful fantasies. However, like any echo, she was at the same time "always so far away," because in becoming an echo she no longer was really there as a separate object. Johnny, however, was able to recognize his desire for the therapist to echo him, and his observing ego—in his words, his rudder world that steered him through life—frequently permitted the therapist to become more than an echoing primitive introject fused with his primary process world. He could gradually let her become an advanced creative echo, an interpreter capable of adding new dimensions to the communication.

Early in the treatment, Johnny brought to the hour his record player—a kind of free-associating machine, as it were, which permitted total fusion between inner fantasy and external reality. The record player represented an extension of the child's delusional omnipotent control over his environment, which he sought to create in his own image, as well as the omniscient and omnipotentially controlling environment, which told him what to think. He also brought the record "Mary Poppins," his choice of an animated but not truly animated extroject onto which he projected his fears that both he and the object might disappear. He presumably brought the record so the therapist could "tell me the words," a request that grew out of a previous session; he had indicated that his singing of a song was an echoing of sounds rather than meaningful words, as indeed was true of the songs themselves, which ranged from the primary process language of "Supercalifragilisticexpialidocious" to the rational secondary process cautionary tale of the "spoonful of sugar that helps the medicine go down," which is to say, helps the demands of external reality become internalized. However, behind his request for the therapist to tell him the words lay, of course, the need to tell her what words to tell him. She was permitted to speak only if she spoke what he had programmed for her; but to the degree that he acknowledged a need to have her explain his language to him, he was opening up the possibility that, as they reconnected, she could begin to disconnect.

Several years later, however, more firmly differentiated and secure in his own identity, he was able to suggest that "we are going to start a new life in outer space. and bring a telescope, camera, and telephone to call Mommy." With this, Johnny diagnosed and prescribed his own conditions of health, which were quite appropriate for a nine-year-old: to be far enough away to create a new life and still close enough to contact Mommy. This may well be the optimal improvement to be expected in the treatment of certain schizophrenic conditions.

Case 4

We now turn to a somewhat different clinical illustration. Don, an eighteen-year-old schizophrenic adolescent, possessed speech and sometimes used a convincing obsessive façade of secondary process thought. During the last few years of treatment he emerged from his former social isolation, in which he had been unable to make use of school or community facilities, and had remained alone in a darkened room communicating with his delusional objects. He improved sufficiently to finish high school and to maintain a number of college courses, drive a car, and attempt social contact with people.* The main delusional object of his inner dialogues and "pluralogues" was a Mr. Punishment (7), who changed his color like a chameleon as he gravitated back and forth between primary and secondary processes.

Don, who is still in treatment, has recently been engaged in building an obsessive-compulsive cognitive structure by means of which he can learn to differentiate between his internal and external world, so that he can begin to bring about a compromise between his impulses and the demands of reality. He tried to build a system to help him cope with his awareness of the need for appropriate delay mechanisms. He literally worked on his treatment day and night, and during a time away from treatment he composed a document entitled *Constitution of the Inner World*, which contains ten amendments as well as a ten-day truce pact. These documents, essentially an intrapsychic Bill of Rights, describe how a schizophrenic deals with his impulses, in this case the seemingly insatiable compulsion to masturbate:

> It has been decided that Don shall stop doing the habit for a period of ten days. This will be an experiment to determine whether or not the habit is the cause of the anxiety and nervousness. I hereby agree to such terms.

This document was signed by Don, later to be witnessed and endorsed by his therapist, to whom he brought this as well as the second document, *The Constitution of the Inner World*, with the subtitle, "Don, President and Ruler—Amendments." We see here this schizophrenic adolescent's philosophy of life: he is the ruler of his own world, who dispenses with the usual power apparatus needed to achieve power leverage in the real world. By emptying it of outside influence, he can maintain the integrity of his megalomanic inner world which is dominated by the pleasure principle. Yet he presented his ideas by using the language of the outer world. One is reminded of Leary's slogan for the hippies: "Tune in, turn on, and drop out." However, to maintain his megalomaniac delusional *Weltanschauung*, Don needed to make rules which reflected his way of thinking, delaying, and dealing with conflicting impulses. As we read his rules, we find that they are inner replicas of outside conditions, even though, like dreams, they go beyond what is possible in the waking world; nevertheless the basic material is derived from the real world, from day residuals. Don's inner world was actually a shadowy replica of the outside world, just as Don's *Constitution*

---

* This case was treated by one of the authors with the assistance of concomitant casework carried out by Mrs. Beatrice Cooper, M.A., who focused on reality issues.

represented a distorted version of the conditions of psychotherapy, revealing how he internalized the words of the therapist. While he may say whatever he wants in the therapeutic hour in the "green-light" room, he also knows he must still keep to some limits and cannot act out what he thinks. He thus worded his statement as follows:

1. All private thoughts and actions shall be kept between Dr. E. and members of the inner world only.
2. Each force, punishing or rewarding, is permitted to demonstrate the reason for believing what is best. All forces have equal rights in expression.
3. No severe punishments are permitted at any time. Spanking hard for real is hereby forbidden except in light demonstrations. All actions are for use only in fantasy and private unless they are important in helping a person gain a victory or a rewarding life.
4. All heroes shall be elected by the majority vote of the inner world. No person or reality can be used for any purpose in the inner world except honorary heroes such as the Beatles, or if their names are changed to names used in fiction or television.

We want to call special attention to the "4th amendment," inasmuch as it makes clear the precarious balance of the boy's capacity for object constancy, the nature of his object relations, and the parallel nature of his level of communication in which he still tries to maintain the denial of the existence of the separate object. Don developed this *Constitution of the Inner World* when he was alone at night, working through what had transpired during the treatment process. He reviewed the implicit demands and conditions of treatment and started to "meet" people, but only on condition that they be fantasy people. He developed an inner dialogue with their differing points of view—fantasy figures who played roles he had assigned to them—in a fashion similar to that of the younger child who assigned the singing role to his therapist. He gathered these people around him and "chaired" the meeting. By giving each introject the right of discussion, he hoped to delay the impulse to masturbate, and he did so for several hours. He started his meeting at 9 o'clock in the evening and delayed until midnight, when he succumbed happily and masturbated, having worked out in these meetings of the inner mind an unassailable alibi of a group decision, as it were. The truce was broken, but the discharge of the impulse had been delayed for three hours. One might also say that the masturbatory act had been preceded by the foreplay of the dialogue of the introjects, who "protested too much."

In this essay we are not concerned with the issue of masturbation, the expression of instinctual desires, or Don's use of his penis as a reassuring transitional self-object, but we are concerned with the method Don used to resolve an internal conflict and its relationship to the nature of schizophrenic language and communication. We may ask why the internal conflict during these evening hours was not resolved by permitting Dr. Ekstein, or the parents, or any other "real" people from the outside world to be at the meeting even in fantasy. Why are these figures that Don gathered around not really internalized representations of objects of the external world, but are rather internal representations of ealier unstable introjects, now represented as free-floating, dreamlike personages in his inner fantasy world? We only know that it was easier for Don to reach what appeared to be a compromise with the requirements of the external world. In fact, he circumvented them by creating a "ghost parliament," in which no one from the real world could really communicate by challenging the inevitable breaking of the truce, which was after all put a token identification with the perceived demands of therapy.

We see how he dealt with his "pursuit of reality" (Ch. 2, this vol.) and how he stopped short of reaching that very reality, in his inability to let the external object become other than a replica of his internal representations. Reality testing was not yet an inner condition for him, beyond this token gesture, and his system of communication reflected this situation: the use of secondary process language was a token gesture and a token identification—a "ghost language" spoken by a plurality of one. This limited capacity for reality testing merely maintained the precarious balance with the outside world, which was experienced as but a shadowy reality of his inner ideas. Of dreams it is said that the latent dream thought can pass the censorship only if it ventures forth in the disguise of the manifest content. In Don's life the real person can pass by the censorship only if he reappears in the patient's dream world in disguise, in a temporary merger with the delusional object.

Don's future progress depends upon whether he can enter into a true dialogue with the therapist—the real person—and his fantasy characters, which would enable him to acknowledge the existence of a separate person and to accept the conditions for a real exchange with outer reality. We have seen that Don's inner world has to some extent come to resemble the outside world, but it is still only a delayed echo, merely imitative and sterile, and without the spirit of genuine identification. His acceptance of the interpretations is more a caricature of the psychoanalytic process, not too different from the imitating devices that Nanny utilized in internalizing the mother figure whom she then used as an internal steering device.

While it is true that these children differ in important respects, we wish to point out certain similarities. Bühler's Organon model can be used as a basic blueprint, except that we have to account for the fact that the language structures of such patients cannot be characterized as stable structures, as was originally maintained during nineteenth-century faculty psychology. Instead of rigid systems, we find that dynamic notions of process give us better insight into the language, communication, and thinking problems of these patients.

Before the acceptance of the object and the emergence of the concept of self, we have an example of the original struggle between impulse and delay carried out on a primitive level. "Here Nanny goes," is in the service of the impulse, while "Here Nanny stays" seems to be characteristic of beginning delay functions. Nanny made these precursors of self-observations away from the therapist and as a delayed echo of the therapist's echoing behavior; hence they represented a somewhat more advanced level of communication than the immediate echolalic repeating of whatever is heard. They reflect the beginning of some experience of self as differentiated from the environment, as if the child had now left the empty, autistic, objectless world through the total fusion with the therapist, which enabled her to begin to discriminate between the animate and the inanimate. At the same time the child not only observed concretely the impulse and the delay—i.e., "Here Nanny goes . . . stops"—but also, via the auxiliary ego of the therapist, began to experiment with the somewhat more abstract notion, "Nanny shouldn't do that," as if in preparation for the future when she would be able to attach that notion which implies some modicum of autonomy and control to her impulsive behavior.

With Danny, the more advanced autistic-symbiotic child, we saw how the more stable symbiotic attachment to the object enabled him to use the therapist as an extension of himself, as an extroject to act out the inner situation, which was but an empty delayed echo of an earlier emotionally meaningless, hence echolalic system of communion with the mother. With Johnny, a borderline schizophrenic child whose fluctuating ego functioning at times led to regression to autistic levels of object relations even though the remaining psychic structures continued to function on a more advanced level, delayed echolalia occurred in the form of self-echoing, as his more critical ego functions observed the intrusion of primary process fantasies over which he exerted some autonomy by "echoing" them, much as the neurotic patients feels his problems are under his control if he labels or names them. In addition, Johnny assigned the role of echo to the therapist as an aid in his struggle against the autistic withdrawal into primary process fantasies away from external reality, and to strengthen his active mastery over the passively experienced regression and eruption of impulses.

We can now see the relationship between echolalia, delayed echo-lalia, and the "4th amendment" in Don's "ghost parliament." Nanny, for example, observed in sound her impulsive acts and their delay via the echolalic means described above. Don put down in writing the observation, "Here Don goes masturbating" and the delayed pseudo-echoing of the outside world's implicit demand for delay. He put down "rules" for his inner world which were a token acknowledgment of the outside world—advanced echoes, so to speak, that fused the impulse with the delay mechanism. Don's essential communication, though seemingly couched in symbolic language, was actually determined by primary process thinking. He excluded reality objects except as an echo of the inner introjects, which had achieved a frozen and immutable psychotic object constancy.

Schizophrenic communications of the more psychologically advanced child contain within them the equivalent motivation of more primitive echolalic speech, expressing both the search for and the autistic defense against the fusion experience. Even though language is acquired for seemingly interpersonal interchange, it fails to become a permanent acquisition brought about by lasting internalizations. The illness makes it impossible to bring about these enduring internalizations which depend on stable object relations. Without these, secondary process language does not develop. Words are then experienced as a kind of "sell-out device," as a fourteen-year-old schizophrenic girl said who complained that the words she used failed to express what she meant on the three different levels of her brain.

The systems of communication which these children use and by which they establish a life line—the "connecting" security line—have ingredients of our thinking, but they are to a large extent attached to the appeal and holding-on aspects of language. Their language is oriented primarily toward conveying an appeal—to join with them in their regression—and not to conveying a thought. It is under the sway of the regressive tendency to restore the early mother-child unity which can dispense with symbolic communication. It is the therapist's ultimate function to translate preverbal experiences into language. Eventually he must interpret, even though the patient initially may want to destroy the representational meaning.

We finally come to what we can do to strengthen that function of language which is task-oriented, solution-oriented, and resolution-oriented; which permits learning and mastery of reality to take place, so that instead of a chasm there will be a viable bridge between self and external reality. That bridge is, of course, the advanced capacity for communication. The language of the schizophrenic is burdened by the primary functions of appeal and of holding on, and is dominated by the need for communication implies the existence of separation between self and object. The schizophrenic struggles with us against the acceptance of our language. Such a child seems to say: "I talk in my language; my language is *the* mother tongue, the child-mother tongue. I have changed the rules of grammar completely and have distorted them in such a way that they restore the early relationship between mother and me, where the object was not an object, where the self was not a self but where self and object are fused in a symbiotic arrangement which is maintained in my thought disorder which dispenses with reality testing." As a matter of fact, words fuse with their referent and become object-symbols, no longer cathected as object representations (Wexler, 15).

Thus the schizophrenic, if we may state it in the language of the philosophy of science, is opposed to the position of radical empiricism, which insists that there is meaning only where there is opportunity for operational verification. We suggest that there are two extremes of communication: that of the radical empirical, a position reiterated by Sidney Hook (11) who insists on operational verification and would force out of language all those aspects that describe the inner psychological world of people, sick and well; and that of the schizophrenic child who is in the diametrically opposite position so that in his system of communication there is no place for reality testing and verification.

The linguistic philosopher, Waismann speaks about the chasm which exists between "soul and soul." Could he have meant the distance between self and object representation? How can this chasm be bridged without a stable separation, which is the problem we face in communicating with the schizophrenic child who has not yet cathected outer reality. We develop a compromise language, a kind of Esperanto of the mind, which does not quite rule out reality testing but neither insists on it nor prohibits it. In this compromise language we do not probe too deeply and we do not force the patient back to reality testing, because this would prevent contact. On the other hand, he could not reach us if he were unable to talk our language just a little bit. But this neutral language—this Esperanto for the separated minds, this bridge between the two kinds of language—is made possible through metaphor. Metaphor becomes a link between the language of inner and outer reality, and brings about primitive understanding, tolerable contact under optimum conditions (3, 8).

At times our patients are people who echo us but who do not think like we do. They establish their precarious identity not via *cogito ergo* sum, but as Edelheit (5) phrases it, in terms of *resono ergo sum*: I echo, therefore I am; but parenthetically we might add: "But am I, or am I you, since I echo?" Sometimes the therapist must play crazy in order to echo the schizophrenic's language, and in the countertransference he, too, may at times ask this question (Ch. 8, this vol.), in his quest for understanding via the suspension of disbelief he temporarily gives up outer reality testing for inner reality communicating. Despite the fact that the patient's system of thinking follows a different order from ours, we can talk with him because we find certain coincidental points between his way of thinking and our way of thinking which permit a kind of vague and primitive understanding. Carnap (2) spoke about the possibility of two people understanding each other, in spite of the fact that the inner experiences which are at the basis of their thoughts can never be compared, in terms of the availability of coincidental points. He likened such different inner sensual experiences to one in which two persons, each viewing a different map of the world, would visualize the earth differently. One might see it in the global form pictured on his map, while the other might envision the earth in terms of the flat map he was viewing. Nevertheless, they could understand each other to some extent since they would find certain points of coincidence on each map, and thus could establish relationships of similarity—complementary *Gestalten*, an important aspect of all interpretation (7).

We would like to sum up our comments on the psychotic child's struggle with language by citing Waismann (14), a linguistic philosopher identified with the Vienna Circle, known to us through the names of Carnap, Schlick, Wittgenstein, and others. He says:

> What, then, are we to say in reply to the question how far language serves the purposes of communication—as a bridge built by the mind to lead from consciousness to consciousness? Is it really established that every thought which is expressed in this language is intelligible to everyone else who uses it? In the face of the examples just given, such a view can hardly be advocated. Is everyone, then, in possession of a private language comprehensible to him alone? Not that either. It would be truer to say that our language is suited equally to the purposes of communication. On the whole we manage to make ourselves understood passably. But there are cases, for instance, in conveying certain rare moods and states of minds, where it is doubtful how far language really bridges the chasm between soul and soul.
>
> It is perhaps convenient to think of the vast domain of language as a photograph taken with a long-focus lens. A certain area of such a photograph would be sharp, corresponding to the area of language in which words are adequately fitted for purposes of communica-

tion. Such is the language of physics. But beyond this as beyond the sharply focused area of the picture, clearness, definiteness gradually decrease, till the edges of the picture, like the uttermost attainments of language, are blurred into indeterminacy.

REFERENCES

1. Bühler, K. (1934). Sprachtheorie. Jena: Fischer.
2. Carnap, R. (1928). The Logical Structure of the World and Pseudo-Problems in Philosophy. London: Routledge & Kegan Paul, 1967.
3. Caruth, E. & Ekstein, R. (1966). Interpretation within the Metaphor: Further Considerations. J. Amer. Acad. Child Psychiat., 5:35-45.
4. Chadwick, M. (1928). Die Unterscheidung zwischen Ton und Sprache in der frühen Kindheit. Z. psa. Päd., 2:369-383.
5. Edelheit, H. (1969). Speech and Psychic Structure: the Vocal-Auditory Organization of the Ego. J. Amer. Psa. Assn., 17:381-412.
6. Ekstein, R. (1965). Historical Notes Concerning Psychoanalysis and Early Language Development. J. Amer. Psa. Assn., 13:707-731.
7. —— (1966). Children of Time and Space, of Action and Impulse. New York: Appleton-Century-Crofts.
8. —— & Wallerstein, J. (1966). Choice of Interpretation in the Treatment of Borderline and Psychotic Children. In: Ekstein (1966), pp. 148-157.
9. Freud, A. (1965). Normality and Pathology in Childhood: Assessments of Development. New York: International Universities Press.
10. Freud, S. (1895). Project for a Scientific Psychology. In: The Origins of Psychoanalysis. New York: Basic Books, 1954, pp. 347-445.
11. Hook, S., ed. (1959). Psychoanalysis: Scientific Method and Philosophy. New York: New York University Press.
12. Kubie, L. S. (1953). The Distortion of the Symbolic Process in Neurosis and Psychosis. J. Amer. Psa. Ann., 1:59-86.
13. Mahler, M. S. (1968). On Human Symbiosis and the Vicissitudes of Individuation. New York: International Universities Press.
14. Waismann, F. (1965). The Principles of Linguistic Philosophy. London, Melbourne, Toronto: Macmillan. New York: St. Martin's Press.
15. Wexler, M. (1960). Hypotheses Concerning Ego Deficiency in Schizophrenia. In: The Outpatient Treatment of Schizophrenia, ed. S. Scher & H. Davis. New York: Grune & Stratton, pp. 33-43.

CHAPTER TWENTY-FOUR

To Sleep but Not to Dream: On the Use of Electric Tape Recording in Clinical Research*

> Let us learn to dream, gentlemen, then perhaps we shall
> find the truth . . . but let us beware of publishing our
> dreams before they have been put to the proof by the
> waking understanding.
>
> KEKULÉ

It is methodologically naive to attempt to demonstrate the usefulness of electrical recordings in psychotherapy research by comparing data obtained with and without such recordings. The data of psychotherapy consist of the kind of phenomena in which the interaction between the data and the recorder (human or mechanical) must be taken into account in the description of the phenomena, somewhat analogous to quantum physics where "an account of the functioning of the measuring instruments is indispensable to the definition of the phenomena . . ."(1)

Data obtained from interviews with different instruments of observation can furnish complementary rather than comparable information.

---

* Elaine Caruth is co-author of this chapter.

328

Both patient and therapist have a different phenomenological field under the different conditions of the presence or absence of recording instruments. For example, the therapist might feel greater freedom to let go of higher critical ego functions and merely experience the process with the patient, in the knowledge that the electrical recording can function as a kind of critical and observing alter ego, albeit a delayed one. This might be particularly true with research where the accurate recording of data for later analysis is of importance. Energy and affect might also be released from memory and critical functions and be totally devoted to the empathic and interpretive functions of the moment. Subsequently, the therapist may use the recording to fill in the manifest content for an understanding of the underlying meanings, of both his own and the patient's communications. On the other hand, the presence of the electrical recording might be conceived of as an inhibiting constricting factor, an externalized auxiliary superego, as it were, spying upon and ultimately exposing the therapeutic interaction. The recording device thus becomes a part countertransference object. For the patient, who has initially been informed of the use of the recording equipment, its presence may well be perceived in a fashion primarily dependent upon the current transference configuration as well as upon the actual physical arrangement of the recording instrument.

It is obvious, therefore, that the value of electrical recording cannot be fully assessed by comparing a situation in which recordings are used with one in which it is not, without investigating the question as to how the manner of recording changes the data. However, it is possible to demonstrate the usefulness of this technique within the situation in which it is used. That is, given different kinds of data obtained within one design which includes both electrical recordings and dictated notes beyond the verbatim account of events, it is possible to analyze the data furnished by these two methods employed simultaneously. We can then compare the kind and amount of information derived from the two recording techniques.

We would like to present a dramatic instance in the treatment of a schizophrenic boy. The information obtained from the recording was strikingly different from the therapist's subsequent recollections and furnished a unique insight into the process during one hour. The particular transference and countertransference problems evoked in this boy's treatment have been described elsewhere (Ch. 8, this vol.). The transference needs of this boy to maintain the therapist as an inanimate-like echo of his own introjects created in the therapist the experience of intense drowsiness. At such times, the therapist's behavior resembled the echo-like behavior and verbalizations of the autistic child whose only means of maintaining contact is through the mimetic devices of echopraxia and echolalia. The sleepiness was seen as a countertransference reaction in which the individuality of the therapist as a separate object was momentarily lost in the service of the adaptive function of maintaining contact, albeit of this primitive nature and on a regressed level.

Sometime later in the treatment of this same boy, the experience of drowsiness culminated in a momentary sleep episode in which the therapist experienced certain dream-like activity. However when his recollections were compared with the transcribed tape recordings, a completely different aspect of the therapeutic process was revealed. This instance of falling asleep had been initially understood as that final autistic position which the echoing had been an attempt to ward off. It had thus been seen initially as a kind of quasi-psychotic countertransference reaction in which the therapist momentarily became the kind of reassurance-echoing symbiotic object that the patient had been seeking. Subsequent insights derived (described below) from the tape recordings revealed the sleep episode as an adaptive maneuver by which the therapist freed himself from the echoing role to become once more a separate interpretive object. His regression was thus in the service of the professional interpretive self, saving its individuality and separate identity in a temporary island of sleep.

In this hour the boy began to ruminate obsessively about his masturbatory experiences and to describe in detail his orgasms (accompanied by explosive, violent fantasy interaction with the delusional object) experienced after periods of temporary, self-imposed abstinence. At this time in the treatment, he was almost totally preoccupied with his attempts to control his masturbation, to master his psychosis. His initial efforts to do so were made because of his conviction that this was the therapist's goal and arose, therefore, from his wish to please the therapist. Inevitably he first misperceived the goal of control as one of suppression, just as he desired to wipe out and suppress the psychosis; the therapist, on the other hand, sought to help integrate the psychotic elements into a stronger ego organization (2).

As he listened to the boy's ruminations about his masturbation, they seemed at first a kind of "magnificent confession" to the therapist. However, when understood as an association to earlier material in which he had revealed his feelings of conflict about his mother's impending marriage, the defensive aspect of these preoccupations became clearer as a kind of "magnificent obsession" with the underlying conflicts over the imminent marriage. The train of associations led from his descriptions of his attempts to abstain from masturbation to a more impulse-ridden description of masochistic beating fantasies. This boy, torn between both positive and inverted oedipal conflicts, thus communicated both the rage against and the masochistic homosexual love for the future step-father. The step-father was perceived as an aggressive dangerous intruder who had done away with the boy's real father in order to marry his mother. The therapist brought to the hour an awareness of these underlying conflicts from the boy's earlier communications.

As the boy continued with his sexual ruminations, the therapist momentarily seemed to fall asleep. In his recollections of the incident he can recall only that he remarked seemingly out of context of the description of the masturbatory activity, "What about those two men who couldn't rescue you more and the wife and murderer in one party." The therapist remembers this response as out of context and meaningless; he recalls it as a dream-like fragment. The dream-like quality is indisputable and, like all dreams, had its day residue. During the hour the therapist had had occasion to reflect about his attendance at a production of *Hamlet* the night before at which the boy's mother and fiancé had also been present.

In listening to the taped recording of the incident, however, it is almost impossible to discern the sleepiness and momentary dreaming of the therapist. From this point of observation, the therapist's response seems merely a dramatic shift in level of interpretation but one still in close contact with the underlying conflict being stressed by the patient. The boy's obsessive preoccupations are defenses in a conflict very similar to that of Hamlet. The two men, respectively the therapist and the future step-father, have, in fact, not been able to rescue the boy but, instead, the future step-father has become symbolically the father-murderer about to steal the wife. The therapist experiences himself as a kind of Polonius at this moment, a helpless witness to the internal drama.

It appears now that the echoing and dream-like behavior, more experienced than observed, was, as it were, a piece of inner reality, more than outer reality. It has some similarity to certain hypnotic phenomena in which regressive ego states in the service of adaptation are also observed. This experience may be directly compared to the hypnagogic and hypnopompic experiences explored by Silberer (3). The sleepiness in this instance was primarily an adaptive response that enabled the therapist to free himself from the echoing role and speak spontaneously from his unconscious recognition of the boy's material. It was as if he could only *not* echo when he could free himself from the conscious countertransference through the seeming falling asleep. There was also, of course, a defensive aspect to the falling asleep. This may be understood as a paradoxical defensive reaction to the boy's love play. The patient's sexual preoccupations, in which he described in detail his masturbatory activity, served also as a kind of expression of his transference desires but elicited in the therapist the defensive reaction of falling asleep and thus escaping from the seduction.

The analysis of this material fully highlights the complementary information obtained from the electrical taping and the therapeutic minutes. Neither alone tells the full story; to listen to the tape we would not be aware of the subjective experience of falling asleep, only of a shift in the level of interpretation. Nor is this shift too drastic, as it is disguised in the semantics of the secondary process, even though the content of the interpretation is derived from the primary process. The tape reveals the adaptive strength of the therapist, the awareness of which he repressed. The therapist's subjective experience as revealed in his therapeutic notes alone would deprive us of this understanding of the adaptive value of the experience where for him there was truth, if not "in vino" at least in sleep. The question arises, of course, as to why the therapist is allowed only to dream the truth rather than experience it. We might speculate upon this as an instance of adaptation to the necessary identification with the psychotic patient's ego organization and mode of functioning. It is often said that the psychotic represses reality, and in this instance we see the therapist attempting to repress his interpretive interventions. He represses the content but not the act of interpretation; a compromise between the wish to be like the patient and the wish to help him. Empathic interpretation has regressed to interpretable empathy in the service of protective distance.

In a previous publication (Ch. 8, this vol.) we suggested that work with these patients requires persistent scrutiny of the data; their evaluation and re-evaluation, their assessment and re-assessment, until finally they seem to tell the story by themselves. In our first look, we described the defensive and regressive aspects of the countertransference in which the therapist experienced the inanimate echo-like features of the role imposed upon him by certain features of this patient's psychotic transference.

In our present assessment of more recent data, we have been impressed with the adaptive function of the sleep-like states experienced by the therapist. As part of the re-evaluation of this patient, subsequent to the publication of the first communication, Card 12 of the Thematic Appreciation Test* was administered. The response to this card is frequently used to develop an understanding of the transference paradigm. This boy told the following story:

Hypnotist hypnotizes a subject. Subject is sleeping. Sure enough, subject does everything he says. Subject is asleep. Hypnotist says,

---

* Administered by Dr. Mortimer M. Meyer.

"Repeat after me everything I say." Subject has to do it. Hypnotist walks away and leaves subject there and hypnotist gets ready for next thing. This is not a stage. He looks in mirror and practices and puts himself into sleep. Subject wakes up and says, "Ready for the show," and hypnotist says, "I am asleep, asleep, asleep." The Hypnotized Hypnotist.

This fantasy communication reads like a prescription that the patient might have written for his own treatment, a prediction of what he will do to the therapist, while our communication describes the show that the "hypnotized hypnotist" puts on as he feels, "I'm asleep, asleep, asleep."

REFERENCES

1. BOHR, NIELS. *Atomic Physics and Human Knowledge*. New York: John Wiley & Sons, 1958, 91.
2. EKSTEIN, RUDOLF & CARUTH, ELAINE. "The Working Alliance with the Monster." In *Children of Time and Space, of Action and Impulse*. New York: Appleton-Century-Crofts, 1966.
3. SILBERER, HERBERT. "Symbolik des Erwachens und Schwellensymbolik ueberhaupt." *Jahrbuch für psychoanalytische Forschungen*, vol. 3, 1911.

CHAPTER TWENTY-FIVE

The Onion and the Moebius Strip:* Rational and Irrational Models for the Secondary and Primary Process**

It has been said that "man is the measure of all things" (4). We might add that he is both the producer as well as the product of his environment. As a matter of fact, the difficulty of distinguishing between man and his environment has occupied many current writers in psychology as well as in modern physics, where, for example, Niels Bohr has written, "The present day situation in physics brings forcefully home to us the old adage that we are actors as well as spectators of the grandest drama of existence" (2). Our tools of observation are inextricably linked to our capacity for comprehension, and an explanation, like a model, describes one phenomenon in terms of another more familiar phenomenon. However, "if . . . there does not exist in the environment of the individual, or among *the items of his mental equipment* [italics added], some familiar pattern which would correspond to the new situation, then no amount of explaining will explain. . . .

---

* A one-sided surface made by taking a long rectangle of paper, giving it a half twist and joining the ends. Any two points on the Moebius strip may be connected by starting at one point and tracing it back to the other without lifting the pencil or carrying it over a boundary. (The Moebius strip draws its name from the German theoretical astronomer and mathematician August Ferdinand Möbius [1790-1868].—Ed.)

** Elaine Caruth is the author of this chapter.

Thus, what may strike us today as a perplexing innovation may be regarded as an excellent model by the next generation" (2).

Our generation can truly be said to be struggling with many "perplexing innovations." Twentieth-century science has introduced a non-Newtonian world which is no longer predicated upon a simple deterministic model of causality, is no longer measured according to the axioms of three-dimensional Euclidian geometry, and can no longer be inferred and predicted by the logical methods of John Stuart Mill. Today's world is a world of probability rather than determinism, and of the science of geometrodynamics, the geometry of space-time which is investigating "the extent to which all physical phenomena can be interpreted as aspects of geometry of a curved empty space-time" (2). (The model of this world is a four-dimensional one developed on the basis of Einstein's special theory of relativity and differing from the familiar Euclidian geometry.)

Twentieth-century medicine has succeeded in returning the "dead" to life, has kept "internal" organs functioning while being maintained externally, and has made yesterday's fantasy world of Jules Verne and Buck Rogers the everyday world of today's reality. The "pure" scientific and mathematical discoveries of the nineteenth century and earlier have become the applied scientific advances of the twentieth.

Parallel developments have occurred in the field of psychology. Nineteenth-century man, a descendant of the age of reason and enlightenment, was considered a rational, logical creature until Freud's advent at the end of the century. The ubiquity of the irrational unconscious forces of the instincts and the forces of repression utilized by consciousness, were recognized and became then the focus of psychological investigation. However, early psychoanalytic formulations, primarily in the area of what Freud has designated as psychoeconomics, were based upon a model, the thermodynamic model, of a closed physical system derived from deterministic Newtonian principles; original formulations within the context of the topographic model of the personality emphasized the dichotomy between the unconscious instinctual forces dominated by the pleasure principle and repressive forces utilized by the conscious personality and ruled according to the reality principle.

More recent advances in psychoanalysis developed out of Freud's formulation of the tripartite model (13), which has facilitated the development of modern-day ego psychology. The growth of personality is seen now in terms of the development of increasingly higher levels of psychic organization and differentiation of function, superimposed upon one another so that different levels of functioning are always potentially available to the individual. Thus, the dream world of the normal and the waking life of the psychotic have become linked; both are seen as manifestation of the primary-process functioning of a more primitive psychic organization, a kind of functioning dominated by the pleasure principle and relatively uninfluenced by reality considerations. Earlier models now begin to appear either insufficient or inefficient to accommodate the complexities of these more recent developments and investigations of heretofore less thoroughly explored areas of psychic structure and functioning. It begins to appear that there may be required different kinds of models for different kinds of mental phenomena, not necessarily to replace but to supplement earlier models.

There have been many parallel developments in scientific understanding of the psychological and physical world of man. Advances in both areas have been predicated upon the ability to give up a pseudo-scientific allegiance to the data of common sense and direct experience in order to apprehend and subsequently comprehend what has, in the past, been regarded as unknowable—the depths of man and the expanse of the universe, as well as the intricacies of the subatomic world. For example, it has been pointed out (22) that one of the stumbling blocks to the understanding of elementary particles is that some of the things to be learned run counter to common sense, just as the understanding of unconscious material is more difficult because unconscious processes are, to quote Fenichel, "directed according to the primary process—unburdened by the demands of reality, time, or logical consideration" (12). It would appear that the seemingly irrational world of modern physics has met its parallel in the seemingly irrational aspects of the intrapsychic world of man.

The worlds of contemporary physics and inner man are remarkably alike. In the world of infinity, a part may be equal to the whole (14); while in the "unconscious," the "object and a part of the object are equated" (12). When the individual is functioning on the level of the primary process, either in dreams and nightmares or in psychotic states, time does not flow in orderly fashion, nor do objects maintain their constancy of size. And what about the world of modern physics? As for time:

> There was a young lady named Bright
> Who could travel much faster than light.
> She departed one day,
> In a relative way,
> And came back on the previous night.

And as for objects:

> There was a young fencer named Fisk
> Whose lunge was exceedingly brisk.

> So fast was his action,
> The Fitzgerald contraction*
> Reduced his épée to a disc.

—a truly vivid description of an oedipal nightmare with an admixture of masturbation guilt and castration anxiety!

As a matter of fact, it would be difficult to more graphically portray a nightmarish schizophrenic episode than has been depicted in a short story called *And He Built a Crooked House* (16). Based upon the fantasy of what would happen if a house designed as a tesseract—a fourth-dimensional cube projected onto our third-dimensional world—were to be constructed. To excerpt briefly:

> . . . they climbed a fourth flight of stairs but . . . found themselves not on the roof but standing in the ground floor room where they had entered the house . . . he threw open the front door and plunged out (and) found (himself) up here in the lounge . . . (he went downstairs and found himself up on the roof) . . . somehow (the ground floor room) managed to be in two different places at once. . . . They saw him wave his arms semaphore fashion. The (man and woman) joined him and followed his stare with their own. Four rooms away, they saw the backs of three figures, two male and one female. The taller, thinner of the men was waving his arms in a silly fashion. (The woman) screamed and fainted again.

One is reminded of Renée's terrifying description of her episodes of unreality in *The Autobiography of a Schizophrenic Girl* (19) and of a more recent literary description of a psychotic episode (in Green's *I Never Promised You a Rose Garden*) in which the author writes:

> A black wind came up. The walls dissolved and the world became a combination of shadows. Seeking for a shadow of firm ground on which to stand, she was only deceived again when it warped away like a heat mirage; she looked towards a landfall and the wind blew it away. All direction became a lie. The *laws of physics* and *solid matter were repealed* and the experience of a lifetime of tactile sensations, motion, form, *gravity* and light was invalidated. (She did not know whether she was standing or sitting down, which way was upright, and from where the light, which was a stab as it touched her, was coming. She lost track of the parts of her body; where her arms were and how to move them.) . . . His coming was absurd, frightening, interesting, funny, *non-Newto-*

---

* The effect of relativistic contraction of all fast-moving objects due to the contraction of space itself.

nian; he was flying. He was prone on the air, his expression utterly blank, as if he felt obliged to live out his life as a trajectory" (15). [Italics added]

This feeling of weightlessness, a characteristic quality of this fiction-alized patient's psychotic episodes, brings to mind our recent astronaut's space walk (although with different accompanying affect), and has also been described by a seven-year-old borderline schizophrenic patient who experienced similar feelings of weightlessness, wondered why his arm would rise up when he dropped something from his hand, and found in the movie *Mary Poppins* the externalized representation of all his own inner fantasies of drifting away and disappearing.

Even the timeworn mind-body dilemma, the self-created, perhaps "delusional" monster of philosophical psychology alluded to by Freud in 1888 when he wrote, "We possess no criterion which enables us to distinguish exactly between a mental process and a physiological one" (13), has its parallel in physics. Thus Tobias Dantzig (4), a mathema-tician, has pointed out, "A principle of relativity is just a code of limitations"; and frankly admits that, "there is no way of ascertaining whether a certain body of facts is the *manifestation* of the *observata* or the hallucination of the *observer.*"* And yet this is the very expe-rience so commonly associated with the treatment of schizophrenia, the same topsy-turvy, Alice-In-Wonderland quality so insightfully described by the mathematician Lewis Carroll, that leaves one truly wondering "who dreamed the dream" (9), reflecting thus a kind of inverse inde-terminacy principle in which the observer, namely the therapist, is himself influenced by the data—i.e., the patient—he is observing, respectively treating.

Carroll's psychological insights were not confined to "Alice in Wonderland." In a lesser-known short story, "The Purse of Fortunatus" (3), he has utilized that curiosity of topology—the Moebius strip—to construct a fantasy about a wondrous purse of which it can be said that:

> . . . whatever is inside that purse is outside it; and whatever is out-side it is inside it. So you have all the wealth of the world in that little purse!

—a fantasy not too dissimilar to the alloplastic omnipotent fantasies of our schizophrenic patients who fluctuate between encompassing—devouring—the world and being encompassed—devoured—by it.

---

* We might truly ponder here that, "The more and more we know of less and less, the nearer we come to an ultimate maximum" (17).

The example of the Moebius strip, this one-sided surface on which the outer surface is continuous with the inner surface, so that there is no way of differentiating between inside and outside, furnishes an excellent metaphor to describe the psychic organization of the schizophrenic or the dreamer, that is, of one whose functioning is on the level of the primary process. For with the schizophrenic, there is also no clear-cut demarcation between inside and outside, between the I and the non-I, between conscious and unconscious, between sleep and waking states or between inner and outer reality. Thus Reich's use of the onion as a metaphor to describe the systematic layering of defense and impulse in the personality organization of the neurotic is clearly inapplicable to the psychotic patient. The essential problem in schizophrenia has been described in terms of the inability to move beyond the undifferentiated stage of symbiotic fusion with the mother and the consequent lack of capacity to differentiate that which is self and inside from that which is nonself and outside. In such instances the only defense available against the symbiosis is the autistic position which ultimately restores in fantasy the undifferentiated oneness with the world, or, in terms of the proposed model, as one travels along the inner surface, one suddenly finds one's self on the outer surface; one does not know who dreamed the dream, one cannot maintain the difference between subject and object. The use of the Moebius strip as a model of the psychic structure of the psychotic patient throws light not only on the intrapsychic structure of the personality, but also on certain so-called interpersonal aspects of schizophrenic functioning. Such a model suggests that the interpersonal and the intrapsychic cannot be differentiated, as is demonstrated all too well in schizophrenic attempts at suicide and/or homicide, wherein self and object are fused, and the murderous rage at the bad object can be directed outwardly or inwardly indiscriminately.

Let us examine now the heuristic value of the conceptualization of the Moebius strip not merely as an analogy, but hopefully as a model for the structure of the primary-process psychic organization and see if it may not help clarify a specific clinical issue.

Distance and distance devices have been described by Ekstein (7, 11) and Wexler (20) as significant in the treatment of the borderline and schizophrenic child and adult. The concept of distance was first developed around the parameter of the relationship between patient and therapist. Subsequently, it was elaborated in more differentiated fashion and was referred to a number of dimensions along which distance could be measured and along which it could vary independently, such as distance from secondary-process thinking, etc. Distance devices, such as metaphoric communication, borrowed fantasies, etc., were thought of as a kind of psychological ballast that helped maintain the necessary interpersonal homeostasis in order to permit the therapeutic process to proceed and allow the patient to relinquish the previously established pathological intrapsychic homeostasis or psychotic adjustment. Distance was assumed to be an arithmetic, potentially measurable construct which in the earlier stages of investigation could be described in quantitative terms of more or less, even if not yet actually capable of being translated into numerical indices, which was the ultimate goal (6).

If we think, however, in terms of the proposed model from the field of topology—a nonmetric rubber-sheet geometry concerned only with nonquantifiable questions such as, "where, between what, inside or outside"—the term distance would then have to be reconsidered and redefined, perhaps as separation—that is, as the existence of a two-sided relationship with a clear-cut demarcation, separating both sides, be they patient and therapist, or inside and outside, etc. Distance devices might best be renamed separation devices, that is, artificial means of maintaining such a separation in these patients, who must constantly struggle against the one-sided, undifferentiated, fused inside-outside relationship.

Furthermore, this model suggests that in the field of personality traits and measurements, we cannot resort to the usual methods of rating and measurement. We know all too well the unreliability of intelligence testing with schizophrenics, recently described as a function of fluctuating cathexis of inner and outer reality (Ch. 2, this vol.). Perhaps this very fluctuating cathexis may be described as the inevitable result of the progression along the Moebius strip, so that one may start with questions about outer reality and end with answers about inner reality. However, if we do deal with measurable dimensions, it may be that we can find better models in non-Euclidian geometries just as the great advances in mathematics and subsequently physics were made by giving up the so-called "self-evident" parallel postulate. In Riemannian space, parallel lines do meet, just as our psychotic patients eventually may fuse in any personal relationship. And just as such patients may attempt to fuse with the object through the mechanism of introjection, which "is an attempt to make part of the external world flow into the ego" (12), we find that in the world of mathematics

> . . . an exercise in imaginative geometry that will help . . . understand such unusual things as curved space and space closed in itself . . . (is to) try to transform your body mentally into a double apple with a channel within . . . the entire universe, including the earth, moon, sun and stars, will be squeezed into an inner circular channel" (14).

We can turn again to the literature of mathematical fantasies for a description of the countertransference problems in the treatment of schizophrenia, where our patients openly wonder why they will not turn into us or we into them. For example, the above-mentioned seven-year-old borderline schizophrenic boy, after a violently aggressive, destructive hour, spent the subsequent visit scrubbing at the walls, almost a literal clinical representation of Lady Macbeth muttering, "Out, damned spot." As he scrubbed away in panic and terror at all of the office furniture and walls, he indicated his concern that his bad thoughts had made the office dirty, had made the therapist dirty and like him had, in fact, made her into him. When this was interpreted to him, he could only wonder why it was that the doctor would not turn into him nor he into her. It takes a long time for the therapist of the schizophrenic to be allowed into his patient's world, and once inside he must struggle equally long to be let out and to take his patient with him, and for a period he may truly ponder whether he be Jonah or the whale, since both roles are equally assigned to him by his patient. This particular little boy played out and acted out such fantasies as well as other variations of this theme, such as alternating between being the helpless teeny mouth and the devouring monster with huge teeth.

In "A Subway Named Moebius" (5) we read about a subway system which was suddenly turned into a Moebius strip by the addition of a shuttle which thus caused a car to travel for many years, suddenly disappear, travel for many more to only reappear with its passengers unchanged. And what therapist of a schizophrenic has not at times pondered whether or not his patient will emerge unchanged from the many years of treatment? As long as the therapist has only the choice of Jonah or the whale, he deals with the unique transference and countertransference problem that there is really little difference between the two positions since neither allows him to be a separate human object, that is, neither permits a two-surfaced relationship between him and the patient. Thus, this seven-year-old schizophrenic child, who has verbalized his fear openly that his therapist is like a whale who may swallow him, not only voices and plays out this feared wish (and wished-for fear) of becoming the therapist, but also at times shows no awareness of where he begins and she ends so that he starts to bandage his finger but unconcernedly switches to hers in the middle of the action. We had a sore finger. Symbiosis revisited. Togetherness—schizophrenic style. Our castration anxiety assuaged but in no way resolved.

In summary, the widening understanding of the irrational aspects of mental life, of man's inner space, has many parallels in the widening understanding of man's outer space and the subatomic world of modern physics. Twentieth-century physics has opened the door to a non-Newtonian world, twentieth-century psychology has opened the lid on a nonrational psychic world. In both instances it is profitable that self-evident assumptions and common-sense formulations and judgments be abandoned. Many of the resulting insights and discoveries in both fields have sufficient similarity as to suggest that in the field of psychoanalytic psychology it also is time to begin to think of exchanging old models for new, and of replacing antiquated analogies for modern-day metaphors. If we need to turn to mathematics and physics to formulate our models, we may need a Newtonian model to describe the everyday rational world of sense experience, and a quantum one to derive our formulations concerning the nontangible irrational world of man's innermost life. Such criticisms then of psychoanalysis, as the oft-repeated one that it is meaningless and unverifiable to have phenomena mean the same and the opposite simultaneously, can be referred to the analogous physical paradox of the wave-particle theory of matter.

The relationship between the use of numbers and man's physical anatomy has long been acknowledged. It may be that parallels can also be drawn between man's psychic anatomy and his utilization of "modern mathematics," and that ultimately man may be truly considered the measure of all things, an observation implicit perhaps in Einstein's own words when he wrote, "How can it be that mathematics, being after all a product of human thought, is so admirably adapted to the objects of reality?"

REFERENCES

1. Arlow, Jacob A., & Charles Brenner. *Psychoanalytic Concepts and the Structural Theory*. New York: International Universities Press, 1964.
2. Bohr, Niels. In Tobias Dantzig, *Aspects of Science*. New York: Macmillan, 1937. p. 135.
3. Carroll, Lewis. The Purse of Fortunatus. In Clifton Fadiman (Ed.), *Fantasia Mathematica*. New York: Simon and Schuster, 1958.
4. Dantzig, Tobias. *Number, the Language of Science*. New York: Macmillan, 1954. p. 17.
5. Deutsch, A. J. A Subway Named Moebius. In Clifton Fadiman (Ed.), *Fantasia Mathematica*. New York: Simon and Schuster, 1958.
6. Ekstein, Rudolf & Meyer, Mortimer M. Distancing Devices in Childhood Schizophrenia and Allied Conditions: A Project Concerning Quantitative and Qualitative Aspects of "Distancing in the Psychotherapeutic Process." *Psychological Reports*, Vol. 9, 1961. pp. 145-146.
7. —— & Wallerstein, Judith. Observations on the Psychology of Borderline and Psychotic Children. *Psychoanalytic Study of the Child*, Vol. 9, 1954, pp. 344-369.
8. ——. The Opening Gambit in Psychotherapeutic Work with Severely Disturbed Adolescents. *American Journal of Orthopsychiatry*. Vol. 33, 1963. pp. 862-871.

9. —— & CARUTH, ELAINE. Psychotic Acting Out—Royal Road or Primrose Path? In Rudolf Ekstein, *Children of Time and Space, of Action and Impulse: Clinical Studies on the Psychoanalytic Treatment of Severely Disturbed Children and Adolescents.* New York: Appleton-Century-Crofts, 1966.

10. ——. Puppet Play of a Psychotic Adolescent Girl within the Psychotherapeutic Process. *Psychoanalytic Study of the Child,* Vol. 20, 1965. pp. 441-480.

11. —— & WRIGHT, DOROTHY. The Space Child—Ten Years Later. *Forest Hospital Publications.* Des Plaines, Illinois, Vol. 2, 1964. pp. 36-47.

12. FENICHEL, OTTO. *The Psychoanalytic Theory of Neurosis.* New York: W. W. Norton, 1945.

13. FREUD, SIGMUND, as quoted by: Stanley Edgar Hyman. *The Tangled Bank.* New York: Atheneum, 1962.

14. GAMOW, GEORGE. *One, Two, Three—Infinity.* New York: Viking Press, 1961.

15. GREEN, HANNAH. *I Never Promised You a Rose Garden.* New York: New American Library, 1965. pp. 90, 114.

16. HENLEIN, ROBERT A. *And He Built a Crooked House.* New York: Street and Smith, 1940.

17. MEYER, JEROME S. *Fun With Mathematics.* New York: World Publishing Company, 1952.

18. REICH, WILHELM. *Character Analysis.* New York: Noonday Press, 1961.

19. SECHEHAYE, MARGUERITE. *Reality Lost and Regained: The Autobiography of a Schizophrenic Girl.* New York: Grune and Stratton, 1951.

20. WEXLER, MILTON. Psychological Distance as a Factor in the Treatment of a Schizophrenic Patient. In Robert Lindner (Ed.), *Explorations in Psychoanalysis.* New York: Julian Press, 1953.

21. WHEELER, JOHN A. *Geometrodynamics: The Geometry of Space-Time.* New York: Academic Press, 1964.

22. WILKINSON, D. H. Towards New Concepts in Elementary Particles. *Turning Points in Physics.* New York: Harper, 1961.

CHAPTER TWENTY-SIX

The Relation of Ego Autonomy to Activity and Passivity in the Psychotherapy of Childhood Schizophrenia*

Act from thought should quickly follow. What is thinking for?

W. H. AUDEN

A useful approach to the understanding of the issues of activity and passivity in psychoanalytic theory and technique is to distinguish between ego activity and passivity, and motoric activity and passivity. The active ego, specifically the autonomous ego, can mediate between demands of id, superego and reality, and retain freedom of choice in the resultant behavior. However, the ego can be overwhelmed and considered liable to passivity to all three.**

Motoric activity can reflect ego autonomy, as in goal-directed behavior, or it may reflect ego passivity, as in automatic behavior like echopraxia and echolalia. Similarly, motoric passivity (or inactivity) may reflect ego autonomy, as in the very potent yet motorically pas-

---

* Elaine Caruth is the co-author of this chapter.

** This viewpoint represents a synthesis of the views of Rapaport (18, 19) and Hart (13, 14).

sive "acts" of civil disobedience, like those of Martin Luther King or Gandhi, or it may reflect the presence of ego passivity. A good example is the paralyzed obsessive who vacillates and cannot act—Buridan's ass who starved between the equidistant bale of hay and pail of water.

The healthy autonomous ego is capable of a greater or lesser degree of motoric activity in relationship to objects, to reality orientation and to instinctual expression. It is capable of establishing an optimal balance between active and passive modes of behavior and the inner degree of ego autonomy. The normal child's behavior tends to show relative consistency between the inner and outer state. When psychologically helpless and inundated by either inner or outer stimuli, he tends to be motorically inactive; when psychologically active, he tends to be more physically active or else engaged in behavior oriented towards future activities, such as school work or study.

When we deal with the schizophrenic child, however, we are faced with the lack of an autonomous ego and we come closer to Orwell's world of 1984. Black is white, up is down, active is passive. This world is characterized by the rules and logic of primary-process thinking which follows a different "grammar." Inside and outside are not clearly differentiated; self and object may fuse but seldom integrate (17); non-Euclidian geometry and non-Newtonian physics can reign (Chapt. 25, this vol.) in defiance of secondary-process laws of space and time.

Unsuccessful in mastering the individuation-separation task, the schizophrenic child is still struggling with early problems: restoring the positive symbiosis in the absence of the object and maintaining separation in the presence of the object. These patients frequently fear the act as destroying the object and self representations which are still so closely fused that they can maintain their separation only through artificial "distance devices" (Chapts. 5, 8, 25, this vol.). Paradoxically, as we will see in the following case, they often maintain their closeness through what appears to be separation.

Carol is a deeply troubled borderline adolescent girl embroiled in a masochistic, suicidal, depressive reaction. Carol barricades herself in her room, writing suicide notes to her family and isolating herself from all contact, except the minimum necessary to continue high-school studies. She comes voluntarily to the therapist fully aware of her need for help and of some of the irrational elements in her pervasive feelings of inadequacy, worthlessness and rejection. Yet she gives the initial impression of coming involuntarily, against her will, even under force, although, in fact, her parents are so frightened of this child that they literally cannot exert any control except by cajoling and pleading. Also, she overtly gives the impression of sullenness, bitterness and resentment, and quickly demands to know how she can be helped if she does not talk. She has had several earlier "encounters" with therapy, the last terminating disastrously. The therapist had responded in anger to her expression of anger, after having previously berated her for not trying because she did not talk enough. Thus, she now presents herself with all of her inner helplessness exposed. Without choice and passively, she submits to the counter-cathectic forces which forbid any impulse expression; her worst fears have previously been confirmed that giving vent to her aggressive impulses leads to the loss or destruction of the object. She experiences the defense against the destructive impulses as ego dystonic, and she becomes, in a sense, a slave to her own projected superego. As the transference develops, however, there is an additional weakening of the defenses, and she begins to experience the counter-impulse of giving in to the destructive forces, equated with talking. At this point, she flees treatment.

Some time later, the mother, strengthened through her own treatment, has been able to reassert control to the extent that Carol no longer locks herself up. The mother can also insist that Carol return to therapy. The girl is now literally forced to come to treatment. One is immediately impressed by the fact that externally there is little difference between her present behavior and her earlier behavior when she had come under her own power. Now her silence is no longer ego alien, but rather can be experienced as a syntonic act. She no longer feels she cannot talk; rather, she can experience it as if she will not talk, that she has freedom of choice. She has relinquished the external activity of seemingly coming voluntarily, which had led to her experiencing the helpless passivity of being unable to talk, or else unable to control the destructive outburst. She has now reached the seemingly passive state of being forced to come, wherein she can feel that she will not talk and consequently not endanger the object. She now experiences as a voluntary act what she had previously experienced as a passive, choiceless symptom.

We are reminded of another borderline schizophrenic child, somewhat younger, who tells us endlessly through his play that without ego autonomy, there can only be the subjective experience of helpless oscillation between being passively driven to destroy the world, or else being passively destroyed by it. His play reflects the shifting dominant phase of the conflict between the wish to inflict and the wish to suffer aggression. He veers between being a "teeny mouth" swallowed by the whale puppet in the office or being, like Hansel, readied for cooking and eating by the therapist, and being the monster with big muscles and big teeth with which to eat the therapist. This seven-year-old boy's constantly fluctuating levels of ego states confuse parents and doctors who seek to see in him only the healthy aspects. For them, the healthy aspects mean "active." This is a desperate attempt to deny his more withdrawn periods during which, in fact, he is able to exert some modicum of control over the impulse-driven behavior, even though forced into a kind of autistic fantasy world.

Let us turn now to another adolescent schizophrenic about whom we have written (3) (Chaps. 4, 6, 7, 13, this vol.). Her first attempts to move from a kind of autistic psychotic position into a world of secondary-process functioning, of reality and actuality, were communicated through a series of psychotic acting-out episodes, following which she developed some capacity to move from a primary-process level of functioning to a beginning capacity actually to fulfill tasks and promises on a minimal level. She has achieved now a kind of pseudo-normal facade of seeming adjustment. She is able to handle everyday details of budget, transportation, minimal encounters with peripheral kinds of social experiences, etc. She seeks to maintain this relatively stable balance by persistent and endless variations of counter-cathectic maneuvers. While rendering her seemingly paralyzed and immobilized in outer reality, these actually serve to master and bind the impulse-ridden, primary-process core. She misses appointments, comes late, spends her days in endless preparations that lead nowhere. In the treatment hours, she slowly begins to recover and reconstruct memories that were previously reconstructed through the psychotic acting out (6) (Ch. 14, this vol.). But she must restore these memories and at the same time defend against the regression to helpless impulsing of earlier days. Thus, she begins to experience a pervasive feeling of paralysis, of inactivity and inability to accomplish in external reality, which culminates finally in a conviction of being a ghost, both dead and alive (Chapt. 13, this vol.).

As she is safely immured in this kind of frozen position, she begins to communicate to us what it is that is defended against. She approaches this through her characteristic distance device, the use of borrowed TV and movie fantasies. In the 578th hour (Ch. 14, this vol.), she relates the story of a street cleaner, rummaging in the sand for trash, who comes upon a part of a statue of a Roman soldier that was destroyed in the earthquake that wiped out Pompeii. As the statue is removed to a museum, it becomes alive and menacing. Thus, she tells us of her attempts to immobilize her own destructive power, which, like the earthquake, are so violent they can destroy the world. And she tells us also of her fears that she cannot maintain this control. She begins slowly then to recall an actual earthquake, which is followed by her memory of a subsequent nightmare about this earthquake in which her little dog is killed. In a succeeding hour, she arrives announcing that she has a burden that is both a mystery and a miracle. She is

like the old woman who never was, she is a ghost, one that is both
dead and alive at the same time, a sleepless ghost that is made out
of flesh and blood. She comes now to remember that this little dog,
which she both loved and hated, suffered because of her guardian's
neglect, clearly revealing that she is striving to ward off the actual
memory of having herself threatened and mistreated the dog, which
we know from the history.

We can now understand the meaning of her current preoccupation
with a variety of trivia and minutiae that literally paralyzes any positive
action by her. We see developing a kind of psychotic obsessionalism
that, although seemingly in the service of her primary-process relationship to time as infinite and unchanging, serves also to develop
inner structure that helps control the drive organization. This very
process of reconstitution and restitution makes possible the kind of
symbolic reconstruction of which she is slowly becoming capable, and
demonstrates the complex vicissitudes of the activity-passivity conflict
that can occur with such a patient. Initially, she appears passively
overwhelmed as she reports the borrowed TV fantasy of the menacing
statue that has suddenly become alive, a kind of borrowed external
representation that serves as a *screen delusional fantasy*. Subsequently,
she is able to recall her own *screen nightmare*, no longer borrowed, of
the volcanic eruption (of which she knows not whether it be inner
or outer) which defended against the actual memory of her violent,
aggressive acts against the dog, prior to his subsequent death from
unrelated causes.

To the extent that the reporting of the delusional material is in
the service of restoring the function of remembering, we can see that
the passivity referred only to certain aspects of the ego. Simultaneously
it was also in the service of those aspects of the ego which had not
been overwhelmed, and aimed at the restoration of active, secondary-
process memory function. As this is restored, the girl comes, two hours
later, to a more conventional screen memory, the aunt's mistreatment
and rejection of the dog. This becomes an acceptable substitute screen
idea for the unacceptable memory of her own violent rage which had
led to her abuse of the dog.

Thus, now that she has achieved the capacity to still the helpless,
driven activity of earlier days, even though in such massive measures
as to achieve a living paralysis, she can begin to remember. We can
hope now that the soft but persistent voice of an autonomous ego (to
paraphrase Freud) will have begun to be heard; for if she can still the
act, she need not fear so desperately the primary thought which can
still turn so quickly into an uncontrolled act.

In subsequent visits to her therapist, she begins to play with the thought that she can moderate the acts without having completely to suppress them. She begins to exert mastery over the loss of the object when it is no longer present by instituting a kind of peek-a-boo game with the therapist. She knocks on his exit door, as if to show that she can still make an entrance only by way of a departure. This in itself is a reconstruction of her own life history with its constant exchange of mother figures, about whom it might be said that she had a more stable relationship in their absence than in their presence.

We would like to end by referring to a rather unique aspect of the activity-passivity issues in the treatment of borderline and psychotic children. All analytic treatment requires of the therapist a constant kind of balancing between a seemingly "active" and a seemingly "passive" position. He must listen and he must intervene; he must understand and he must interpret; he must experience and he must observe and reflect (12), he must identify with and he must confront; he must "regress" empathically with the patient and progress with the analysis; he must accept the endless dalliance of the patients for whom time is interminable and he must press for the working alliance that implies finite goals. But with these children, the nature of the regression—to a symbiotic fusion, to primary-process archaic levels of functioning, to fragmented and discontinuous contact and communication—creates special countertransference problems which at times seem to echo and make him an echo of his patients (Chapts. 8, 16, 24, this vol.). His task becomes then to sleep but not to dream (Ch. 24, this vol.), to mirror but not to echo, to accept the symbiosis but not to become attached to it, to enter the autistic wonderland bu to reserve passage for a return.

It is for such reasons that the treatment of these children within a research program can not only enrich but facilitate it. Such patients provide the therapist with the opportunity for the continued search for understanding that requires his own integrative and synthesizing functions to make the necessary empathic regression (Chapter 24), truly in the service of a therapeutic and autonomous ego, which is to say, of an active psychic organization.

REFERENCES

1. ANDERSEN, HANS CHRISTIAN. "The Red Shoes." In: *The Fairy Tales*, 1835.
2. EKSTEIN, RUDOLF. Discussion of "Transference and Countertransference" by A. Aberastury et al. Presented at 2nd Pan Amer. Psychoanalyt. Cong., Buenos Aires, Argentina, August, 1966. Unpublished.
3. ——. "The Opening Gambit in Psychotherapeutic Work with Severely Disturbed Adolescents." *Amer. J. of Orthopsychiat.*, 1963, 33:862.
4. ——. "Puppet Play of a Psychotic Adolescent Girl in the Psychotherapeutic Process." *Psychoanalyt. Study of the Child*, 1965, 20:441.

5. —— & CARUTH, E. "Distancing and Distance Devices in Cchildhood Schizophrenia and Borderline States." *Psycholog. Reports*, 1967, 20:109.
6. — & CARUTH, E. "Psychotic Acting Out: Royal Road or Primrose Path." In: *Children of Time and Space, of Action and Impulse* by R. Ekstein. N. Y.: Appleton-Century-Crofts, 1966.
7. —— & CARUTH, E. "The Working Alliance with the Monster." *Bull. of Menninger Clin.*, 1965, 4:189.
8. —— & WALLERSTEIN, J. "Choice of Interpretation in the Treatment of Borderline and Psychotic Children." *Bull. of Menninger Clin.*, 1957, 21:199.
9. ERIKSON, ERIK H. *Childhood and Society*. N. Y.: Norton, 1950.
10. ——. "Reality and Actuality." *J. of Am. Psa. Assoc.*, 1962, 10:451.
11. FENICHEL, OTTO. *The Psychoanalytic Theory of Neurosis*. N. Y.: Norton, 1945.
12. GREENSON, RALPH. "Empathy and Its Vicissitudes." *Int. J. Psychoanal.*, 1960, 61:418.
13. HART, HENRY H. "The Meaning of Passivity." *Psychiat. Quart.*, Oct., 1955, p. 595.
14. ——. "A Review of the Psychoanalytic Literature on Passivity." *Psychiat. Quart.*, Apr., 1961, p. 331.
15. KNIGHT, R. P. "Borderline States." *Bull. of Menninger Clin.*, 1953, 17:1.
16. LINDNER, R. M. "The Jet Propelled Couch." In: *The Fifty-Minute Hour*. N. Y.: Rinehart, 1955.
17. MATTE-BLANCO, IGNACIO. "Expression in Symbolic Logic of the Characteristics of the System UCS." *Int. J. Psychoanal.*, 1959, 40:1.
18. RAPAPORT, DAVID. "Some Metapsychological Considerations Concerning Activity and Passivity." *Archivos de Criminologia Neuro-Psiquiatria y Disciplinas Conexas*, 1961, 9.
19. ——. "The Theory of Ego Autonomy: a Generalization." *Bull. of Menninger Clin.*, 1958, 1:13.

Index